Advance Praise for *Mistreated*

"*Mistreated* is a powerful read, an incredible insight into American health care, a mix of poignant personal memoir by a son, the clinical perspective of an experienced surgeon, and the vision and understanding that comes from being the CEO of one of the largest and best health care organizations in the country. Robert Pearl is all those things, and with *Mistreated* he proves he is also a wonderful writer."

—Abraham Verghese, MD, professor of medicine, Stanford University, and author of *Cutting for Stone*

"Robert Pearl argues that the troubles of the American health care system begin with a problem of perception: conceptual misunderstandings that warp priorities and distort choices. *Mistreated* is a brilliant and original analysis from one of medicine's most insightful leaders. The doctor is *in*."

—Malcolm Gladwell, bestselling author of *David and Goliath*

"Pundits like to speculate about the future of health care, but Dr. Robert Pearl has been busy creating it . . . at scale. As CEO of the nation's largest medical group, he and his colleagues at Kaiser Permanente have created a system serving 10 million members that is low cost, but with nation-leading quality outcomes and high patient satisfaction. They haven't just bent the cost curve, they've wrestled it into submission. If you want to understand how to fix health care, listen to him: he knows."

—Chip Heath, coauthor of *Switch* and *Decisive*

"Relying on his long history as one of the country's most innovative and powerful physician-leaders, Dr. Robert Pearl lays bare the shortsightedness of the broken US health care system: why we resist better science, newer technology, and reform. He offers a vision of how to improve our medical care, informed and tested in his own real world practice."

—**Elisabeth Rosenthal,**
editor in chief of *Kaiser Health News*

"*Mistreated* is a timely and necessary book on how to fix our broken health system from one of our most important voices in health care. Dr. Robert Pearl's diagnosis isn't pretty. Morale in health care is low, costs are unmanageable, and health and survival are often worse than in other high-income countries. But Pearl is a leader who transformed his own health system to have very different results for patients and clinicians alike. And he offers that experience to show everyone the way."

—**Atul Gawande, bestselling author of** *Being Mortal*

"Drawing on psychological research and his diverse roles as physician, business professor, and chief executive, Dr. Pearl diagnoses the problems of the American health care system and offers simple yet important solutions. In a health care system undergoing rapid changes, *Mistreated* is an essential and trusted guide to the future."

—**Ezekiel J. Emanuel,**
author of *Reinventing American Health Care*

"*Mistreated* is the honest conversation we need to have about the beautiful but broken craft of medicine."

—**Marty Makary, MD,** *New York Times*–**bestselling**
author of *Unaccountable*

"A respected expert gets personal. The result is a gripping drama set in our troubled health care system—and happily a roadmap for fixing it."

—Ceci Connolly, president and CEO of the Alliance of Community Health Plans

"This is an important book. With clear and engaging examples, *Mistreated* reviews the flaws in our traditional fragmented health care system, showing that context and perception matter more in health care than logic and data. This powerful insight can help our nation transform American medicine and make it the best in the world. A must-read for anyone who has ever been or will be a patient—and that is all of us."

—Alain Enthoven, professor emeritus, Graduate School of Business at Stanford

"*Mistreated* provides a poignant and powerful portrait of what causes our health system to fail despite our best intentions. Starting with the painful story of his father's untimely death due to medical error, Dr. Pearl honors his father's memory by teaching us how to build a system that creates health and prevents harm."

—Ian Morrison, PhD, author, consultant, and futurist

"Dr. Pearl combines facts, evidence, and real-life experiences that demystify the complex American health care system and offer ways to improve it. His vast and varied experiences in medicine lend particular weight to his ideas for constructive change."

—John Iglehart, founding editor of Project HOPE

MISTREATED

MISTREATED

*Why We Think We're
Getting Good Health Care—
and Why We're Usually Wrong*

ROBERT PEARL

PUBLICAFFAIRS
New York

PublicAffairs books are available at special discounts for bulk purchases in
the U.S. by corporations, institutions, and other organizations. For more
information, please contact the Special Markets Department at Perseus Books,
2300 Chestnut Street, Suite 200, Philadelphia, PA 19103, call (800) 810-4145,
ext. 5000, or e-mail special.markets@perseusbooks.com.

Book Design by Timm Bryson

The Library of Congress has cataloged the printed edition as follows:
Names: Pearl, Robert, author.
Title: Mistreated : why we think we're getting good health care and why we're
    usually wrong / Robert Pearl.
Description: First edition. | New York : PublicAffairs, [2017] | Includes
    bibliographical references.
Identifiers: LCCN 2016057376 (print) | LCCN 2016059335 (ebook) | ISBN
    9781610397650 (hardcover) | ISBN 9781610397667 (ebook)
Subjects: LCSH: Health services administration. | Medical
    Informatics—Management. | BISAC: MEDICAL / Health Policy. |
MEDICAL / Public Health.
Classification: LCC RA971 .P387 2017 (print) | LCC RA971 (ebook) | DDC
    362.10285—dc23
LC record available at https://lccn.loc.gov/2016057376

First Edition
LSC-C
10 9 8 7 6

In loving memory of my father, Jack Pearl

CONTENTS

PREFACE

America has the greatest health care in the world. At least, that's what people say. It's a claim made often and by a variety of influential leaders, from high-ranking politicians to hospital administrators to corporate executives. And despite the rancorous politicizing of the health care system, when it comes time to actually visit a doctor or hospital, the majority of Americans agree. Seventy-six percent of patients describe the quality of care they personally receive as good or excellent. When their doctors speak, they listen, trusting that they are in the best of hands.

There's just one problem. When independent researchers crunch the numbers and compare nations, American health care ranks nowhere near the top of the list. In fact, among developed countries, the United States has the highest infant mortality rate, the lowest life expectancy, and the most preventable deaths per capita.

Several years ago, I set out to understand the strange division between our positive perceptions of health care and the reality of the current system. The closer I looked, the more questions and contradictions I encountered.

As a nation, we spend 50 percent more on medical care than any other country, and yet we rank seventieth globally in overall health and wellness. We pay US physicians far more to intervene during a heart attack than to prevent one in the first place. We have the best-trained doctors on the planet, and yet their avoidable mistakes kill nearly 200,000 Americans each year. And as consumers, we demand the latest technologies from our banks, telecom providers, and retailers, but we passively accept last century's technology in our hospitals and medical offices.

While searching for answers to these and other mysteries, I was fortunate to collaborate with my colleague and a respected neurologist, Dr. George York. We were interested in a different but related topic: Why do smart people do dumb things in their jobs, relationships, and everyday lives?

As part of the research, we combed through the latest brain-scanning studies and decades of psychological literature to uncover a surprising connection, one that helps explain some of the most puzzling contradictions in American medicine.

Scientists have demonstrated that under the right conditions, our brains undergo a shift, causing us to perceive the world around us in ways that contradict objective reality. I'm not talking about illusions or magic tricks. Rather, it's something that is decidedly more serious and prevalent than you might think, especially in the world of medical care.

As you'll soon see, our health care system functions in an environment unlike any other. There's nothing comparable to it in American culture, society, or industry. The rules are different, the stakes are elevated, and the perceptions of everyone in it—from doctors to patients to US presidents—get radically distorted, leading to behaviors that prove hazardous to our health.

What's most problematic about this neurophysiological process is that the changes in our brains occur subconsciously and therefore beyond our awareness or control. This reshuffling of perception is entirely independent of our personal values, beliefs, or intelligence.

To help shed light on this phenomenon, some of the studies described in *Mistreated* come from recent psychological and medical literature. Other studies referenced in this book are decades old and familiar to many. I've chosen to cite them here for three important reasons. First, this type of research can no longer be performed. Newer ethical restrictions are designed to protect research subjects from experiments with the potential to cause psychological damage. As such, these classic studies are the best examples of mistreatment available. Second, their findings have been reviewed and validated dozens of times. Finally, when they are combined with recent brain-scanning studies, something never done before, all of us can better understand why the American health care system fails us time and again.

When we hear the word *mistreated* in the context of medical practice, we associate it with botched surgeries and flawed individuals who act dishonestly, out of greed and with a blatant disregard for the well-being of others. Although those individuals do exist, they are the exception.

This distinction is crucial. If character flaws were the central challenge facing American medicine, the solutions would be much simpler. We would select different medical students and isolate the sociopaths. But health care's most common failings aren't individual. They're contextual, systemic, and therefore much more problematic. Transforming the conditions of American medicine will be difficult but possible. These chapters contain real case studies that demonstrate what's possible and help light the way.

Mistreated incorporates a variety of patient anecdotes and personal stories, included with the hope of holding your interest through the more academic and policy-focused sections of this book. As the song goes, "a spoonful of sugar helps the medicine go down."

Accounts of the patients profiled herein come from several sources. In almost all cases, real names have been altered—and when necessary, some medical details modified—to protect individual identities. The exceptions are three patient vignettes, originally filmed (with their permission and their doctors' approval) as part of an educational series created by the Council of Accountable Physician Practices, an organization for which I serve as chairman. Other stories and information found in this book come directly from my work as a contributor to *Forbes*, in which I explore the intersection of business and health care.

Throughout my career, I've had the opportunity to observe American medicine from many different angles: as a physician and a health care CEO, as faculty at both the Stanford University School of Medicine and the Stanford Graduate School of Business, and as the son of a man who died too young from a series of medical errors. My conclusion is that the American health system is sick. We have excellent physicians who are burned out, unfulfilled, and in some cases, terribly depressed. We have a number of billion-dollar pharmaceutical companies raising drug prices upward of 5,000 percent, operating without fear of public backlash or legislative overhaul. We have already unaffordable health care costs that continue to rise at twice the rate of our nation's ability to pay. And even after the implementation of the Affordable Care Act, millions of Americans remain uninsured.

Last year, while writing this book, I visited the Accademia Gallery in Florence, Italy. Long lines of people waited outside to see Michelangelo's remarkable seventeen-foot-high marble statue of David, on his way to the battlefield, wearing no armor and carrying but a slingshot with five rocks as weaponry. As a surgeon, I stood for more than half an hour admiring the sculptor's knowledge of anatomy, a remarkable feat achieved five centuries ago and during a time when it was against the law to dissect the human cadaver. Each muscle had been masterfully chiseled from marble block. Even the basilic vein on the back of David's forearm was perfectly placed.

Two features, however, were out of proportion, both with clear intent. First, David's head is notably oversized, signifying the importance of discernment and choice as he sets out to face the biblical giant Goliath. Second, his hands are huge, a nod to the importance of action. In the moment, I was struck by how apt this metaphor is for American health care. As individuals and as a nation, we need to see what is happening, decide to do something about it, and take action.

Adjacent to *David* is another set of the artist's sculptures known as the *Four Prisoners*, all four of them unfinished, their figures seemingly trapped inside their marble casings. The first is titled *The Awakening*, with the head of the statue struggling to free itself from the block. The second, *The Young Prisoner*, has a youthful face with a single leg freed. The third, *Atlas*, is carrying a huge weight on his shoulders and head. Finally, *The Bearded Slave*, the most finished piece, appears to emerge from the marble almost entirely free.

In the same way that Michelangelo sculpted the progressive liberation of his forms, *Mistreated* outlines the steps necessary to transform American medical practice. The first step will be the awakening, becoming aware of how we as patients are mistreated. From there, we will need youthful optimism and a collective confidence that our problems can be solved. That will be followed by years of hard work. And by the end, I hope that we will have freed American medicine from the outdated cottage industry it resembles today. I invite you to come along on the journey.

Chapter One

VICTIMS OF CIRCUMSTANCE

Palo Alto is a charming bayside town in the heart of Silicon Valley. Named after the soaring California redwoods that dot its landscape, Palo (stick) Alto (tall) is home to Stanford University Medical Center, where I trained as a surgical resident and where I remain on the clinical faculty.

It's springtime, the year 2000, and all across the state the California poppies are in bloom. The silky trumpets of our state flower burst with color, carpeting the hillsides in yellows, oranges, and golds. Hummingbirds float under bright blue skies. If you listen closely, you can hear their little wings flapping dozens of times per second as they lap nectar with admirable precision.

The sights and sounds of the world outside contrast with all that I can see and hear inside the Intensive Care Unit of Stanford Medical Center. Under muted lights, I listen to the rumble of medication carts and nurses chatting in the hallway. The steady chirp of the heart-rate monitor pulses and blends into the whir of the respirator, which is currently forcing oxygen through the endotracheal tube doctors have placed down the nose and into the lungs of my father, Jack Pearl.

He's unconscious, his blood pressure low. Bacteria race through his bloodstream. My father, the handsome and strong dentist with steady hands, smooth skin, and sharp green eyes, hardly resembles this shriveled, pasty man lying on the hospital bed, his hair disheveled and lips parched. My father is in septic shock, the result of an infection that has spread through his lungs to his entire body.

This bed, one of sixty-seven in the ICU, is where my father will remain unresponsive for the next four days. My younger brother, Ron, who looks every part the doctor, stands beside me. He inherited our father's smooth skin, light brown hair, and passion for medicine. Ron is the chairman of the anesthesia department at Stanford Medical School. He oversees the operating rooms and is responsible for the nationally renowned medical care provided to ICU patients like my father. Ron's colleagues, fellows, and residents care for our dad as we hover near his bedside.

My brother and I understand the significance of our father's diagnosis. We realize the serious obstacles the care team must overcome to reverse his life-threatening condition. Ron and I speak to each other in the language of doctors and, between each care-team check-in, we ask his physicians about respirator settings and blood-culture results. I think back to when Ron and I were both residents here years ago, taking care of complex and acutely ill patients together. This feels very different, surreal, terrifying.

We take turns sitting at our father's bedside and calling our sister in New York with updates. We know, medically, what's happening to our father. But how our father got here remains a complete mystery to us.

I step outside for a break and take deep breaths of fresh air. The fountains that line the plaza of the medical center ripple and glisten under the midday sun. Doctors, nurses, and hospital staff mingle at nearby tables, enjoying their lunches, making conversation beneath the umbrellas. I realize that, for them, it's just another day.

The Past Twenty-Four Hours

My father and I played golf yesterday, as fathers and sons do. Conditions on the course were idyllic. The round flew by and my father's skills were on full display. Although his long-game wasn't quite as long as it used to be, his putting and chipping abilities more than compensated. He shot an eighty-three, joking that he couldn't wait to get a few years older so that he could "shoot his age."

Ron joined us for dinner later that evening at my house in Los Gatos, about thirty minutes south of Palo Alto. We talked about the good times we had growing up and the challenges of American medicine. My dad reminisced about family vacations and the joy he experienced through his dental practice. We made plans to get together that summer at our father's condo in New York City. Afterward, my dad drove back to my brother's house to get some sleep.

Early the next morning, as my brother got ready for rounds, he found our dad lying unconscious on the living-room floor. Immediately, he called 911. His next call was to the hospital, notifying the physicians that our dad would be arriving in a few minutes and that he'd require immediate admission to the ICU. The ambulance and my brother arrived within minutes of each other. The care team stood by, ready.

The Next Twenty-Four Hours

After a day at our father's bedside, amid the constant beep of medical equipment and the rush of personnel coming in and out of the room, Ron and I are tired and very much on edge. We've exhausted the vocabulary of medical dialect with a meticulous succession of "what ifs." We fidget and shift in our chairs. It's amazing how quickly time moves when you're the doctor providing care. And it's eerie how slowly time passes when your father is the patient, and all you can do is watch and wait.

When there's nothing more to contribute to clinical discourse, Ron and I break the silence with words of comfort. We agree it's fortunate this happened so close to Stanford's hospital. I understand how lucky it is my father was downstairs from a critical-care expert, not back in New York by himself. Of course, none of these insights comfort me or disarm our fears about what might happen next. Even if everything goes perfectly and our dad lives, his recovery will be long and difficult at best.

Every day in American hospitals, friends and families wait nervously by the bedsides of their loved ones, hoping everything will be okay. They pace about the hallways and huddle in the sitting areas, waiting for answers and assurances. Amid the commotion and the unknown, the world of medicine can feel intimidating and alien to outsiders.

As a physician and surgeon, I'm comfortable with this world, at ease in the Operating Room and inpatient units with their rituals, sights, and sounds. Through my training and clinical work, I have learned how to deal with death, pain, and fear. But this is my father. Nothing in my training prepared me for this moment.

I know the members of the care team are doing everything they can. And if you put almost anyone else in that bed, Ron and I would enjoy the camaraderie of once again working together as doctors and brothers to save the life of a patient. But in this most familiar of settings, we're outside our comfort zones. Standing at our father's bedside, we're not physicians consulting on a complex medical case. We're two sons wondering if our dad will live until tomorrow.

The Greatest Generation

My father was the youngest child of poor immigrants from Belarus. In the early part of the twentieth century, his parents fled the pogroms of Russia, though not together. Each sailed to the United States looking for a new life. There, they met each other and married. My grandmother crossed the Atlantic as a teenager, alone, with only the name of an aunt as reference. She arrived in America completely naïve about the realities of this new land. Unable to speak a word of English, she had assumed everyone in America spoke Russian and that the streets were literally paved with gold, just as those back home had promised.

My grandfather picked up some English before arriving, helping him land a pair of jobs in New York City to support himself and, eventually, his new family. He was a tailor, like many immigrants of his generation. He'd bring home leftover scraps of garment, piecing and sewing them together at night into new clothes for extra income, all in the tireless pursuit of the American dream.

At home, my grandparents spoke in Yiddish, making plans for the future, trusting always that in this country anything was possible. If they had little else, they had each other and their family. As parents, they held firm to the conviction that if their children studied hard and took advantage of the opportunities of this great nation, the future would be bright. This was the world my grandparents knew, equal parts hardship and optimism.

In the early twentieth century, however, hardships weren't just economic. Health care in the era before vaccinations meant doctors could do little to prevent or treat some of the most life-threatening diseases.

My father's only sister, Mary, died from measles at age six. Although he was too young to remember her, my father talked often about the grief Mary's death caused his family. Losing a child is one of the most painful events a parent can experience, and it would haunt my grandparents for the rest of their lives. In their day, when life was guaranteed to no one, there was little time to mourn. As my father and his brother, Herbert, grew up, they honored their parents' wishes. They studied hard in school and worked multiple jobs during nights and weekends. Both went on to pursue careers in health care.

My uncle Herb took to medicine and became a general surgeon. My father gained acceptance at Columbia University en route to dental school at New York University.

Shortly after earning his dental license, my dad enlisted in the 101st Airborne to fight for the Allies during World War II. As a captain in the army, he could have asked for a safer assignment, perhaps caring for new recruits on this side of the Atlantic. But that's not who my father was.

As a member of the "Screaming Eagles," my father parachuted behind enemy lines in the Battle of Normandy. There, he and members of his unit were captured by the Germans. Inside a truck transporting a dozen or so American soldiers to the closest Nazi prison, my father led a daring escape. For two days, he guided his unit through hills and forests in the dark of night, hiding beneath the brush at daybreak, promising each other they would survive.

The soldiers were eventually reunited with their battalion, returning to America not long after. Radio stations across the country aired stories of the unit's bravery. My mother, so proud of her husband's heroic efforts, obtained a copy of the story on vinyl. When I was a child, she played it for me on the phonograph in the den. Growing up, I had no doubt my father was a great man.

After the war, my dad opened his dental practice in Queens. A few years later, he and my mother bought a home in the suburbs of Long Island, and together they raised a family. My father, the son of poor immigrants, the war hero, the successful dentist and loving father, spent his life working hard to fulfill the American dream that his parents had begun. Throughout his life, he earned the esteem we as a country ascribe to the "greatest generation."

Life Goes On

After practicing for forty years and at the age of seventy-two, my father hadn't lost his dental skills one bit. He simply retired, wanting to pursue his other interests. He was always passionate about art. In his thirties and forties, he painted and sketched. In his fifties and sixties, he toyed with sculpture. Now in his seventies, he combined his former profession and his artistic passion, employing a variety of dental tools to smooth and shape acrylics. Away from his practice and the canvas, he loved spending time with his wife, his children, and his friends. And, of course, he loved having more time to work on his golf game.

In 1994, my parents sold their Long Island home, opting for a condo back in Queens. Shortly after, they purchased a second home in West Palm Beach and, like many of their friends, enjoyed the best of both locations. Springs and summers in New York, then off to Florida just as the leaves began to fall and the nip of autumn settled across the boroughs. And when spring returned to New York, so would they, soaking up the vibrant culture of the Big Apple.

For most of his life, my father was the picture of good health, full of energy and strength. But in his sixties, his energy ebbed. Doctors diagnosed him with a hemolytic anemia, a condition that destroys red blood cells before the end of their normal life span.

His hematologist prescribed a variety of medications in hopes of slowing the destructive process. He ordered repeat transfusions to restore my dad's red-blood-cell count to normal. Unfortunately, his body continued to destroy the cells, and his blood count fell week after week, draining his strength. The time had come for a more aggressive approach. So, a surgeon removed his spleen. Surgery was the right thing to do. The procedure does not always solve the problem, but in this case, the operation was a success and my father's blood count normalized. His vigor returned, and I was overjoyed to have my father restored to full strength.

As the years passed by, however, the unfailing certainties of time caught up with him. My father developed mild hypertension, atrial fibrillation, and cataracts, the types of chronic medical problems commonly associated with aging. He saw a team of physicians: an internist, a cardiologist, a hematologist, and an ophthalmologist. His physicians were skilled, and each condition was properly treated. Every Sunday night, my father would fill his plastic pill box with the exact medications he needed. Seven pills in the Monday compartment, seven in the one labeled Tuesday, and so on for the entire week.

Whenever I'd visit him, whether in New York or Florida, he'd ask me to accompany him on one or more of his physician appointments. I gladly obliged. As his doctors sat down to take a patient history, clipboards in hand, they always began with the same question.

"What medications are you taking, Dr. Pearl?"

I'll admit I was surprised to hear this. At the time, our medical group had already implemented an electronic health record, although not as sophisticated as the one we use today. I took for granted how easy it was for our thousands of physicians to access this information on their office computers and in their exam rooms. I was jolted by the realization that these well-trained physicians from renowned academic programs seemed content to rely on the memory of a man in his seventies to tell them what kinds of medications he was taking and the exact dosages.

Fortunately, my dad was a fastidious man, as most dentists are. Whenever the doctors asked him about his prescriptions, he would reach into his pocket and unfurl a tattered piece of paper containing a handwritten list of all his current medications. When prescriptions changed, he'd dutifully cross out the old medication or dosage, and write in the new one.

Finally, a Clue

Back in the Stanford Medical Center, Ron and I are waiting for our father's blood culture results, which take two to three days to come back and during which every hour feels like a lifetime. First, the bacteria need to grow. Then the technician needs to perform a diagnostic analysis to determine the exact variety. Finally, the lab has to complete tests to establish which antibiotics are likely to be effective.

Two days after my father's admission to the ICU, the resident helping with his care shares what they have learned. "Your father has a pneumococcal infection," he says, assuring us the antibiotics he's taking are appropriate for this particular bacterium.

As doctors, Ron and I know this particular organism well. The "pneumococcus" is a common cause of pneumonia. In the past, it was a frequent cause of death. Thankfully, modern antibiotics such as the ones my father are on reduce that likelihood.

But these antibiotics are a treatment for a condition my father didn't need to suffer from in the first place. And this is where his medical history becomes very important.

Years before, the removal of my father's spleen helped return his blood count to normal and restore him to good health. The surgeon who performed the procedure did so with masterful skill and without postoperative complication.

But medicine is a tricky craft. Many of the procedures we perform have downsides that can surface years later. A patient with his spleen removed, for example, is at risk of developing severe infection. One specific bacterium that's particularly problematic for people without a spleen is the pneumococcus. Without a spleen to filter this pathogen out of the bloodstream, the pneumococcus can infect a patient's entire body.

Every surgeon who removes a person's spleen, and every doctor who cares for that patient afterward, knows there's an increased risk of pneumococcal infection. They also know that every person whose spleen has been removed should receive a pneumococcal vaccine. This vaccine allows the body to fight this organism more effectively. And without a doubt, every one of my father's excellent physicians knew he needed it.

But after calling around, I discovered the hard truth. My dad's doctors in New York assumed the ones in Florida had given him the vaccination. The physicians in Florida assumed the ones in New York had done so. The medical specialists believed the surgeon who removed my father's spleen had administered it. And all the specialty physicians thought my father's internal medicine doctor had taken care of it. In the end, no one had.

After four days in Stanford's ICU and another ten days in the hospital, my father is alive but extremely weak. He's barely able to feed himself. Days of bed rest have rubbed the skin of his heel raw, which will result in a deep ulcer on his foot, making it difficult for him to walk for months.

Before his collapse, my father was the most energetic person I knew. But as he takes his first steps outside the medical center, it's as though he has aged an entire decade. We encourage him to take ten steps that day, hoping he can do twelve tomorrow. We're thankful to his critical-care doctors who saved him from death. Still, the toll this experience has taken on his body will sap our father's strength for the rest of his life. We know he will never again be the man he was before.

The Wounds Time Can't Heal

My father, like millions of other patients in our country, suffered a life-threatening complication because of an avoidable medical error. His experience reflects the contradictions that plague American medicine.

We train superb physicians who can accomplish the remarkable when patients become extremely ill, pulling them back from the brink of dying. And yet we in the medical community fail to consistently follow basic steps such as washing our hands between patients, a practice that can prevent infection, the number-one cause of death among hospitalized patients.

Similarly, as doctors, we demand the most advanced medical devices money can buy, yet we undervalue simple information technologies with the power to prevent fatal medical errors. Electronic health records keep and provide details on the totality of a patient's care, information that is essential to achieving superior outcomes. And yet in the United States today, about 50 percent of all doctors still rely on paper medical records.

These paradoxes extend to the lives of our patients, too. Americans live in a constantly connected world and value the conveniences of modern technology. Using their smartphones and computers, they can schedule airline flights, check their financial statements, and communicate with friends around the world. Yet as a medical community, we deny people these same types of services, placing an undue burden on the lives of busy families all throughout our country. I'll give you a personal example.

After being discharged from the Stanford Medical Center in late spring of 2000, my father spent the summer living at my house in Los Gatos. He worked hard to regain his strength. But despite the frequent elevation of his foot, along with a variety of medications and even a surgical procedure on his heel, the ulcer persisted. So when he returned home to New York that fall, he met with a wound specialist who scheduled a standing weekly appointment.

Because of the problem with his foot and his overall weakness, my father couldn't drive. My sister therefore ferried him to and from his appointment every Wednesday for six months. During most visits, the specialist would quickly inspect the wound, offer her evaluation, and tell my father what to do for the next seven days. For what amounted to ten minutes of medical care each week, my sister would have to drive nearly two hours to our father's apartment, take him by wheelchair to the car, drive him to the doctor's office, get him into the waiting room, and reverse the steps on the way back. My sister, who was at the time CEO of a Planned Parenthood affiliate, never once complained about missing half a day of work each Wednesday. She would have gone to any lengths to help our father. But she shouldn't have had to.

On most visits, my father's physician needed only to assess the wound and make sure it was healing properly. For that, my sister could have visited our dad at night, taken a digital photo of his foot, and e-mailed it to the doctor for thorough review at her convenience. I doubt this idea ever crossed the doctor's mind. Physicians are not trained in medical school to worry about the inconveniences they place on patients or their families. And in their practices, they find that insurance companies are rarely willing to pay for the kind of "virtual visits" that would have saved my sister more than a hundred hours of missed work.

My father paid a high price for the medial error he suffered. Sadly, his health care story is not unique. Whenever I speak at health care conferences about my dad's experience, people nod knowingly. I'm always amazed by how many from the audience will line up afterward to share similar stories and frustrations about the care their loved ones received. Just about every family seems to have had an experience like ours.

The Loss of Compassion

By 2002, about a year and a half after returning to his home in New York, my father was able to walk short distances and drive to the grocery store. One morning, a driver rear-ended his car. My father suffered severe and disabling back pain. To provide relief, his doctors recommended a series of cortisone injections around his spinal cord. To prevent bleeding from the injections, they took him off the anticoagulation medications he was on for his atrial fibrillation. Before he could complete the series, he suffered a massive blood clot in his brain. Once again, he was back in the hospital, this time in Florida.

As soon as I got the call, I flew in from California and rushed to his room. My heart sank when I saw him. As a physician, I had seen hundreds of patients just like him: a breathing tube down his throat, a feeding tube through his nose, his hands and feet tied to the bed, restraining him as he fought to remove these painful foreign objects.

That night and the following morning, doctors came one by one into his room, each recommending a different surgical procedure or medical treatment that could prolong his life. One physician wanted to perform a tracheostomy, putting a hole in my father's windpipe. Another recommended a permanent feeding tube. A neurosurgeon suggested removing a piece of skull to decompress his brain.

By this point, my siblings and I all knew our father could never again return to his former self. None of these solutions were what he would have wanted, and none would have allowed him a reasonable quality of life. So, as the doctors came by to recommend various invasive procedures, we thanked them all but declined. And when there were no more suggestions to be made, no procedures left to recommend, the doctors stopped coming altogether.

From that moment on, we never saw another physician in our father's room. No one came by to check in on the family or ask how we were doing. None of his doctors dropped in to offer a word of support. I felt abandoned by these healers in our time of greatest need.

Throughout much of history, there was little doctors could do to help their patients. They simply lacked the tools, medications, and knowhow we have today. Perhaps that's why doctors of the past became such skilled practitioners of empathy and compassion. For centuries, painters have depicted images of doctors at the bedsides of their patients, deep in thought and ever-present. These depictions created ideals of compassion that remain frozen in our memories. But those days are gone now.

In today's health care system, ruled as it is by economics, there's no "billing code" physicians can use for the time they spend comforting a family or holding a patient's hand when death is inevitable. Doctors get paid for intervening, not for moments of compassion. Today, the insurance reimbursement system dictates how care is delivered. It has eroded personal relationships, devalued empathy and kindness, and undermined the very mission and commitment that led most doctors to practice medicine in the first place.

Death is no stranger to physicians. I have lost patients to cancer, infection, and trauma. Each death is painful. But to see someone die prematurely from a medical error or preventable problem is something else entirely, especially when that someone is your father.

In January 2003, a few days after being transferred from the hospital to a skilled nursing facility, Jack Pearl died in his sleep. He was eighty-three years old.

Analyzing the Symptoms

Physicians learn in their training that to make the right clinical diagnosis, they must first analyze the patient's symptoms and then look for a pattern. Diagnosing what ails our health care system is no different. This particular "patient" has a number of troubling symptoms, many of which have increased in severity over the past few years:

- The cost of American health care is nearly twice that of any other nation. Today, the United States spends close to $3 trillion each year, approximately $10,000 for each man, woman, and child.
- Despite the high cost of medical care, our clinical outcomes are below average. Among the seventeen wealthiest countries, the United States ranks dead last in life expectancy for men and second to last for women. Comparing the most advanced nations in the world, the United States ranks last in infant mortality.
- American doctors and hospitals invest millions in fancy medical equipment—from surgical robots to proton-beam accelerators—but US health care trails almost every other industry in the adoption of information technology. As a result, fewer than 15 percent of all patients can use e-mail with their doctors, and even fewer can review their own medical information online or schedule a "video visit."
- We pay doctors and hospitals based on the number of services they provide rather than the quality of care they deliver to their patients. Consequently, American patients undergo a very high volume of unnecessary tests and procedures.
- The quality of a patient's care and his or her access to it varies dramatically based on such characteristics as race, ethnicity, and socioeconomics. As a result, Latinos and African Americans on average experience clinical outcomes that are 20 percent worse than other ethnic and racial groups in their communities.

Were American health care a patient, we would diagnose it as suffering from "multiorgan failure" and put it in the ICU for further testing. Very few of the test results would be normal. And even before all results came in, we would need to begin aggressive treatments. Once the patient was stabilized, attending physicians would work to identify the exact underlying etiology of the problem, a key step in preventing further deterioration.

Without understanding the root cause of system failure, the patient's problem will only get worse.

Mistreated was written for the purpose of helping people understand what ails the American health care system and how to improve it. By the end of this book, I hope readers will recognize the symptoms, understand the underlying problems, and embrace better solutions.

I think most health care professionals, academics, and policy experts will find this book educational and helpful in their work, although a few are likely to label the book controversial, disagree with its assessment, and differ with its conclusions. I will be interested in—and open to—their feedback. But they aren't the audience for whom this book was written. *Mistreated* is for the patient in all of us. My hope and belief is that once all Americans begin to see the true problems endemic in our health care, and once we understand the threat they pose to our families and ourselves, we will demand change. And once enough people do, we can reverse the damage, for good.

In trying to identify the shortcomings of our health care system, it's tempting to point our fingers at a short list of familiar villains: negligent doctors, ineffective politicians, and overpaid drug-company CEOs. And yes, they're out there. But they are not the fundamental problem.

They're what we call in medical practice "opportunistic infections," problems that turn up in the context of other diseases. Ridding the system of their misdeeds is not the ultimate solution. It won't significantly change the underlying pathology.

To understand the root cause of a broken health care system, we need to go back in time, decades in the past, and reexamine what may be the most famous research project ever conducted on the subject of mistreatment.

Palo Alto, 1971

In the basement of Jordan Hall on the campus of Stanford University, one student is forcing another to clean a toilet with his bare hands. The student on his knees is wearing what looks like a potato sack inscribed with a four-digit number near the chest. The student standing over him is dressed like a prison guard. Actually, he's dressed like a caricature of a prison guard, aviator sunglasses and all.

This scene took place in one of the most analyzed experiments in all of psychological literature: the Stanford Prison Experiment, funded by the US Office of Naval Research and carried out by a psychology professor named Philip G. Zimbardo.

Zimbardo wanted to understand the effects of prisons on human behavior and how to improve the conditions of incarceration. So, over the summer of 1971, he and a team of researchers placed a classified ad in the local paper: "Male college students needed for psychological study of prison life. $15 per day for 1–2 weeks beginning Aug. 14."

After interviewing a few dozen students, making sure to accept only those who were psychologically normal, Zimbardo flipped a coin to randomly select nine student prison guards and nine student prisoners. The rules for the guards were simple: maintain control of the prison without hitting or assaulting prisoners in any way.

The experiment devolved into chaos almost immediately. Inside the prison (Jordan Hall), the inmates and guards adapted to their new roles very quickly. By day two, prisoners in one of the cells (a converted teacher's office) complained of unfair treatment by the guards. In protest, they fashioned a blockade, propping their bed frames against the door to prevent the guards from getting in. Meanwhile, prisoner number 8612 began to "scream, to curse, to go into a rage," according to Zimbardo.

To restore order, guards doled out severe psychological punishment. In the coming days, many of the prisoners, some of them convinced they were no longer part of an experiment, began to internalize their roles. They stopped resisting and became passive victims of the abuse. Solitary confinement, sexual humiliation, and institutional disorder ensued. Zimbardo was forced to abandon his experiment in less than a week.

In his 2007 book, *The Lucifer Effect*, Zimbardo asked, "If you put good people in a bad place, do the people triumph or does the place corrupt them?" He went on to write, "We want to believe in the essential, unchanging goodness of people, in their power to resist external pressures."

Of course we do. As ethical individuals and principled human beings, we tell ourselves we'd never do anything to harm another person, regardless of the circumstances. There's comfort in believing that good people, raised by good parents and with strong morals, can withstand the negative forces of just about any situation. But that's not what science teaches us. Through the Stanford Prison Experiment and dozens of similar research studies, we've learned that our environment has a far greater impact on our actions than our upbringing or personal beliefs.

Zimbardo's subjects weren't sociopaths or horrible individuals. They were regular students, assigned to one group or the other based on a coin toss. Their personal values and ethics likely weren't so different from yours or mine. But this experiment, along with many others we'll explore throughout these pages, demonstrates that context—the circumstances we find ourselves in, the instructions we are given, the threats made against us, and the rewards we're offered—can and often does shift our perceptions of reality without our even recognizing a shift has happened. Context has a profound impact on what we see, hear, and feel. It has the power to change our behavior.

As difficult as it is to believe, numerous studies have shown that the majority of us would act the same way as the Stanford students if placed in an identical situation. Under the right conditions, most people would act in ways they could never imagine. That is just as true for doctors, patients, politicians, insurance executives, and anyone else. Recognizing the powerful and pervasive influence of context on perception and behavior is fundamental to understanding the failings of American health care.

Widow-Makers

In 2004, one of America's largest hospital chains paid $450 million to settle complaints that its doctors performed unnecessary heart surgeries on hundreds of healthy people in one of its Northern California facilities.

Patients experiencing symptoms that *could have been* cardiac in nature were referred to specialists who performed the recommended radiological studies of the heart vessels. And even when their arteries were determined to be relatively normal, physicians recommended surgical operation. These patients didn't need surgery, of course, but they underwent it nonetheless.

How could this have happened? The media blamed a handful of greedy administrators and unethical doctors. But before we accept this conclusion, we would need to be convinced that Redding, California—more than any other location in America—attracted doctors of moral turpitude and malicious intent. There's no evidence this was the case. As such, we need to search for another explanation, something that goes much deeper.

Heart surgery is not a minor operation. These are long procedures. The surgeon begins by using a power saw to split the sternum, right down the middle of the chest. The patient's heart must be stopped and later restarted. In the interim, a heart-lung bypass machine takes over the heart's role of pumping blood through the body. This mechanical process is far from risk free. It has been associated with long-term memory loss and neurological damage due to the risk of small blood clots being embedded in the brain.

Even in otherwise healthy people, this procedure brings with it the dangers of infection, bleeding, and death. This is risky business. That's why the doctors who recommend and perform this operation are highly trained. They know what to look for in the radiological results, and they know their way around an operating room. The training and background of the physicians in Redding were no different.

Show these same X-ray studies to most heart surgeons across the country and they would see relatively normal vessels without any significant narrowing. But that's not what the doctors in Redding saw. Even for patients whose radiological findings were essentially normal, these physicians were convinced that surgery would help them avoid a heart attack at some point later in life. In the doctors' minds, these heart surgeries were equivalent to removing a patient's appendix to ward off appendicitis down the road. They believed this so much that one surgeon labeled not operating as "widow-making."

Unless the cardiac surgeons and cardiologists in Redding were sociopaths, we can assume that they did not consciously decide to operate on patients with normal hearts. Instead, based on the lessons of recent brain-scanning data, we can assume that what they saw was different than what they would have seen had they been working in another hospital somewhere else in the country. The very minor abnormalities found on most X-rays were perceived by the Redding doctors as indicative of major pathology. And unless all of these physicians were incredibly dishonest, uncaring, and unethical—consciously deciding to put their patient's lives at risk for their own gain—it is more likely that the context in which they practiced distorted their perception, just as it did for the students in the Stanford Prison Experiment.

In the basement of Jordan Hall, context shifted the perception of the guards so that, for no logical reason, they saw the prisoners as unruly criminals. Through this lens, the harsh treatment of their fellow research subjects seemed appropriate. Put the students in Palo Alto in a different context, such as a fraternity party, and they would have seen their peers as friendly and fun to be with.

In the same way, the doctors in Redding saw minor abnormalities in the blood vessels to the heart as problematic, even life-threatening. From their perspective, operating seemed reasonable, even beneficial. That's why, when confronted with the medical evidence of their wrongdoing, the surgeons showed no contrition. Rather, they were convinced that what they'd done was best for their patients. Even the Redding hospital's head of medical ethics believed it—so much so, in fact, that he brought his own father to the hospital from Chicago to be diagnosed and operated on by the facility's doctors.

Psychological literature is replete with examples of normal people willing to do abhorrent things to others simply based on the context of their surroundings. In situations filled with personal fear, or when given the opportunity for individual reward, research subjects throughout history have been willing to inflict severe pain, even death, on strangers.

A decade before Zimbardo's experiment and a year after the trial of Nazi Holocaust organizer Adolf Eichmann, one researcher wanted to understand how millions of German soldiers could commit so many heinous acts during World War II. So, Yale University psychology professor Stanley Milgram recruited hundreds of men from New Haven to participate in an experiment under the guise of a study about "memory and learning." In it, Milgram hooked an actor up to a fake electric-shock machine. In order to speed up his learning, participants were instructed to turn up the voltage each time the actor made a mistake. If they hesitated, they were once again given the instruction to proceed. After applying 300 volts, some research subjects refused to go further and quit the study. However, two-thirds followed instructions, ultimately turning up the dial to the highest and most lethal level.

As Milgram explained in his 1973 article "The Perils of Obedience": "I set up a simple experiment . . . to test how much pain an ordinary citizen would inflict on another person simply because he was ordered to by an experimental scientist. Stark authority was pitted against the subjects' strongest moral imperatives against hurting others, and, with the subjects' ears ringing with the screams of the victims, authority won more often than not."

For decades, these classic experiments have been used to explain societal behavior and a variety of atrocities. In *Mistreated*, they are applied for the first time to the failures of American health care.

Put cardiologists and cardiac surgeons in a relatively rural hospital like Redding, one that depends on heart-procedure volume for the survival of not just the hospital but the entire community, and perceptions begin to shift around surgical indications. Operate on healthy patients and your mortality rates plummet, reinforcing your self-perception as a leader in your field. Add senior surgeons who tell you that these slightly abnormal vessels are potentially deadly, and you begin to see the next set of studies differently. Over time, those doctors who are more conservative or operate only on patients with severe disease are perceived as lower in quality. This shift in perception affects everyone in the group. No one consciously decides this is what should happen. But it happens.

In many ways, faulty perception spreads like mass hysteria. In 1962, several dozen workers in a textile mill suddenly become severely ill. Many required hospitalization. The details of the medical findings were reported in the *Annals of Internal Medicine*. These individuals described being bitten by an insect that caused them nausea, vomiting, dizziness, and numbness. Research conducted by the US Public Health Service's Communicable Disease Center and onsite physicians found no evidence that the workers had been bitten by any type of bug capable of producing these symptoms. All of the reported problems reflected subconscious shifts of perception, the result of spreading anxiety and fear.

More recently, in 2006, an analogous epidemic struck Portugal when more than three hundred students from fourteen schools reported symptoms consistent with a life-threatening virus. The students described and showed symptoms ranging from difficulty breathing to dizziness and rashes, the same symptoms experienced by characters on a popular teen television drama called *Morangos com Açúcar* ("Strawberries with Sugar"). On the show, these symptoms resulted from a terrible underlying disease. And in real life, the fear of spreading the "disease" led to school closures throughout Portugal. Investigation by the Portuguese National Institute for Medical Emergency found no evidence of an infectious disease etiology or any other medical cause.

These experiences are different from those we might encounter with "groupthink," rationalization, or malingering. In such cases, the people harboring the faulty idea could, theoretically, figure out what was happening through deductive reasoning. In the cases of mass hysteria, the symptoms were just as physical as if the people had the actual disease they reported. In that context, what they felt was distorted and experienced as if it were real. But try as you might, you would not be able to convince them that they were wrong, at least not until you put them in a different context. When it comes to American health care, the same is true for doctors, patients, hospital leaders, and drug-company executives.

The Perception Problem

Across the United States, the leading cause of death for hospitalized patients isn't heart attack or stroke, but infection. And one of the leading causes of hospital-acquired infection is the result of doctors, nurses, and other hospital staff failing to wash their hands as they go from one patient's room to the next.

This common oversight can spread a life-threatening bacterium called *Clostridium difficile* or *C. diff.* This bacterium can contaminate surfaces in hospitals and remain infectious for up to six months. Once a patient is contaminated, *C. diff.* attacks the gastrointestinal tract, leading to massive diarrhea and bowel damage that can require surgery. This makes decontamination of hands, rooms, and hospital surfaces an absolute necessity.

It's estimated that *C. diff.* causes more than 400,000 infections each year and 14,000 deaths in the United States. Every American physician who cares for patients in a hospital knows about the hazards of spreading infection. Yet at least one-third of the time, doctors fail to wash their hands between patient visits.

Asked why they don't wash their hands every time, doctors will offer a litany of excuses. They'll talk about how rushed they are or explain that they don't touch every patient they see. They all know about the consequences of *C. diff.* infection, but, to a person, they will deny being responsible for the rising rate of unnecessary deaths in American hospitals.

Logically, we know people are spreading the germs and that it could very likely be the doctors who do not wash their hands. But that's not how individuals who skip this step see the situation. Like the participants in Zimbardo's study, they are not bad people who want to harm hospitalized patients. And they're not ignorant, either. Give doctors a written test on how *C. diff.* is spread, and all will know the correct answers. But in the rush of the morning, amid the anxiety of racing from one inpatient room to the next, context shifts their perception. In spite of the mandatory training they have undergone, they don't see their actions as contributing to the problem. The process is neither conscious nor logical. But based on observational studies, this same perceptional shift happens to the majority of doctors in this nation.

The Duality of Doctors

For more than fifteen years, I've had the privilege to lead the largest medical group in the country, with over 10,000 doctors and 34,000 medical staff. I've also had the opportunity in my role on the clinical faculty at Stanford Medical School to train close to a hundred residents and teach thousands of medical students, both in clinical medicine and health care policy. As chairman of the Council of Accountable Physician Practices (CAPP), which includes physicians from twenty-eight different medical groups, I have met hundreds of doctors of all ages and backgrounds from a variety of practices and geographies.

I can assure you that regardless of where they practice or when they graduated from medical school, these are dedicated, compassionate people wanting to do what is best for their patients. It doesn't matter if they're millennials or baby boomers, cardiologists or family practitioners. America's doctors are smart, highly motivated, ethical individuals. They're capable of inventing new approaches to the provision of medical care that can improve clinical outcomes for their patients. They are the best and brightest our nation has to offer, motivated by a passion for helping others. They can transform the American health care system for the better.

I've observed American physicians on volunteer trips in foreign countries, caring for the poorest and sickest patients on the planet. I have met with medical first-responders in Haiti after the 2010 earthquake that killed more than 160,000 people and with the doctors who risked their lives in Africa to treat patients dying from the Ebola virus. On such trips, I have seen doctors working eighty to one hundred hours a week, from early in the morning to late at night, without pay and in some of the most dangerous and hostile conditions imaginable. They volunteered for one reason: there were people in trouble who needed help, and they had the ability and skill to lend a hand. In spite of the pressures and demands placed on them, their joy and personal fulfillment was profound and inspiring.

However, this fulfillment from helping others, once intrinsic to the medical profession, is crumbling. One-third of all doctors are dissatisfied with their professional lives and over one-half would discourage their children from following in their footsteps. Many are counting down the days to retirement. Physicians across the nation are frustrated by the challenges of running their offices and tired of fighting with insurance companies to get paid for the work they do. American medicine once was and should be one of the most fulfilling professions. Today, it's not. Something is deeply wrong.

Observe from a distance the American physician volunteering in Liberia, outfitted in a bulky suit designed to prevent infection as she toils in 100°F heat, knowing full well she is about to risk her life. Compare her experience with that of the doctor perched in a comfortable chair in his beautiful wood-paneled office with air-conditioning and a handsome salary. You'd be surprised who is more satisfied.

In 2014, while researching an article for *Forbes*, best-selling author Malcolm Gladwell told me, "I don't understand, given the constraints physicians have in doing their jobs, and the paperwork demanded of them, why anyone would want to become a physician."

Indeed, observational studies demonstrate that physicians in community practice spend as much as half of their day completing insurance forms, entering computer data, and performing clerical work. In medical offices and hospitals across our land, mundane tasks combine with perverse economic incentives to push doctors further and further away from the reasons they chose a career in medicine.

As paperwork and financial pressures compete with doctor-patient relationships, frustrations intensify on both sides of the stethoscope. More and more, there is a duality to being a doctor. There's the fulfilling and awe-inspiring personal side of treating patients, making diagnoses, and saving lives. And then there's the fatiguing and frustrating impersonal side. The personal side offers a profound sense of satisfaction. It reminds doctors of why they get up in the morning. The impersonal side sends doctors home exhausted. These day-to-day frustrations present a significant threat to the health of our nation. So, too, does the culture of medicine.

The medical community prides itself on being scientific, pragmatic, and precise. Scratch away at these virtues and you'll find that the way doctors practice medicine is wildly inconsistent. Despite its empirical roots, the culture of medicine is mired by the doctor's conviction that he or she knows best how to deliver care to patients. It should be no surprise, then, that research indicates a large variation in clinical outcomes from one doctor to the next. This inconsistency in clinical practice has a major impact on patient health. In fact, when you compare results, physicians in some medical groups have reduced their patients' chances of dying from a stroke, heart attack, or cancer by 30 percent or more when compared to others.

You might think that every doctor would want to learn from and emulate those achieving the best results. But they don't. Like the doctors in Redding and the ones not washing their hands, even physicians with poor clinical outcomes perceive that they are delivering excellent medical care, in spite of what objective observation might indicate.

Doctors are caught up in all sorts of contradictions. For reasons we will explore in greater depth, they eagerly embrace new drugs and purchase sophisticated machinery that hardly moves the needle on overall patient health. Yet they ignore and fail to act on some of the biggest and most straightforward opportunities to save more lives. A decade ago, the Institute of Medicine reported that 98,000 people die in hospitals each year due to medical error. The most recent research indicates that the true annual mortality statistic may be closer to 200,000 avoidable deaths when you add (1) doctors who fail to communicate effectively with their colleagues, (2) doctors and nurses who dole out the wrong medications, and (3) doctors who are responsible for causing or spreading hospital infections. And yet most physicians can't see the opportunities for improvement sprouting up all around them.

The perceptions of American patients are just as inexplicable and paradoxical. Half of American adults have a negative view of the health care industry in general, but nearly 80 percent of all patients reflect positively on the health care they personally receive. Once again, the math doesn't add up. Both conclusions can't be right. The data comparing the United States with the rest of the world demonstrate that we're not all getting great care. But among doctors and patients alike, perception trumps data.

As was discovered with the students in the Stanford Prison Experiment, context shapes how patients see the world around them. In the context of health care, patients choose their own doctors and entrust them with the health of their family. The medical acumen and ability of doctors can be awe-inspiring, their work sophisticated and curative. At the same time, there will always be some doctors whose skills lag behind those of their colleagues. Few patients are aware when this is the case. Having chosen their physicians, and with their health in the hands of these experts, it's no surprise that patients see their doctors as the best available. And when patients see their doctors as outstanding, they perceive the medical treatment they provide as excellent. From a statistical and comparative standpoint, however, that's frequently not the case.

Designed to Fail

In business schools, professors are known to put forth an axiom that goes something like this: "Tell me the design of the system, and I'll tell you the outcome you will get."

They're usually right, and nowhere is it truer than in medical practice. The design of our health care system—how it's structured, reimbursed, technologically supported, and led—determines how the people in it will behave.

When you design a health-insurance reimbursement system that financially rewards doctors for providing patients with more care (as opposed to better care), that's exactly what doctors value and do. And when third-party insurers pay for patient care regardless of the outcomes, patients also assume that more care is better, even when research and data demonstrate that's not the case. And when we pay physicians more to take care of heart attacks or strokes than to prevent them in the first place, they value emergency intervention dramatically more than disease prevention.

Even with good intentions, a system's design can lead to harmful consequences. Professor Zimbardo conducted the Stanford Prison Experiment to improve the lives of those incarcerated. He never imagined his study would result in the inhumane and degrading treatment of innocent people.

This correlation between the design and its outcomes inspires a question: If Zimbardo could create an environment that led good students to do terrible things, is it possible to shift the environment of health care in ways that would lead highly motivated, mission-driven doctors to provide better care to patients like you and me?

I believe it is possible. But before we can focus on the solution, we need to fully understand the real problems.

Over the next three chapters, we'll examine the design of health care and its consequences through several different lenses, including those of the doctor, the patient, and the other major health care players (insurance companies, national medical societies, and drug manufacturers among them). In the second half of the book, we'll look at what direction American health care might go and focus on why most of the solutions we've tried in the past led to dead ends. We'll break down the changes implemented via the Patient Protection and Affordable Care Act (ACA), the first step in a long journey to fix the broken US health care system. We'll examine what's likely to change in the years ahead and provide a four-point plan to address health care's next biggest set of challenges. Finally, we'll look at how health care's most promising solutions will affect the patient.

Along the way, we'll go inside America's Emergency Rooms (ERs) and watch courageous doctors battle an orphan disease. We'll travel to Flint, Michigan, and examine the mindset of government officials who ignored a horrific medical development that threatened the lives of children. We'll visit the laboratories where researchers face insane pressures to "publish or perish," opening the door for drug companies to interfere with independent medical studies. We'll travel the world to learn from countries that have succeeded where the American system has failed. We'll meet the community organizer who helped shape our nation's most transformative health care legislation and the businessman-turned-political-newcomer who is likely to reshape the landscape once more.

As we visit these diverse places and meet the men and women who embody American medicine today, I invite you to follow the common thread that connects all parts. That thread is the profound and powerful relationship between the structure of US health care and the subconscious perceptions of everyone in it.

Without doubt, the environment in which care is delivered and received is unlike any other—a potent context that alters our senses in ways that don't always align with objective reality. Understanding this relationship—the connection between context and perception—helps explain the paradoxes of American health care and allows us to identify the underlying etiology of its problems. It also shifts the blame. Today, we accuse individuals for the majority of problems facing health care. In doing so, we overlook and fail to call out the deeper systemic problems.

Seventy years ago, the founder of The Permanente Medical Group, Dr. Sidney Garfield, wrote about moving medical practice from "sick care to health care." We have an opportunity in America today to fulfill that vision now and in the future, but only if we are willing to see what's really happening, confront what is wrong, and demonstrate the courage to do something about it.

An essential place for us to begin this journey is inside the mind of the physician, understanding both the mission-driven side and the part that's riddled with intense fears.

Chapter Two

What Doctors See

The human body maintains a delicate balance between too much and too little of just about everything it needs. A healthy body, one with just the right balance, operates with clockwork precision, bringing oxygen, nutrients, and infection-fighting cells to tissues and organs with each beat of the heart. But it remains, always, a delicate system. With not enough liquid, blood pressure begins to fall, kicking the heart into overdrive as it struggles to push sufficient blood to vital organs. With too much liquid, fluid backs up. Like a clogged pipe, the lungs flood, swelling the feet and reducing the flow of oxygen to the heart and eventually the brain.

Our bodies walk a perpetual fine line. What exactly tips them one way or the other isn't always clear, even to experienced clinicians. That's why medical students, residents, and newly trained doctors work hard to master this tightrope act.

In school, doctors spend their days and nights learning the intricacies and solving the mysteries of the human body. Through rigorous practice and years of training, physicians can decipher medical secrets by looking into the eye, listening to the heart, and palpating the abdomen. Over time, they gain the competence to cut open the body with a scalpel, insert scopes into the different orifices and cavities, prescribe powerful medications, and remove damaged tissue to eradicate disease. It's an awesome privilege and a responsibility afforded only to those who have earned the title of "doctor."

In the right circumstances, physicians can accomplish amazing things. Modern technology grants them access to the latest and greatest scientific advancements, from human genomics to the totality of published medical literature. Using computerized systems and mobile devices, doctors can instantly peruse massive quantities of data and a wealth of diagnostic information. Over the past twenty years, physicians have used this information and its insights to radically enhance the quality of care they deliver, reaching levels previously thought impossible.

In today's world, many patients who undergo total joint replacement (a procedure that replaces a damaged joint with a metal, plastic, or ceramic device) are out of bed and walking within hours, and home in less than a day. It's remarkable, given this surgery once kept the patient in the hospital for a week.

Meanwhile, children with inherited life-threatening conditions such as cystic fibrosis are living longer and more normal lives, creating the demand for specialists who can treat them in adulthood—a need that simply didn't exist back when long-term survival was impossible. And only a generation ago, certain types of childhood leukemia were uniformly fatal, whereas today, care providers can save thousands of these children each year, with some institutions achieving cure rates as high as 70 percent.

But of all the areas of medical practice, our progress in the fight against heart disease is the most astonishing. Physicians have helped patients improve their heart health through diet, exercise, and medications to the point where heart disease is no longer the leading cause of death in certain parts of the United States and the world. With advanced surgical methods, doctors can now replace heart valves without ever opening the chest cavity. All across the United States, surgeons have reduced death rates after heart surgery to the low single digits.

Looking back, the progress we've made and the speed at which we've advanced the medical frontier has been awe-inspiring. To the outside observer, physicians can appear all-knowing, all-seeing, and all-powerful. Inside the physician's mind, however, the world of health care looks very different.

Despite the bounty of treatment options available and the promise of greater cures to come, there lingers inside each doctor a persistent and underlying sense of terror. The best physicians know that any intervention or medication capable of saving a patient's life is also capable of harming or even killing the patient. Maintaining the delicate balance of the human body—that constant undulation of too much and too little—requires a combination of judgment, skill, and luck.

For doctors, the worst days aren't those that require the longest hours or involve the most demanding patients. They're the days when something goes wrong. Few physicians can imagine anything worse than making a mistake that harms a patient. But that consequence is the ever-present reality of medicine. Practice long enough, it'll happen. Even the most highly skilled and fastidious doctors have missed a life-threatening diagnosis, caused a major infection, or committed a technical error.

This fear that doctors carry with them isn't just some form of self-protective paranoia or the dread of being sued for malpractice. It's the fear of violating that deeply embedded, core principle of the profession: *Primum non nocere*, or "First, do no harm." When something goes wrong, the physician's distress runs deep. The refrain "if only" echoes through the brain. There are sleepless nights filled with tossing, turning, and painful reflection. *How could I have missed that diagnosis? How could I have cut that blood vessel? Why did I recommend that treatment?*

Welcome to the mind of the physician, filled with scores of medical facts and endless self-doubt. Although doctors brim with a certain kind of confidence necessary to solve the most complex problems, this feeling belies the ever-present fear that making a mistake is never a question of "if" but "when."

Doctors are given the privilege to ask the most intimate of questions and the trust to touch the patient's skin with their hands. They have the curative expertise to safely pierce the human shell with needles and knives. In return, they hold themselves to near-impossible standards and expectations. As patients, we all should feel keenly grateful for our doctors' medical mastery, while understanding that, sometimes, bad outcomes arise from good intentions.

Drawing Blood

In the summer of 2011, the overhead paging system rang out above the din of a bustling Northern California hospital. Hospital operators use color codes to communicate urgency to physicians. In this case, it was a code red, the most urgent alert, indicative of a life-threatening problem. A rush of activity swiftly ensued.

As nurses and doctors raced to the Emergency Department, they soon began to swirl in choreographed chaos around the eighty-two-year-old man lying on the gurney in front of them. Barely aware of the medical frenzy happening beside him, the man felt disoriented and afraid. In the ambulance ride over from his home in San Jose, he complained of weakness and trouble breathing. As an experienced nurse slipped an oxygen mask over his face, she bent down to reassure him, "You can breathe now, Stanley."

In that moment, Stanley's breathing steadied, but he was far from okay. Soon after, his blood pressure slipped and his pulse quickened. If you could have seen the inner workings of his body, you would have marveled at how hard it was laboring to correct itself, trying to restore what physicians call homeostasis. As the doctors scrambled to save him, the digits on the pulse-rate monitor next to Stanley's bed rose. His heart fought to maintain adequate perfusion, but no matter how hard it tried, it couldn't keep up. Blood flow slowed first to his kidneys, then his intestines. This was his body's last defense and Stanley's only hope. Without immediate intervention, his brain and the heart itself would have been the next to go.

Expedited lab tests and vital signs appeared on the computer screens in the treatment room, confirming that Stanley was in septic shock. Bacteria raced through his body, just as they raced through my father's, infecting Stanley's organs and impeding their function. Sepsis disrupts the delicate balance of life like few other medical problems can. It accounts for only 2 percent of all hospital admissions but one in six hospital deaths.

Sepsis was progressively shutting Stanley's body down. Without enough blood returning to the heart, it couldn't provide adequate circulation to all of his vital organs. For three hours, the team of doctors in the room worked masterfully and frantically to rip Stanley back from the clutches of death. As their hands and minds raced, they fought to stabilize his blood pressure, hoping to improve it just enough so that they could move him up to Intensive Care on the second floor. Even if Stanley survived, the doctors realized he would face months of rehabilitation.

Stanley's diagnosis of sepsis was clear to the care team in this hospital—and would be to just about every physician in the nation—just as my father's sepsis was apparent to the ICU care team at Stanford. Stanley's clinical condition and diagnosis sat at the obviously critical end of a wide spectrum. Not everyone with sepsis comes to the ER in extremis.

For younger, healthier patients, sepsis can come out of nowhere, appearing mild in its earliest stages but becoming vicious and deadly a day or two later. For these patients, the difference between life and death depends on whether the care team recognizes that a crisis looms on the horizon, before the destruction begins.

Nancy, a forty-nine-year-old mother of three, still doesn't know how she contracted the infection that almost took her life. "It was the weekend before Christmas and I had been out shopping for presents that Saturday with our nine-year-old," Nancy said, recalling that she felt sluggish hours later at her dance class. There was a flu going around, and she thought that could be the problem. That night she tossed and turned.

"I had the chills and couldn't stop shaking. I finally woke up my husband, George."

George, a physician, took her pulse and found it a little fast. Nancy's foot was slightly red, so George figured it could just be a skin irritation from her dance class or from hours of walking around the mall. But better safe than sorry, George drove to a nearby pharmacy and left Nancy in bed to rest.

He wrote out a prescription for a first-generation antibiotic to treat what doctors call cellulitis. When he returned home, Nancy propped herself up and pulled back the covers. Her leg had turned bright red, all the way up to her knee.

"Get out of bed now," George insisted as he helped her to her feet. "We're going to the Emergency Room."

An ER physician saw Nancy immediately and confirmed the diagnosis of cellulitis. That much was clear. He treated her condition just as any other doctor would by inserting an IV line, drawing blood cultures, and administering antibiotics.

After drawing the blood culture, however, the ER physician did something else, something that likely saved Nancy's life. He ordered a blood-lactate test. This laboratory study is neither costly nor risky nor difficult to obtain, so you wouldn't think there'd be much to it.

But what's strange is that this crucial and often life-saving step is one that many doctors in many other hospitals would have skipped.

Physicians always order a blood-lactate level for patients like Stanley who come to the ER with an obvious systemic infection. And the test results always come back grossly abnormal, confirming the diagnosis. Nancy, while clearly sick but not nearly as compromised as Stanley, had a blood-lactate level somewhere between normal and abnormal, the so-called intermediate range. So, the question with Nancy became: What to do next?

As soon as her results came back, the Emergency Department physician in this particular hospital triggered the same stat page used for Stanley. With that page, physicians from a variety of specialties rushed to the ER and began aggressive treatment. And if all doctors in every ER consistently ordered the test and provided immediate, intense therapy, they would save enough lives each year to fill a pro football stadium. But they don't.

Understanding why they don't teaches us a valuable lesson about the psyche of physicians and the role perception plays in American health care.

If Nancy's husband, George, had taken her to a different hospital, even in the same community, the approach would be different and intensity of care would be much less. The emergency physician would diagnose her cellulitis just as quickly but would assume the infection was confined to the leg. That physician would put her on a slow-drip IV, order antibiotics, and admit her to the hospital. No blood-lactate test would be ordered or performed. On the medical floor, she would be judged as low risk. The next morning, the discharge planner would come by Nancy's room to make arrangements for her to go home.

At that point, Nancy would be moderately sick, but stable. Later that day or early the next morning, however, she would "crash." Her blood pressure would bottom out, her pulse would race ever more rapidly, and the window of opportunity would close. Without the initial blood-lactate test result and without emergency physicians willing and trained to respond aggressively, Nancy's chances of making it to New Year's Day would have been 20 to 30 percent lower.

The question you might be asking yourself right now is why wouldn't all physicians order this test whenever they see a patient with a worrisome infection? After all, the test is safe and relatively inexpensive. The answer is complex. It requires us to look deeper inside the mind of the doctor and examine this deadly disease more closely.

A Powerful Killer

Sepsis is one of the oldest known diseases, given its name by Hippocrates some 2,400 years ago. It has claimed the lives of millions of people, including *Superman* actor Christopher Reeve and Pope John Paul II. The disease process of sepsis has killed two US presidents: William Henry Harrison in 1841, after only a month in office, and James Garfield in 1881. Although many believe Garfield was assassinated—and indeed he was shot by a would-be assassin—he actually died from systemic sepsis after doctors (with unwashed hands) tried but failed to dislodge the bullet.

Sepsis can begin in seemingly innocuous ways with something as simple as an insect bite or a bladder infection. Regardless of exact etiology, it's a powerful killer, responsible for more deaths annually than AIDS (acquired immunodeficiency syndrome), prostate cancer, and breast cancer combined. Sepsis affects more than 1 million people in our country and, every year, wipes out 210,000 Americans, equal to the population of Rochester, New York.

If any of this comes as a surprise to you, well, you wouldn't be alone. Most Americans (nearly six in ten) have never even heard of sepsis. And if you are perplexed by the lack of name recognition for an illness that's both lethal and common, Dr. Emmanuel Rivers can relate.

Dr. Rivers, who goes by Manny, is an emergency and critical-care physician at the Henry Ford Medical Center in Detroit. He was one of the first physicians in America to encourage health care providers to adopt aggressive protocols for the early detection and treatment of sepsis. In his seminal 2001 *New England Journal of Medicine* article titled "Early Goal-Directed Therapy (EGDT)," Manny brought the concept of rapid and aggressive sepsis treatment into the Emergency Department, where the fight against this deadly infection is often won and lost.

The life-saving potential of Manny's EGDT approach was off the charts. But upon its release, the article didn't have quite the impact Manny imagined.

Now, if he had discovered a new cancer drug with even half the life-saving potential of his sepsis protocols, here's how his story would have gone: *Doctor from Detroit invents a breakthrough treatment, every single oncologist in America rushes to prescribe it, mortality rates plummet, Dr. Rivers hoists a slew of awards, graces magazine covers, and becomes the envy of all his peers.*

But that's not what happened. Although his breakthrough sepsis protocols could have saved hundreds of thousands of lives by now, doctors didn't rush to adopt them. In fact, even a decade after publishing his study, Manny was still having a very difficult time convincing everyone to follow his teachings. Instead of being lauded by his peers and praised by the media, his data and recommendations came under fierce attack. There are reasons for that, very few of which conform to logic.

The Orphan Disease

Some fifteen years after his groundbreaking EGDT findings, Manny offered one reason that this deadly disease continues to flourish in the halls of American hospitals.

"Sepsis is an orphan disease," he says. "It is not owned by the major players out there like heart attacks, cancer, and stroke."

You see, sepsis affects many parts of the body and is treated by physicians from multiple specialties. All play some role in fighting sepsis, but sepsis belongs to no one specialty. Therefore, all of these experts perceive other causes and diseases to be more important to their day-to-day practices.

Cardiologists dedicate their careers to coronary health and are largely concerned with heart attacks. Some of their patients will get sepsis, but it's not the cause of death they worry about most. Oncologists spend their days fighting cancer and, for them, chemotherapy is the Holy Grail. And though sepsis is a known complication of many cancer-treatment drugs, most oncology patients die from the spread of their cancers, not from sepsis. And so it is for all specialties involved in the battle against sepsis.

Perhaps if this orphan disease only affected the heart or the kidneys or the intestines, one of the specialty groups would adopt it as its own. But for specialists in America, sepsis is a secondary concern, not their life's passion.

And because no one "owns" sepsis, there is no national society that makes recommendations or does extensive research on it the way the American Heart Association does for cardiac disease. There's no massive, national network of sepsis champions raising hundreds of millions of dollars or putting advertisements on TV the way neurologists have rallied behind stroke prevention and detection. There's no major support from drug or device companies to fund university research on sepsis the way there is for drugs that are easily marketed to such single-specialty groups as gastroenterologists, pulmonologists, or hematologists.

As Manny lamented, "Some people dedicate their lives to conditions of the heart and others to the lung. Sepsis is the orphan disease that falls through the cracks."

That doesn't have to be the case. In California, one dedicated physician—armed with a computer—managed to fight sepsis like no one ever had before.

Virtues and Vices

Dr. Diane Craig has been a colleague of mine for over two decades. Soft-spoken and calm, Diane is self-assured but never arrogant. She's a big thinker, a problem solver, and an incredible leader. If you met her, you'd instantly recognize why her colleagues hold her in such high esteem.

Throughout Diane's career, she has fueled transformative ideas and sparked meaningful change.

About twenty years ago, for example, Diane began to radically alter the way doctors in hospitals provide medical care. After studying physician workflows and clinical outcomes at her facility in Santa Clara, California, Diane realized that the traditional model wasn't working. Back then, doctors saw patients at the hospital in the morning before heading to the office for the next eight hours. As one might imagine, a lot happened while the doctors were away. It made more sense, she thought, to have dedicated physicians available to care for hospitalized patients throughout the day.

So, thanks to Diane and her colleagues, the role of "hospitalist" emerged. It wasn't easy to make the switch. Doctors liked dabbling in both inpatient and outpatient medicine, and so they resisted at first. From idea to implementation, the process of getting this specialty up and running took close to two decades. Most people don't have that kind of stamina. But as these specialized doctors honed this new expertise, patient care improved and overall mortality rates dropped dramatically.

Today, Diane is recognized across the country as one of the pioneers in developing the hospital-based physician model of care. The role of hospitalist is now a major specialty nationwide, considered the gold standard for providing the best care in hospital settings.

Diane is proof of the positive influence physician leaders can have on their colleagues and the stubborn culture of American medicine. Having solved one problem, Diane was eager to move on to the next.

For most of the 1990s and early 2000s, the hospital mortality rates where Diane practiced fell significantly, reaching levels much lower than you would find almost anywhere else in the country. But when the rate of improvement began to level off, Diane started looking for new answers. That's when she met the sepsis problem head on.

Her efforts began with a new ally: computerized patient health records. Diane's mind runs on hard data. And when her hospital installed a comprehensive electronic medical-record system (and connected it with other systems in the hospital network like the lab and pharmacy), she was eager to take advantage of its sophisticated analytics and digitized patient information.

As she dove into the data, she was surprised to learn that a common assumption made in most hospital settings was dead wrong. She found that many of the well-known killers (heart attacks, cancer, and stroke) were no longer the leading causes of death among hospitalized patients. Contrary to what most thought at the time, sepsis was the number-one killer, ten times deadlier than heart attacks. But that discovery was just Diane's first step. The best physician leaders are like detectives: each clue motivates them to uncover another.

As Diane and her colleagues culled through hundreds of medical records, looking specifically at patients who died from sepsis, they discovered that only about half of them arrived at the Emergency Department extremely sick, like Stanley. The other half seemed relatively healthy upon admission, like Nancy. And in most cases, the treating physicians underestimated how sick these individuals really were.

Then Diane did something no one else had done before in the fight against sepsis. She started matching pairs of patients using electronic health-record data, meaning she would identify two patients of similar age with similar symptoms and equivalent degrees of illness. For example, she looked at two patients in their thirties who had kidney infections, one who lived and one who died from sepsis. She then matched two patients in their forties with cellulitis of the leg: one lived, one died. Tracing each patient's care back to the very beginning, she and her team tried to identify the first branch point in their care. And that is when she discovered the importance of the blood-lactate test, along with the value of early, aggressive treatments based on the test results.

"The most important step in lowering the mortality from sepsis," Diane explains, "is making sure that the Emergency Room physicians order a blood-lactate test for every patient at risk, even those who are not yet extremely sick."

Every Emergency Room physician can tell you that a blood lactate above 4 millimoles per liter (mmol/L) means the patient is in serious danger. Just to give you a reference point, Stanley's lactate count was 8.8 mmol/L. Emergency doctors also know that a normal level is 1 to 2 mmol/L, no cause for alarm.

But when it comes to patients in the middle, those with "intermediate" lactate levels, most ER physicians aren't sure what to make of the results. Diane Craig's findings have erased all doubts.

"Examining hundreds of records of patients who died from sepsis, we found that even a level as low as 2.5, which is considered trivial in many hospitals, was a huge red flag," she said.

This was a seismic discovery. If a lactate level just 0.5 above "normal" could be life-threatening, then how many diagnoses were doctors missing? How many seemingly healthy patients were actually just hours or days away from death? Diane and her team determined that the majority of patients who die from sepsis have an initial blood-lactate level in that intermediate range.

Armed with this insight, Diane's mission was clear. She would use Dr. Rivers's EGDT recommendations to create protocols for all "intermediate" patients. She and her colleagues concluded that whenever individuals had two symptoms consistent with a significant infection—even minor symptoms such as a fever and an elevated pulse rate—sepsis had to be considered a threat. In each case, regardless of how healthy the patient seemed, a blood-lactate test had to be performed. And if the results came back in that intermediate zone, aggressive treatment would need to begin immediately.

Under Diane's leadership, the physicians in Santa Clara were quick to embrace the new approach, and from that moment on, any combination of worrisome symptoms and a lactate level of 2.5 or more triggered a "sepsis alert." Now, whenever that alert echoes through the PA system (or, more recently, on the iPhones doctors now carry), highly trained clinicians race to the ER just as fast as they did for Stanley.

And to help ensure that doctors followed this approach every time, Diane printed the information on laminated cards and attached them to lanyards so that every doctor and nurse could wear them around their necks. And, over time, she placed best-practice alerts into the electronic health-record system and built specific protocols into its order-entry function.

With her guidance, her persistence, her laminated cards, and her alerts, Diane changed the hospital's environment for the better. Instead of tolerating major variations in practice, she used objective data on clinical outcomes to change expectations for how doctors provide care.

The results spoke for themselves. Diane and her hospital team drove sepsis mortality rates down to 40 percent below the national average.

With those results, you might assume that every emergency physician in the United States would be convinced to follow this approach. However, Dr. Rivers estimates that only about one-half of the hospitals in the United States have put in place effective sepsis protocols, with maybe another one-fourth "working through" the issue. The remaining one-fourth of hospitals "have nothing."

So we're back to the same question. Why the hesitation to order this simple test?

Physicians and Fear

In 1981, researchers Amos Tversky and Daniel Kahneman asked their subjects to help the United States prepare for a hypothetical outbreak of a disease that if left untreated would kill six hundred people. Participants in one group were told that a treatment would save two hundred lives. Seventy-eight percent of the research subjects in that cohort favored moving forward. Another group was told that in spite of the treatment, four hundred people would die. In this case, less than 25 percent of the participants opted to administer the treatment.

Obviously, the result was the same in both scenarios: two hundred lived and four hundred died. But the two groups saw the consequences very differently. It's a powerful example of how the human mind magnifies loss compared to gain. Our brains respond to the possibility of killing someone with intense emotion. In fact, it is felt to a far greater degree than when we are presented with the opportunity to save a life, or even multiple lives. And when we are personally responsible for killing someone, the gap between the two sets of actions expands even further. Here's where the doctor's mindset comes into play with sepsis.

Aggressive sepsis treatment is intense and potentially fatal. As described in Manny's EGDT findings, the first step is to place what is called a "central venous line." That means the physician punctures the patient's neck with a large needle, threads a plastic tube down near the heart, and administers powerful antibiotics. Placing the central line comes with some major risks, including the possibility of damaging the underlying lung. And that's just the beginning. With the tube in place, the physician then administers massive volumes of fluid, as much as two to three quarts in the first hour. This much fluid can flood the patient's lungs and overwhelm the heart's ability to pump—literally drowning the patient.

This is a terrifying thought for a physician. Even if this approach could save nine out of ten lives, the fear of killing one patient this way can be overwhelming.

Psychologists and ethicists have studied this same phenomenon through hypothetical scenarios. For example, would you throw a switch to redirect a runaway trolley—and possibly save the lives of dozens onboard the train—if it meant killing a worker on an adjacent track? Now, if you said yes, would you push someone onto the track to stop the runaway trolley? The majority of people would throw the switch. But results from different experiments show that when an individual must directly inflict harm to save lives, the subject's reluctance increases by as much as 50 percent.

The scenario is similar with sepsis. Based on Dr. Craig's data, doctors who treat every person with an intermediate lactate level as aggressively as they would a patient with full-blown sepsis will save more lives. In fact, ordering the test and starting intense treatment immediately when lactate levels are only slightly abnormal lowers the mortality rate by half. But when you are the one directly inflicting the harm, the consequences feel different. The death you might cause feels far more significant than the multiple lives you might save by acting immediately. This is where perception and objective information don't align, creating intense anxiety for the physician. On the one hand, doctors have read the literature closely and understand the science. On the other hand, the thought of personally harming a patient is devastating. The best solution for the doctors: Don't order the test in the first place. That way, you don't have to decide whether to treat the patient aggressively. *Primum non nocere*—first, do no harm.

This isn't a malicious or negligent or conscious decision. Rather, the thought of killing a patient alters what the doctor sees. And in these borderline situations where sepsis may be present, the doctor perceives the patient as not being sick enough to require testing for potential sepsis. The physician still admits the patient and, in doing so, hands the decision of whether to order the blood-lactate test and aggressively treat the individual over to someone else, usually the admitting physician or specialty consultant.

The Conformity of Fear

Nearly half of all companies do not survive their first two years, according to the Bureau of Labor Statistics, proof that failure is a fairly common occurrence in business. Read the headlines of business publications or hang out in Silicon Valley long enough, and you may even get the sense that failure is something of a badge of honor. In medicine, however, failure is always negative. It comes with serious consequences, both for the patient and the physician.

When I compare the experiences of the students I teach in the Stanford School of Business with those in the Stanford School of Medicine, their worlds contrast vividly. In business school, students are encouraged to dream big and innovate. Future doctors, on the other hand, are expected to check their creativity at the classroom door. In no uncertain terms, medical school professors lay out their expectations for students: memorize the medical terms, learn the recommended clinical approach by rote, and repeat.

The goal of medical training is not to challenge conventional wisdom. It is to learn "the right way"—often presented as the only way—to provide medical care. This long-reigning pedagogy ensures that yesterday's truths remain tomorrow's answers, at least for much longer than they should.

Future physicians are taught to embrace conformity by memorizing the right answer for every clinical question posed, although "taught" may be too soft a term. On rounds and in the Operating Room, young physicians are "pimped," an intimidating process through which attending and senior physicians fire questions at medical students and junior residents. Those who get the answers wrong are often belittled. The only defense? Commit to memory and recite exactly what they read in the textbooks. There's no thinking outside the box in these situations, no coloring outside the lines.

In medical school and residency training, you learn to protect yourself from criticism by conforming to the practices of others. Doctors who follow the rules and use the same approaches as everyone else rarely face severe consequences when something untoward happens. But when doctors go against the grain and something goes wrong, they risk their licenses and careers.

So, if your teachers and colleagues wouldn't obtain a blood-lactate test for a patient with a low-grade fever and a slightly elevated pulse, you would be well protected when you don't either. But if you order the test, get "intermediate" results, and damage the patient's lung trying to insert the central venous line, there will be no one to save you from the fallout.

Deeply embedded in the physician psyche is the "community standard" of care. It's described and held up as the right way, the only way to provide care, and it prevails well beyond medical school. Follow the community standard, even when you know it's suboptimal, and your colleagues will stand up for you. Violate the community standard, even when you know it's the right thing to do, and you risk a malpractice suit. Worse, you'll be separated from the herd, forced to fend for yourself—alone and unprotected.

To reinforce this culture of conformity, academic programs and some community hospitals convene monthly "morbidity and mortality" conferences. There, the most senior physicians judge the mistakes and complications that arise from treatment. In these emotionally charged settings, doctors are grilled by their peers and attending physicians about what went wrong. When errors are deemed major and the explanations unacceptable, a doctor's reputation and career can be permanently damaged.

In the book *Decisive*, authors and brothers Chip and Dan Heath asked Dr. Diane Craig about her experience in helping doctors cope with the fear of harming a patient.

"It takes a while for people to get comfortable saying, 'This patient looks good but I'm going to put a large central IV catheter in their neck and put them in the ICU and pump them full of liters and liters of fluids. And we'll do all this because of borderline test results, even though they look perfectly fine at the moment.'"

Through this lens, we can see why so many physicians and Emergency Departments have resisted the teachings of Dr. Rivers, labeling his approach "controversial."

For completeness, it's worth pointing out that some of Manny's earlier approaches—such as the use of the central venous line—have been found unnecessary for many patients. Doctors today often insert multiple IVs in the patient's arms instead. But over time, Manny's fundamental approach for getting ahead of the disease has proven accurate and life-saving.

When Intermountain Healthcare's sepsis protocols gained near-full compliance in 2010, mortality rates dropped to 9 percent (down from around 20 percent before the implementation of protocols). And in New York state, fifty-five hospitals in a sepsis pilot program observed an 18 percent drop in deaths in just over a year by using the types of protocols Dr. Craig created.

How Doctors See Themselves

Aside from the fear of harming patients, there is another reason doctors resist embracing these types of protocols. Simply put, they don't like to be told what to do. After a decade of training, they believe their answers are the right ones—a self-perception that's reinforced by society.

Regardless of where they travel, in the United States or around the globe, doctors are held in high esteem. I am often amazed by how many people insist on calling me Dr. Pearl out of respect, even though I introduce myself as (and prefer to be called) Robbie. I'm particularly uncomfortable when people in social situations address me using only my professional title, "Doctor."

Outside of religious leaders and elected officials, few others are identified by their profession in this way. This reverence underlies the traditional physician attitude that "doctor knows best." There exists a fine line
(but a big difference) between feeling appreciated and becoming arrogant.
Unfortunately, it's a line the medical profession steps across too often.

You would expect that a doctor working at a hospital with a 25 percent
sepsis mortality rate would want to learn as much as possible about (and
emulate) the facilities that have a death rate two-thirds lower. But they
usually don't. And because American physicians rely so heavily on their
own judgment and skill, the pace of improvement in our nation's overall
health remains slow.

Medicine: An Art or a Science?

Among physicians, there's something of an ongoing debate as to whether
the clinical practice of medicine is more of an art or an applied science.
The stances on both sides reveal a lot about health care and about doctors
specifically.

Like the majority of "A" students, as most physicians were in college,
doctors recognized early in their educational endeavors that every question in chemistry or physics had a right answer. They worked hard in
school to figure out those answers before every test.

Years later, they read medical journals routinely to learn the newest
right answers based on the scientific method. But when faced with data
on their own lagging performance, they often defend their medical intuition and preferred approaches, insisting that numbers don't tell the whole
story and that medicine is an art form with no single right answer.

Medical problems aren't like snowflakes. The anatomy and physiology
of most people are similar, as are their diseases. But because physicians
don't like being told how to practice, they reject the idea of following
consistent data-based approaches. When expected to always order a
blood-lactate test for any patient with even a relatively low risk of sepsis,
many doctors bristle. They complain that the person requiring them to
do so doesn't respect their clinical expertise. They frequently snicker at
these approaches, labeling them "cookbook medicine."

When it comes to style, medicine is an art. Earning the trust of patients and helping them improve their overall health through diet and

exercise requires understanding their specific situation and personality. And, of course, there are some patients with problems so complex or numerous that no evidence-based approach exists. Here, the doctor's clinical judgment is essential. And on occasion, there are situations in which the medical literature is unclear or the recommendation too new to evaluate. These cases require the doctor's unique expertise and judgment, as well, at least until the data can eliminate uncertainty and render an answer.

But for much of clinical practice, there is a best approach, one based on data and evidence. And if each physician followed the available evidence-based guidelines, hundreds of thousands of lives would be saved each year.

As an example, over a decade ago, research made known to doctors helped the medical community determine that four very safe and inexpensive medications could reduce the likelihood of a heart attack in certain patients by close to 40 percent. One was a drug to lower cholesterol, a second to increase blood flow to the kidneys, a third to reduce work load on the heart, and the fourth, an aspirin.

This simple approach was recommended for nearly all patients who had experienced a prior heart attack and for those with aortic aneurysm, peripheral vascular disease, or diabetes.

Logic indicates that based on this evidence and the relative safety of the drugs, physicians would follow this common approach 100 percent of the time. They don't. And this is where the influence of context comes into play.

Physicians who use a comprehensive electronic health record are reminded each time they see a patient with one of these problems to prescribe all of the effective and recommended medications. Those without such a system are likely not to take the time to make sure these drugs have been prescribed. Physicians in a large medical group with consistent quality reports see the gaps and have incentives to close them. Those working alone have to search for the data in their medical records and those of others. That's a lot of work.

In the end, the debate is less about *whether* medicine is an "art" or a "science." It's about *when* medicine should be an art and *when* it must be a science. As Dr. Craig showed, science consistently trumps intuition, and consistently following the best practices saves lives. You might think that the community standard would align with the best medical practice, but most often it is wedded to the past, incorporating a wide variety of options rather than embracing the best one.

Medicine is an applied science that needs to be practiced artfully and never compromised. More often than not, variation in practice harms patients. Organizations such as the Institute for Healthcare Improvement and the Institute of Medicine have demonstrated this time and again.

It Doesn't Matter Who the Best Doctor Is

In the same way that doctors overvalue the art of medicine, patients are convinced that the best clinical outcomes are physician dependent. That's why the most common question I get asked by friends with a medical problem is, "Who is the best doctor for my problem?"

There was a time when this question was important. Until the last quarter of the twentieth century—prior to our current understanding of most medical problems and the advanced medical technologies of today—a doctor's personal skill and intuition were paramount.

Today, individual acumen and technical skill rarely separate the best from the rest. Randomly assign a group of patients to doctors, or even let them search out the "best" doctor for their specific problem, and the differences in clinical outcomes will be negligible.

The most important determinants for making the right diagnosis and achieving the best clinical outcomes are (1) how well individual physicians are supported by information technology, (2) how well their entire medical team works together, (3) how consistently the doctors on that team follow the best national guidelines, and (4) how often the physician treats a particular problem or does a particular procedure.

Thanks to advances in medical understanding, along with sophisticated diagnostic and therapeutic tools, the variation in individual ability among physicians today is relatively insignificant and will become even less so in the future.

When physicians can access comprehensive patient information electronically, when they collaborate on patient care and are supported by data analytics, and when they follow evidence-based guidelines, the likelihood of their patients dying from a heart attack or stroke decreases by as much as 30 percent. That's not what patients or doctors believe, but it is what the data show.

Meet Your New Assistant, Siri

The practice of medicine is continually evolving. New information accumulates at an ever-intensifying pace. In fact, the half-life of medical knowledge is now estimated to be five to seven years, meaning that half of what we learned five, six, or seven years ago is now understood to be wrong. It also means that even the smartest and most knowledgeable doctors need help. Modern information technology can bridge that gap, but only if doctors are willing to embrace it.

At present, there are two schools of thought about how to best use technology in health care. Although both have value, one will have a much more powerful impact on reducing mortality in our nation, and it is not the one most doctors would prefer.

First, meet IBM's Watson, the supercomputer that took down Ken Jennings on *Jeopardy!* Using the power of big data, Watson has the ability to quickly find clinical answers buried in millions of pages of medical records. Watson, a machine that's about the size of a pizza box, is already being used to sift through nearly 1 million new medical studies published in more than 20,000 journals each year.

In the context of how doctors have traditionally seen themselves, Watson isn't a threat. He's more like a "Lifeline" from the TV quiz show *Who Wants to Be a Millionaire?* If you're stumped, Watson may have a suggestion. If doctors don't like his answer, they ignore it.

Watson's capacity and speed are incredible. But he's not really what doctors need. The problem with Watson isn't that he can't do amazing things. His problem is that the amazing things he does rarely add value. Being able to peruse massive amounts of information in relatively short order doesn't make much of a difference for most medical problems. It is a rare patient for whom a thorough review of every article ever written would be necessary. Besides, Watson can't discern which papers should or should not be trusted. Achieving the best outcomes is not a matter of discovering the obscure, but rather providing the right care consistently. The biggest opportunity we have as a nation for saving lives is ensuring that every doctor follows the best available approaches every time.

Therefore, what doctors really need is Apple's Siri. When treating patients, the most common physician error is forgetting a step. Siri's memory is perfect, and she can make certain doctors follow the best protocols available. What's more, her mind is encased conveniently in the body of an iPhone. Unlike Watson, Siri can follow doctors from room to room while delivering more than enough memory and computing speed to help physicians diagnose and treat nearly all problems that patients experience.

Better still, Siri's expertise will grow over time. Using information contained in millions of electronic health records, she can be programmed to calculate the probability that a particular patient in the ER is having a stroke or needs a particular cancer treatment.

Not only is she a powerful source of information, but she can also question the doctor's approaches and make sure the specialist uses the right admission order set every time, even offering up friendly reminders as doctors go step by step through the treatment process.

In the case of sepsis, Siri would insist that every patient with two symptoms consistent with systemic infection have blood drawn for a blood-lactate-level test. And she would have insisted my father receive the pneumococcal vaccine he needed.

Physicians will likely resent having a computer application looking over their shoulder and questioning their judgment. But it's a very small price to pay for the opportunity to save tens of thousands of lives each year, particularly when one of those lives is yours or your father's.

The Context of Age

Studies of generational differences tell us that when a doctor was born is important in understanding his or her outlook on medical practice and where it is heading.

Baby boomers, born 1946 to 1964, are known for their work ethic. Many doctors of this generation have spent their entire careers building up small, solo practices. They value the independence of running their own offices and having their names on the door. Throughout their careers, they have been willing to trade work-life balance for professional success and, more so, for the freedom to treat patients the way they deem most appropriate. Many prefer the stethoscope around their neck to the newer handheld, wireless ultrasound machines. On the whole, they are less likely to embrace new approaches to the treatment of problems like sepsis, particularly when doing so requires them to modify how they've practiced for years.

In contrast, the millennial generation, spanning the birth years of 1982 to 2004, embraces modern technology and prefers to text rather than talk. Having come of age with social media, these people are "sharers," wholly at ease with communicating information in bits and pieces. As such, this could be the generation that ultimately embraces the power of the team and the smart machine over independence and intuition. At the same time, this newest generation of doctors has been accused of being more interested in work-life balance than prioritizing patient care. As such, it remains to be seen whether they will lead the transformation of American medicine or wait for someone else to do it.

Not all generalizations about different generations are accurate, of course. There are plenty of millennial doctors who put in longer hours than their boomer mentors. And Dr. Craig, a boomer, achieved much of her success through analyzing computerized data and embedding treatment protocols into an electronic medical-record system. How doctors of certain demographics will see or shape a better future for health care isn't ultimately dependent on their age. It's dependent on their ability to lead in ways that (1) inspire other doctors to follow, and (2) improve results where it matters, in the lives of patients.

Leadership is the ability to make change happen that otherwise wouldn't. The best health care leaders do this by creating a vision and using it to shift the context and perceptions of others, for the better. In Santa Clara today, a decade after Diane took on the challenge of sepsis, every physician embraces and implements the protocols she created, a tribute to her tenacity and leadership.

The Almighty Dollar

Unfortunately, meaningful change in health care often takes years, even decades. The Institute of Medicine estimates that a new, proven treatment takes an average of seventeen years to make its way into routine patient care.

The doctor's personal fear of change and the culture of medicine account for some of the lag. But few forces in health care alter perceptions or slow progress quite like money.

And it's hard to think of a more pernicious or regressive system of financial reward than that of health care's prevailing reimbursement model.

"Fee-for-service" medicine pays doctors and hospitals for each procedure they perform, each test they complete, and each office or Emergency Room visit they provide, regardless of whether any of it adds value. The consequences are predictable.

Imagine you're planning to update your kitchen. You hire a contractor and opt to defer entirely to his judgment on the kitchen's aesthetics and the source of his materials. Instead of requesting a competitive bid or limiting the remodel to exactly what you want, you agree to a time-and-materials contract. By the end of the project, the contractor has billed more hours than you expected, installed windows and appliances you can't afford, and charged you twice for his construction errors.

Chances are you would never agree to such a lopsided contract for your kitchen. Yet that's exactly what happens when most Americans receive medical care. The reason we do this is as predictable as the consequences: someone else is footing the bill. Once patients cover their deductible and out-of-pocket expenses, insurance covers (and cloaks) most of the costs of medical care.

Outside of health care, most types of insurance (home, auto, and so on) cover unpredictable, relatively uncommon events such as a fire, theft, or accident. In contrast, much of medical care can be predicted based on an individual's disease status. And whether you see high utilization as problematic or positive is based on the context in which you practice and the method by which you are paid.

To explain, let's see what Nancy's sepsis treatment (and medical bills) would have looked like in two different hospital environments.

Let's start with the hospital where Nancy was admitted and effectively treated. Here, Nancy's doctors diagnosed her sepsis early on, treated it immediately and aggressively, and had her home in three days. As a result, her medical costs were moderate. And that was just fine for this particular hospital. That's because its payments come in the form of an annual fee covering the needs of a defined patient population. This medical center does best financially when its doctors intervene early and avoid the need for an ICU admission or a prolonged inpatient stay. It's the same annual fee, regardless.

Now, let's imagine Nancy was taken to the hospital down the street with a fee-for-service payment model in place. There, if she'd developed full-blown sepsis, she would have been admitted to the ICU, where she would have received intensive and ongoing treatment for a potentially deadly problem that might have been prevented in the first place. And as a result, the hospital would bill Nancy dramatically more for her treatment, most of which would be paid by her insurance company. It's not likely that anyone would *want* this for the patient. But these outcomes do in fact work best for the facility's bottom line. There may be multiple reasons that doctors in the Emergency Department would delay ordering the blood-lactate test. But the combination of how they are paid and what is reimbursed shapes perception about what is most important among hospital leaders.

Sepsis costs the US health care system more than $20 billion a year, paid to doctors and hospitals through insurance premiums. The total expense continues to rise. And this problem is not limited to sepsis.

As many as 4 percent of all patients in hospitals are there because of a problem they experienced after being admitted—problems such as pressure ulcers, pneumonia, and increasingly, hospital-acquired infections.

Although the government-run Medicare program for seniors no longer pays doctors and hospitals for these "never events" (serious and largely preventable occurrences), most insurance companies still reimburse care providers twice: once for the original problem and a second time for treating the complications they created. It's the equivalent of paying contractors double after they botch your kitchen renovation.

But without the revenue from patient complications, many hospitals would teeter on bankruptcy. A recent study found that privately insured surgical patients with one or more complications provided hospitals with a 330 percent higher profit margin than those who had none.

Without the right financial disincentives, we would expect both kitchen contractors and physicians, even very ethical ones, to maximize their own economic benefit. They may not do it consciously, but medical decisions are driven by dollars.

If you have any question, just look at back surgery. Some of the procedures available are extremely beneficial, particularly when there is nerve compression and loss of feeling in the legs. But when pain is the main indicator, non-operative treatments often prove just as effective.

Surgery can be relatively simple or very complex. The complex way involves expensive hardware and implants. For most patients, these more extensive procedures add little benefit.

But when surgeons and their hospitals are paid by the number and complexity of treatments they provide, studies show they perform significantly more procedures and use their most expensive equipment more often. Ask physicians whether the economics of health care cause them to perform unnecessary surgeries or recommend more complex or costly treatments, and they will fervently deny it. The numbers tell a different story.

Why It's Hard to See the Problem

Our surroundings and expectations matter a great deal in how we perceive the world around us. That's true for everyone, both inside and outside the walls of health care. To demonstrate the impact of situational context on perception, staffers at the *Washington Post Magazine* watched from afar as busy government workers scurried through a bustling Metro station on an especially cold Friday morning in January 2007. They were looking at people's reactions to a raggedy panhandler in a baseball cap, playing his violin for spare change.

What they observed was shocking. Out of the nearly 1,100 commuters who passed through this particular station stop during the man's performance, fewer than thirty people gave him money. And even fewer stopped to listen. Of those who did, all but one failed to appreciate what they were hearing.

As the article would reveal, this wasn't just any street musician scraping away at a busted fiddle. This was Joshua Bell, internationally acclaimed virtuoso and the man behind the soundtrack of *The Red Violin*.

It was the same Joshua Bell who, three days before his undercover Metro performance, had sold out Boston's Symphony Hall. But, of course, in the context of this particular environment, this wasn't *that* same Joshua Bell, the one who earns tens of thousands of dollars for his live performances. This was a nondescript beggar with an open briefcase who, after forty-three minutes of symphonic mastery, earned just $32 and change.

One passerby told the *Post*, "Yes, I saw the violinist, but nothing about him struck me as much of anything." Given the setting, most people judged one of the best in the world as average or, worse, ignorable. Phrased differently, 99 percent of what the musician earns is based on people's perception of him and the setting in which he performs, not the objective sounds he makes.

Just as the context of the Metro station altered the expectations and perception of passengers, the setting in which physicians practice has a similar impact.

A surgeon who earns double-digit returns from his investment in a "surgicenter" will see surgery as a more beneficial solution than a conservative, nonsurgical treatment. An oncologist who buys and marks up chemotherapy medications will more likely offer the drugs to patients who won't benefit significantly from them.

These are not conscious or logical choices. They are perceptions, altered by situational context. If we observed these actions from afar, most of us would shake our heads in disbelief, just as if we saw commuters walking right past Joshua Bell. However, if we found ourselves standing in the same shoes as doctors or on the platform of the Metro in Washington, DC, most of us would act in the same way.

Lessons from Uber

On a beautiful late summer day in 2015, I was traveling from California to Washington, DC, to speak at a conference organized by the *New England Journal of Medicine.* In a hurry to get from the airport to the hotel, I stood impatiently in a taxi line where only one cab company was permitted to pick up passengers. As I got into the cab, I was greeted by a lingering odor and a sullen driver. Upon arrival at the hotel, I paid the $72 fare, which might have been a few dollars cheaper had the driver not taken a wrong turn.

On the way back to Dulles Airport later that week, I used the Uber app on my iPhone.

Immediately after I requested a ride, I knew how far away the driver was, his name, the make of his car, and his driver rating on five-star scale. I knew that if the wait-time Uber calculated was too long, or if I simply preferred a different type of vehicle, I could cancel the ride with a second tap. When my driver pulled up, his car was in pristine condition, clean and pleasantly scented. He offered me a bottle of water and I connected my Spotify station to his speakers. Because the app asked me where I was going, the directions were sent to my driver's GPS. He took the shortest, computer-generated route, and upon arrival, my credit card (already on file) was automatically charged $38. I had received superior quality, easier access, and more personalized service, all at a significantly lower cost.

From the backseat of my driver's Ford Taurus, I could see the future of American health care.

Uber, now worth more than Hertz and Avis combined, unveiled its prized app in 2009. Reporters soon heralded it as a classic case of disruptive technology. Not long after its launch, the news media were pointing to a groundswell of health care start-ups, all vying to build their own version of Uber, pairing doctors or nurses with drivers, each promising a high-tech spin on the house call of yesteryear. Unfortunately, most of these stories and start-ups missed the point.

Technology is just one component of Uber's success. The smartphone app is foundational, but not revolutionary or even cutting edge. The takeaway for the health care industry isn't that we need to build the next killer app or start driving doctors to people's homes in rush-hour traffic. The greatest opportunity for health care is to accept, and learn from, what Uber did to revolutionize its industry. Uber changed the environment of drivers and, without doing much else, shifted both driver and consumer perceptions of what was expected.

When I thought about the two drivers I met in DC (the cab driver who picked me up at the airport and the Uber driver who took me back), I realized both were working hard to support their families and, to me, they both seemed honest. There was nothing about them individually to explain my two extremely different experiences. The difference was entirely contextual.

One driver happened to be stuck in a broken model that negatively affected his perception of what was expected, and the other worked in an environment that encouraged high-quality, convenient service.

No one should be surprised by these outcomes. If changing the environment affected students in Palo Alto in overwhelmingly negative ways, then why shouldn't a positive environmental shift be able to improve the perceptions and actions of Uber drivers?

And if Uber could change the rider experience by modifying the finances, design, and culture of the taxicab industry, why can't we change the patient experience in health care? If we paid physicians for the quality of their outcomes, wouldn't we expect higher-quality care, fewer medical errors, and a greater emphasis on preventive medicine? And if all emergency physicians worked with someone like Diane Craig, wouldn't we likely see fewer sepsis deaths?

Of course, such changes wouldn't be easy to pull off in health care. They weren't easy for Uber, either. When the ride-sharing start-up created a better model for connecting riders with drivers, both faster and cheaper, the taxi industry hated it. Even today, the old-school taxi powers fight to preserve the monopolistic system they created, pushing for legislation that turns back the clock and restricts competition. The incumbents in the taxi industry could have invested all that time and energy in a more convenient, lower-cost version of their own service. But they decided to fight change instead. Today, they continue to lose customers by the fleet.

As in the taxi industry, the customs in health care began decades ago. These approaches may have worked well in the last century, but we can do better in the current one. As we have seen, the psychology of the doctor in the context of American medicine is change resistant, the same as the cab drivers and the companies for which they work. If health care were like most competitive industries, change would already have happened. However, the combination of strict regulation and entrenched institutions makes that shift difficult. As we will see in future chapters, some providers have already begun to embrace the future, but not many.

Regardless, the future of American health care will be determined as much or more by patients as by physicians. The balance between the patient's desires and fears will determine whether the current health care system—with its shortfalls and limitations—continues along the same sluggish route or changes radically.

Chapter Three

WHAT PATIENTS SEE

Meet Emma, a wavy-haired little girl with big blue eyes and a beaming personality. Emma lives in a modern suburban home with her mom, dad, and brother just outside of San Francisco. On most days, the energetic three-year-old zips from room to room, her blonde locks bouncing as her smile lights up the house.

About five hundred miles south of Emma (and a figurative world away) lives Felipe, a blind man with diabetes, high blood pressure, and cholesterol issues. He lives with his wife, Juana, and their children and grandchildren in a modest home near the US-Mexico border.

Emma and Felipe come from different backgrounds. They've had vastly different life experiences and challenges, too. But as patients, Emma and Felipe have something very important in common.

A couple of years ago, Emma's mom, with nine-month-old Emma perched on her hip, was rushing through her morning routine: packing up her workbag and preparing breakfast while minding the clock. Amid the hustle of getting her family ready for another day, Laura placed a cup of hot water for tea on the counter, just within Emma's reach. As curious babies do, Emma stretched out her arm. What she did next would change Laura's world.

Emma caught the rim of the cup with her finger and pulled the scalding-hot water onto her chest and lap. Her cries filled the house. It was every mother's worst nightmare. In a panic, Laura rushed Emma out the door, got her into the car, and broke several traffic laws on the way to the Emergency Department.

"When we arrived at the hospital," Laura remembers, "I came running through the doors holding her in my arms, shouting, 'My baby has been burned!'"

Dr. Richard Dow, the family's pediatrician, heard about the accident and raced to the hospital to assess Emma's condition. There, he comforted the family and quickly began to coordinate Emma's care in concert with the emergency physicians. They transferred her to the nearest pediatric burn unit, where a specialist was waiting to care for her wounds.

About six months before Emma's accident, Felipe awoke one morning to find that his vision had become blurry. He told his wife, Juana, about it but decided not to see a specialist right away. The next day, the sixty-two-year-old man went completely blind, a consequence of his diabetes.

Even before he lost his vision, Felipe's body had been racing full speed toward a cliff. He'd stopped taking his diabetes medications. He was no longer exercising, watching his diet, or checking his blood sugar. He had stopped taking care of himself, and his body couldn't take it anymore.

For most of their lives, Felipe and Juana have tried to make the most of their situation. Although they never had much, they do have children and grandchildren who love them dearly. They have both worked hard to raise a strong, close family and keep food on the table. But after Felipe went blind, their world came apart.

"I was no longer able to provide for my wife, my children, my grand-children, and even my elderly father who's still alive," Felipe says in Spanish, his speech weighed by grief. "I couldn't go to the store by myself anymore. I couldn't go to the doctor without help. I wasn't able to see the birth of my granddaughter."

Health is a curious thing. When it's good, we hardly give it any thought. We focus on our jobs and errands, our friends and family, our deadlines and daily lives. The responsibilities of adulthood consume us, providing us with a constant flow of more pressing matters. As we hurry to work and orchestrate the comings and goings of our loved ones, our well-being slides further and further down our list of priorities. And sometimes, we wait too long.

When a body suffers damage, it tries to adjust itself, retaining or releasing water, proteins, sugar, and salt as needed to achieve homeostasis. But bodies have their limits. Once the conditions and ailments we've ignored for so long begin to take their toll, the delicate balance tips and the effects can be irreversible.

No matter what he does now or how well he cares for his diabetes in the future, Felipe's vision will never return. And his eyes may not be the last organ to go. If he doesn't find a way to manage his blood glucose and blood pressure, the problems will progress to his kidneys and heart. Felipe could have a stroke or even require leg amputation.

Dr. Edward Greene, an internal-medicine physician, understands the ravages of this disease and has been trying to help Felipe limit further damage to his body.

They meet often and know each other well. That's why Dr. Greene grew worried when, one afternoon, Felipe and Juana showed up more than a half-hour late for an appointment. It was uncharacteristic of them, so he asked what was going on.

Juana explained that since Felipe can no longer drive, they have to take the trolley from their home to San Diego. From there, they make a transfer and wait for a bus. The whole trip takes close to two hours each way. And that's only when the trolley and the bus are on time. That day, they weren't.

Because of the unpredictable commute, Felipe was missing entire meals, increasing his chances of experiencing low blood glucose (hypoglycemia). Dr. Greene could see that traveling for long periods to his office was exhausting Felipe's energy. Juana, meanwhile, was having trouble balancing her work schedule with Felipe's medical needs, putting their family's lone source of income at risk.

"I was constantly being written up by my supervisor. I was worried that I would have to choose between my job and Felipe's health."

Faced with an impossible decision, Juana was at the end of her rope. Something had to give.

———————

When Emma was discharged from the burn unit, the healing process had just begun. Laura would now need to take her to a burn specialist whose office was twenty-five miles away, a good hour in typical Bay-area traffic.

On the morning of their first visit, Laura remembers dressing her daughter, carrying her delicately to the car, and fastening her in. And as the straps dug into Emma's wounds, the little girl cried out in pain. Suddenly, the horror of the situation, and of every moment since the accident, began to overwhelm Laura.

Most doctors don't understand or appreciate the anxiety patients like Laura experience in their health care encounters. In medical school, physicians study forms of anxiety during their psychiatry rotations, but usually in the context of the abnormal—the psychopathology of the human mind.

Having been trained in the medical model, physicians perceive anxiety as deriving from the individual, not from the individual's situation. They fail to recognize the fear and anxiety that patients experience every time they go to see a physician.

To the doctor, asking a patient to wait in a reception area or sit in an exam room for extended periods of time is both reasonable and necessary to maximize office efficiency. Having patients drive long distances or take multiple buses is seen as just a normal part of providing care. Rarely do the consequences of having to miss school or work enter the doctor's consciousness or affect clinical decision making.

On an overcast Monday, Dr. Clyde Ikeda, Emma's new burn specialist, welcomed the little girl and her mother into his office. With a calming presence and caring demeanor, he carefully evaluated Emma's burns, taught Laura how to change the dressings, and explained that he would need to see Emma three times a week for the next four to six weeks, or until Emma's wounds were completely healed. And just like that, Laura's anxiety gripped tighter. She envisioned repeating the steps of that morning every other day for weeks on end.

That's when something rather unexpected happened. Dr. Ikeda said, "If you prefer, we could do most of Emma's visits through video. And if you want, we can invite your pediatrician to join us, as well."

Just like that, the sun came out from behind the clouds. With that solution, Laura could now picture her days at home with Emma instead of on the road fighting traffic. She could see herself carefully washing and leisurely dressing Emma each morning from the comfort of her home, instead of hurrying to cinch her into a car seat. She could care for her daughter and still complete her work from home. Slowly, the weight and severity of this family tragedy began to lift.

"I really needed that," Laura says. "Traveling hours at a time, several times a week, would have been challenging. It would have taken a toll on Emma and our family. Thankfully, Dr. Ikeda put our needs first."

And so the healing process began. On Mondays, Wednesdays, and Fridays, Laura, Emma, and the burn specialist (and sometimes Dr. Dow) would connect through a secure video-conferencing app. From the comfort of their house and with the push of a few smartphone buttons, Laura and Emma were virtually transported to Dr. Ikeda's office, talking face-to-face.

It surprised Laura just how personal the visits felt. There was Dr. Ikeda, inspecting Emma's wounds through his computer screen, evaluating her progress and giving Laura instructions on further care.

But technology offered even more than that. Anytime Laura had a question, rather than having to telephone the office or come in, she'd simply e-mail Dr. Ikeda or schedule another video appointment. And whenever Dr. Dow wasn't taking part in the video visits, he would check Dr. Ikeda's notes on the electronic health record they shared. Even though these two physicians worked twenty miles apart, a common electronic medical record allowed them to seamlessly coordinate and facilitate Emma's care.

For Emma, seeing her doctor "on television" was fun. For Laura, the experience couldn't have been more natural, normal, or satisfying. Instead of driving hours to receive ten minutes of care, the whole process took ten minutes from start to finish. Looking back on the experience, she wonders why anyone would choose to receive care the old way.

"This was life-changing," Laura recalls. "Dr. Ikeda and Dr. Dow turned a terrible accident, a tragedy, into something we could manage. They gave us a beautiful gift."

––––––

It's a Tuesday morning in Southern California. Felipe sits in the dining room, flanked by a small skyline of orange pill bottles—medications for his diabetes, high blood pressure, and other ailments. There's a computer in front of him and from the monitor springs a cheerful, welcoming voice.

"*Hola, Felipe, cómo está?*" It's Felipe's internal-medicine doctor, checking in for their regular appointment. When Dr. Greene realized how challenging it was for Felipe and Juana to come to his office, he decided to try a different solution.

A few years back, Dr. Greene and his colleagues began offering their patients the opportunity to receive care virtually. Not every doctor at the medical center was on board. Some worried the care would be less personal, and as a result, they'd lose their patients' trust. Others worried about being able to navigate the new technology or that making a mistake would open them up to malpractice liability. But Dr. Greene knew that part of being a physician meant improving people's lives, not just treating their physical problems.

"Change is hard for anyone, especially in medicine," says Dr. Greene. "It's hard to get over the barriers, but you have to lead. And often the best way to help others practice differently is to lead by example."

Felipe wasn't the typical high-tech candidate for "telehealth." His blindness, limited experience with technology, and complex medical problems presented a handful of challenges. But clearly, the traditional medical model wasn't working either. With telemedicine, Dr. Greene could counsel Felipe in real time and watch him take his medications. Juana helps Felipe with the technical issues and participates in the discussions when she can.

Dr. Greene hopes more patients like Felipe will soon have access to these life-changing solutions. "This is the future of health care," he says. "It's not sci-fi. It's happening right now, today."

For both Emma and Felipe, and for their families, telemedicine has been a game changer.

"I feel great when I hear Dr. Greene's voice on the computer," Felipe says. "We talk about my health issues and he answers my questions just like I am sitting in his office. My wife no longer has to take time off from work for me. Our family is doing great. I feel as though I can go on living life normally rather than being a burden."

Some experiences in life change us forever. Felipe's doctors can't restore his vision, just as Emma's physicians can't undo the full damage of her burns. Some diseases never go away, and some scars never fully heal. But today's health care providers, armed with technology and compassion, can treat patients in ways that were never possible before.

As Felipe closes his computer, he feels around for his medications and follows his doctor's recommendations. He does his exercises at home in the morning and, in the afternoon, walks around the neighborhood with his friends. He greets Juana when she returns from work, and at night they talk about the blessings of their family. During the moments in between, Felipe holds his granddaughter in his arms and sings her Spanish lullabies, imagining the life that awaits her.

The Health Care We Accept

For most patients, telemedicine would represent a significant improvement over the kind of care they receive today. But what's most remarkable is that Emma and Felipe's stories remain the exception and not the rule in American medicine. It doesn't have to be this way.

After all, the information and mobile technologies used to improve Emma and Felipe's care are at least a decade old. Computers have been connecting doctors with other doctors and their patients' records since the turn of the twenty-first century. Platforms such as Skype have been linking people through secure video since 2003. Meanwhile, the iPhone recently celebrated its tenth anniversary.

If doctors wanted to incorporate these tools and expanded services into their practice, they could. In the same way hotels and restaurants encourage guests to book reservations online, doctors could let patients schedule their appointments digitally. And just as banks and financial advisers allow people to check their accounts online, safely and privately, patients could check their laboratory results through a secure website or app.

The environment of health care causes both physicians and patients to focus on the risks of technology, not the massive benefits. Many harbor legitimate concerns about privacy and fraud, but if the banking industry could effectively address these concerns, why couldn't health care? After all, those with malicious intent are far more interested in gaining access to your checking account than your medical history.

Some physicians worry that the quality of care will suffer with video visits and leave them at risk for committing a medical error. But in doing so, they're overlooking the massive sum of errors and inefficiencies caused by the *absence* of technology.

The cases of Emma and Felipe demonstrate how modern technology improves, not compromises, the quality and convenience of patient care. And for both families, video increases their trust in their physicians and strengthens the doctor-patient relationship. This technology could improve the lives of millions, including patients who travel for work, put in long hours, have children, or simply don't have the time to meet face-to-face with a doctor for every problem they experience. In today's hectic world, doesn't that include just about everyone?

The reality is that today's health care delivery system is not designed around your time or priorities. It is designed to maximize the productivity of doctors. And as the physician's reimbursement rates continue to decline, and as insurance companies continue to refuse to pay for virtual care, none of this is likely to change soon.

With no incentive to change, doctors have every reason to hold on to the ways they have provided care in the past. And that's exactly what most of them do.

More Than Meets the Eye

If you're admitted as a patient to a teaching hospital, you'll likely notice all of the doctors taking care of you are wearing white coats. The color was selected centuries ago, in the pre-antibiotic era, to communicate that the person taking care of you was uncontaminated.

In recent years, these coats have sparked all sorts of controversy among infectious-disease experts. Their concern is that the long sleeves on these clean-looking white garments have the potential to gather microscopic particles and thus transmit harmful bacteria and viruses.

Why then do doctors still wear them? These coats may carry disease but, to patients, they also carry credibility. Recent polls revealed that as many as 70 percent of patients prefer it when doctors wear white coats, noting the professional attire contributes to a greater sense of comfort with (and confidence in) their physicians.

But there's more to the tradition than patient preference. Look closer at the coats and you'll notice something you probably missed. This garb communicates the hospital's hierarchy, as well. The coats on medical students come down to the waist, whereas the residents' coats cut off at the thigh, and those of attending physicians end at the knees. The length of this attire has nothing to do with helping patients understand who's who in a hospital setting. Physicians in today's health care system are expected to introduce themselves to you with their name and title. They wear badges with this information to meet regulatory requirements.

No, the coat lengths were designed to establish relative authority among doctors. In the same way that stripes and stars on military uniforms communicate rank, the length of a doctor's coat establishes to what degree his or her opinion matters.

In medicine, long-standing traditions continue far beyond their logical utility, evidence that health care is influenced as much by culture and past norms as by science.

The Evolution of Fear

With so much of American medical culture rooted in the past, health care reform efforts move in slow motion, especially when compared to other industries. This is understandable, but what's most puzzling is why patients are willing to accept so much less from health care than from just about any other industry.

The answer resides in the psychology and neurophysiology of our brains and can be traced back thousands of years. For nearly all of history, disease, trauma, and pregnancy were dangerous, often lethal, experiences. In that context, coping mechanisms were essential to avoid being overcome with fear.

We know from brain research that people, when faced with extreme anxiety, undergo a subconscious shift in perception. This is mankind's instinctive, neurophysiological response—our ability to cope with perceived threats—and it remains intact from the distant past, hardwired into our brains.

When our ancestors stared down prey that outweighed them by six tons, they either overcame their fears or starved to death. The human brain evolved accordingly. Throughout our evolution, humans have endowed certain individuals with protective powers, be they tribal leaders, religious figures, or healers. As our ancestors faced threats of war, disease, and death, this process of transference came in handy. We put our faith in others so as to manage our otherwise immobilizing fears. And in doing so, we have become reluctant to question our healers.

The problem now, however, is that these same tendencies—once so valuable to our survival—can have a negative impact on our modern lives. Although the trust we place in today's healers underscores the importance of the doctor-patient relationship, and even though it increases our confidence in physicians and facilitates the healing process, it also makes us act in funny ways. To patients, demanding greater convenience or better service seems dangerous.

"Because They Saved My Son's Life"

Each year, the organizers of the annual World Heath Care Congress put together panel discussions sure to spark controversy. Last year's agenda was no exception. Along with two other health care leaders, I had the privilege to participate in a session called "Putting the Consumer First," no doubt intended to liven the ongoing debate in health care circles about whether or not people should be thought of as "consumers" rather than patients.

We planned our presentation carefully, hoping the audience would leave with a deeper understanding of the advantages to twenty-first-century care. With the other speakers focusing on the emergence of retail-based clinics (think: CVS's walk-in "MinuteClinic") and wearable devices (think: Apple Watch), I emphasized the role of such health information technologies as video and secure e-mail in making patient care more convenient, higher quality, and more in tune with our lives today. I also stressed the difficulties doctors confront in trying to provide superior, safe, and rapid medical care without a comprehensive electronic health record.

Not everyone in the audience agreed. During the Q&A period, some doctors raised doubts about the safety of providing care virtually and how difficult it is to get paid for these services. Others complained about how expensive the electronic health-record systems were to purchase and maintain. All in all, however, we three panelists felt good about our presentation, believing we had successfully elevated the importance of these topics and highlighted the contributions these technologies can make to American medicine. We were satisfied with the lively discussion and confident the attendees would at least consider using these new approaches in their practices.

As we exited toward the speakers' area, one of the panel organizers stopped us backstage. She complimented us on our presentation. It really resonated with her as a patient, she said, by virtue of how hard it was to obtain any level of advanced medical care from the doctors who treated her and her family. She noted that even getting her doctors on the phone to answer a simple question was nearly impossible. As she continued, she expressed her pessimism that any of her physicians would consider alternatives to the traditional office visit such as secure e-mail and video, or that they'd ever embrace any of the ideas we presented.

Her statement caught me off guard. I understood that twenty-first-century health care isn't nearly as accessible as it ought to be, but I also knew there were individuals and medical groups in her area offering these solutions. Furthermore, I recognized that this particular conference organizer wasn't your average patient. She had been a health policy expert for decades and is, by all accounts, incredibly savvy about the goings on in the health care industry. Surely she was aware that highly qualified physicians in Washington, DC, could provide her with the convenience and excellence she desired. So I asked her why she didn't just change doctors.

"Because they saved my son's life," she said.

Her remark stopped me in my tracks. I felt terrible. Of course, I had no idea she had a sick child and worried she might have found my question insensitive. When the other panelists left, I asked if she wouldn't mind telling me more about her son. She explained that her pregnancy had been complicated, including difficult obstetrical issues and a premature birth. Thanks to her obstetrician and pediatrician, she said, everything turned out well. It sounded to me as though her doctors had provided her with good care at the time, though I wasn't convinced they'd done anything out of the ordinary. Still, her loyalty and reluctance to change providers was understandable. That is, until she mentioned that her son was going off to college in the fall.

Nearly two decades after her son's birth, the woman wasn't planning to have another child. And her boy, now a man, no longer needed pediatric expertise. Rationally, her reluctance to change doctors and health systems made little sense. Her story reinforces what we now know from the brain research. What we perceive about our medical care reflects our subconscious fears and hopes, much more than it reflects objective thought. As a consequence, the health care decisions we make and the loyalties we hold dear remain steeped in the events, experiences, and even neurobiology of the past.

In Doctors We Trust

What we call "medicine" dates back 5,000 years to India and parts of the Middle East. Indeed, we could trace the healing arts back even further to shamans and other spiritual healers practicing thousands of years before that. It's an ancient craft.

But from the dawn of medicine until quite recently, doctors largely did their patients more harm than good. Although healers didn't recognize it as such at the time, medicine before the modern era was crude. Vaccines didn't yet exist, medical technology hadn't yet boomed, few medications were available, and the profession's most enduring procedure was the ill-conceived practice of "bloodletting." That is, doctors would open a vein with a sharp metal or wooden object to let the patient's blood flow into a waiting receptacle, believing it released "humors," which when unbalanced led to disease. Of course, we now know this practice only weakened the patient and increased the risk of infection.

For more than five millennia of medicine, life was dangerous and death was ever-present. Mothers died in childbirth at rates that would terrify us today. Young children often perished from communicable diseases such as measles and whooping cough. Teenagers were paralyzed by the ravages of polio. Pneumonia, heart disease, and even the flu killed millions of people early in adulthood. Doctors were simply outgunned by disease and the limits of their understanding. Their treatments and approaches were futile at best and deadly at worst.

Somewhere around the 1930s, with the advent and licensing of antibiotics and vaccinations, doctors' harm-to-good ratio shifted. As Americans entered the modern era of health care, our nation's doctors began curing diseases and finding new treatments for old problems. Before long, they were operating on the human heart, transplanting organs, and restoring circulation to the brain to reverse strokes. But even though medical science changed quickly, our subconscious fears, perceptions, and culture didn't evolve quite so fast.

Even today, we rely on the practices and rituals of yesteryear. Take, for instance, the "laying on of hands." First described in biblical texts, this practice of healing by touching has endured throughout antiquity as patients experience the doctor's touch as therapeutic, protective, and, often, essential. There's a biochemical reason for this. Studies show that when a doctor ceremoniously places a hand on our shoulder or wrist, it triggers a release of hormones and brain neurotransmitters that produce a healing sensation.

And as the physician moves the diaphragm of the stethoscope up the back then down, left then right, reminding us all the while to inhale and exhale through our mouths, we grow calmer with each meditative breath. In the context of medicine, touch conveys both compassion and caring, further deepening the trust and confidence we have in our doctors.

As a result, embedded in our subconscious is the powerful image of the doctor sitting at the patient's bedside, touching the forehead to assess fever. Even now, centuries after healers introduced the laying on of hands, the doctor's touch reassures us that we are in a protective, healing environment.

The Context of Health Care's Contradictions

Of course, the laying on of hands is much less medically relevant now than in the past. High-tech thermometers possess far higher acuity than the temperature-sensitive nerves of our hands. Ultrasound machines, likewise, can diagnose a heart murmur with far greater accuracy than the human ear.

As patients, we expect our doctors to have access to high-powered machinery that can heal us in times of crisis. But at a subconscious level, we also expect the hands-on rituals of the past. We want our medical care to be both "high tech" and "high touch." Both have become health care's table stakes.

Today's doctors and patients demand that hospitals be stocked with the most advanced medical technology in the world. Multimillion-dollar scanning and radiotherapy systems carry and communicate the promise of cutting-edge treatments that can diagnose and zap away our problems. And for anyone who needs more than a checkup or a flu shot, these types of technologies are seen as a medical must-have.

And yet, there is one glaring exception. In spite of our demands for the most modern *medical* technology, we as patients tolerate the absence of advanced *information* technology and accept inconvenient systems from the past. No doctor today can practice effectively without an electronic health-record system, and yet nearly half of the doctors in this country still insist on keeping paper records.

For deeper insight into why this contradiction in expectation exists, think back to the Stanford Prison Experiment, to Stanley Milgram's electric-shock study, or to Tversky and Kahneman's research on the hypothetical outbreak of disease. Perception is rarely objective and data based. It reflects the context of our environment and is altered by anxiety, fear, and reward. And when our perception changes, we unknowingly act in ways that seem irrational to outside observers.

In many ways, certain aspects of how doctors practice and their notions about the best medical care are analogous to superstitions. These irrational beliefs usually begin with totally random events that yield a particularly positive or negative outcome. Objectively, we might acknowledge that the two were unrelated, but why take the chance? If you shoot a great round of golf, you might wear that same shirt the next time you're out on the course. Presented with the possibility of another great round (reward), logic disappears. And when, by chance, a good outcome happens twice, perception shifts, and your brain subconsciously embeds a permanent association.

Applying this illogic to health care, imagine a farmer with a high fever some centuries ago. Weary from illness, he falls and cuts himself, leading to significant blood loss. A doctor sits at his bedside and marvels as the patient makes a full and speedy recovery. In his journal, the doctor notes the elimination of tainted blood as one possible reason for the patient's sudden reversal. For the next patient with high fever, the doctor draws a bit of blood. This patient, too, heals up nicely. Pretty soon, this random success becomes standard community practice—a false but logical explanation for the positive outcome.

There is a scientific basis for this shift in perception. It is what physicians label "the placebo effect." From a chemical and molecular standpoint, placebo pills and approaches should be totally ineffective. And yet a variety of research studies have shown that taking a placebo has a very real impact on brain activity and hormone release.

Placebos don't just make people think they are getting better. They have been shown to trigger the release of endorphins in our brains that biologically diminish the intensity of discomfort. A simple sugar pill has been shown to speed up or slow down the human heart, depending on whether the subject believes it to be a stimulant or a depressant. Placebos can even cause our bodies to release a variety of immunological elements that help fight disease.

Putting these pieces of evidence together, we can start to deconstruct and accept the irrational. Patients, both desirous of cures and fearful of disease, assign credit to doctors beyond what is quantitatively measurable. And as a result, they are hesitant to question their physician's recommendations. Patients worry what will happen if they complain about not receiving the convenience they desire.

That is why we sit in waiting rooms for long periods of time without demanding better service, even though we'd never tolerate such delays in a restaurant. It's why we call up the doctor's office during normal business hours and wait on hold, even though we'd never book a flight or hotel that way. And despite all the hassles we're forced to endure, we keep going back to the same physician year after year. In the end, we don't demand the convenience in health care we deserve, fearing that if we complain, we risk making our problem worse.

Irrational fear and the pursuit of reward have consequences beyond inconveniencing us. They also alter our perceptions of health care quality, sometimes leading to decisions that are bad for our health.

The President Is Having Heart Surgery

Today, NewYork-Presbyterian/Columbia University Medical Center in New York City has the nation's number-three cardiology and heart-surgery program in America, according to *U.S. News Health*.

But in the early part of the twenty-first century, it had one of the highest death rates in the state of New York for patients undergoing cardiac procedures. Since 1991, New York's Department of Health has published these risk-adjusted mortality rates from heart surgery.

Using a variety of statistical approaches and data analytics, the department corrects the raw death-rate data to account for the age of the patients, their associated illnesses, the severity of their cardiac problem, and any other complicating factors, such as previous surgery. And with that information, it publishes rankings for doctors and hospitals in the state so that patients can select the best from the rest.

Here's what the report read when it came out in April 2004: "Two hospitals (Columbia Presbyterian–NYP and Westchester Medical Center) had risk-adjusted mortality rates that were significantly higher than the statewide rate."

In other words, if you were thinking about having heart surgery at either NewYork-Presbyterian/Columbia University Medical Center or the Westchester Medical Center in 2004, you'd want to think again. That's because your chances of dying there were statistically much higher than if you chose any of the thirty-five other heart surgery hospitals in the state.

This publicly reported, independent analysis was statistically significant and scientifically based. That's what makes the following excerpt from a *Slate* magazine story so puzzling. It noted that, in 2004, "former President Bill Clinton developed chest pains caused by blockages of several coronary arteries," and that he chose to have his "tests at nearby Westchester Medical Center, where cardiologists suggested that he undergo surgery at Columbia-Presbyterian Hospital in New York City."

As a former president, Bill Clinton could have chosen any hospital in the country. And as an architect of national legislation on health care in the early 1990s, he should have known that this statistically accurate, independent data existed in 2004. Yet he got his diagnostic tests at the second-worst heart-surgery hospital in the state before undergoing a life-threatening procedure at the hospital with the highest death rate in New York.

What's more, the New York State Department of Health report noted that Clinton's surgeon had the worst statistics of any specialist who had performed at least one hundred surgeries a year within NewYork-Presbyterian/Columbia University Medical Center. It was right there in black and white. Any other hospital in New York would have been a more logical, rational, and arguably better choice. But the mindset of the patient—even that of a former president—is affected and influenced more by subconscious and subjective factors than by impartial research and data.

It's possible, given the urgency of the problem, that President Clinton neither checked the data online nor contacted someone with this information. In support of that thesis, the *New York Times* reported shortly after his surgery, "There was no indication that the Clinton family was aware of the state report when Mr. Clinton checked in on Friday with blockages in a number of coronary arteries."

But that doesn't explain what happened six years after his surgery. According to the *Times*, the former president developed complications from his first procedure, thus requiring another. And where did he go for this follow-up operation to address the complications from the previous one? Back to the Columbia campus of NewYork-Presbyterian, the same facility where the problem began.

Hearing this story, we may be tempted to ask: What was he thinking? But conscious thought and deductive reasoning likely had nothing to do with his return to the hospital that harmed him.

When smart people with access to clear data make foolish decisions, all signs point to a subconscious shift in perception. In this case, we can best ascribe the selection to "anchoring bias." Psychologists tell us that having made a decision (even an irrational one), we cling to it. We filter out dissenting information while overvaluing the data points that support our original selection. We don't do so voluntarily, but we do it nevertheless.

When it comes to our health, our brains sometimes do our bodies a disservice. For example, if a surgical procedure goes well for someone we know, we magnify the significance of that outcome and project the likelihood of a good result upon ourselves.

This might have made sense in the past, but the truth is most surgeries these days turn out well. So, knowing someone had a good result tells us very little. In fact, it's possible that your friend's surgeon has a complication rate of, say, 10 percent, whereas patients of other doctors in the area suffered a complication only 5 percent of the time (in other words, half the complication rate of your friend's doctor). In practice, these types of friend-to-friend referrals signify nothing about the probability of a subsequent successful outcome. Rather than trusting the advice of our friends, we would be much better off researching objective data on physician or medical group outcomes.

Now, a quick note to Republican readers who might ascribe to Clinton a unique set of errors in judgment or perception: Don't. Irrationality in health care crosses party lines. In 2013, former president George W. Bush underwent a procedure to place a stent in one of the narrowed arteries going to his heart.

This may sound reasonable. If you have a narrowed blood vessel, it would seem logical for your doctors to open it up and place a stent in order to prevent the vessel from constricting again. Unfortunately, there are no data to demonstrate that this procedure makes any long-term difference in patients like former president Bush.

But when something seems logical, our brains tend to believe that it's true, even when the scientific data say otherwise. Dr. Darshak Sanghavi, a cardiologist and a health care columnist, pointed out that "cardiac stents don't prevent heart attacks, prolong life, improve symptoms, or do much

of anything in people like the former president who have no symptoms."
But when it comes to intervention, we're biased. Our perceptions (those
of both doctors and patients) are that more care is better care.

In an era of unprecedented access to information, you'd think Bill
Clinton and George W. Bush would be two of the most informed health
care consumers around. You'd assume that if anyone would make decisions based on the most unbiased, scientific information available, it
would be these two former commanders in chief.

But former presidents are just as susceptible to altered perceptions as
the rest of us. Amid the threat of disease and death, none of us behaves
like "rational consumers."

Health Care: The Consumer Exception

Whether we like the term or not, in our current culture, we're all consumers. The twenty-first century has ushered in the kinds of choices and
conveniences past generations would have thought impossible.

From our smartphones, we can make purchases based on scores of reviews from critics and fellow consumers. With a few clicks or finger taps,
we can order a pizza or make reservations at an upscale restaurant at any
time from anywhere. Although we sometimes prefer to stroll through the
concourse of a mall, examining items before we buy, more and more we
prefer to do things digitally.

Regardless of how we choose to shop, the existence of so many options,
coupled with our ability to make informed choices, is the essence of modern consumerism.

Health care traditionalists, many of them physicians who completed
their medical-school training decades ago, find the word "consumer" degrading. They argue that acquiring medical care isn't at all like shopping
for an appliance or hailing a cab on your smartphone. They fear that
when patients become consumers, doctors will be relegated to the role of
retail clerk. To medical traditionalists, the people they treat are "patients"
and they hope it stays that way. But whether they like it or not, consumerism in health care is becoming the new reality, just much more slowly
than in practically every other industry.

That's why proponents of health care consumerism are becoming impa-
tient. They question why we can't enjoy the same variety and convenience

in health care that we demand from just about every other product or service industry. If we can schedule a flight or book a hotel room online, they argue, we should be able to make medical appointments in the most convenient way possible. If we can find out our bank balance whenever we want with just a few clicks, they ask, why can't we get our laboratory results the same way? And if our daughter is about to start kindergarten, why do we have to drive to the doctor's office Monday to Friday to pick up the medical form she needs?

The pro-consumer argument calls for a shift away from prioritizing the time, convenience, and preferences of the person giving the medical care toward those receiving it. In their minds, health care needs to parallel the evolution of the car-buying experience.

Twenty years ago, buying a vehicle was fraught with anxiety and discomfort. The consumer was relatively powerless because the dealership had all the information and control. Dealers knew the car's actual cost, the expected margin, the relative demand, and what their competitors were charging. Consumers, by comparison, knew very little. When a salesman assured you that you were getting a great deal, and when you considered how much time it would take to start negotiations all over at a lot across town, you said yes to the price and often regretted it the next day.

Today, car buying is radically different. From the comfort of your own home, you can go online and get the exact invoice price, comparison shop, and check deals from a number of locations, even hundreds of miles away. When you're ready, you buy from the most overstocked dealer who is willing to give you the best price. Maybe you choose to pay a little more for a particular model that's being sold closer to your home, but you make informed decisions based on your personal preferences.

American health care is the auto dealership of the past, void of the transparency, technology, and consumer control we value today. And most of us just accept it.

Building Patient Trust in a Digital World

Not all that long ago, people were more inclined to fear technology than embrace it.

It may be difficult to believe now, but Amazon and other online retailers once had a tough time convincing consumers to use credit cards when purchasing products over the Internet. Slowly, as online security measures tightened and more people started buying books at lower prices, consumers overcame their fears.

Amazon.com has since surpassed Walmart as the world's biggest retailer by market value. Meanwhile, brick-and-mortar stores such as Blockbuster and Borders have become relics of the past. Most of us consider this to be progress. Still, old fears die hard.

Before we worried about having our identities hacked on Amazon, we worried about the safety of ATMs. It was one thing to get money from the faceless device, we thought, but it was another thing entirely to feed our hard-earned cash into a machine. In time, those fears were allayed, too.

Today's tech concerns are primarily about security and privacy. News headlines tell of data breaches in both retail and health care alike, some small and some not. And this is where perception once again trumps data. As a society and as individuals, we tend to worry more about events we hear and read about in the media and our social networks than those that are actually the most dangerous.

Broadcast media, by design, cover exceptional events to boost viewership. For example, planes killed fewer than 1,000 people worldwide last year, whereas car crashes kill an average of 37,000 Americans each year (and over 1 million globally). But when was the last time traffic deaths made national headlines for days or weeks on end? As a result, we overestimate the risk of flying and underestimate the risk of driving.

As mindful citizens, we likewise focus on data breaches, which are important and worrisome. And yet we pay little attention to medical errors that result from a lack of data. Most important, we fail to recognize how the absence of modern technology in the medical arena produces failures of communication and fatal mistakes.

Medical errors are now the third-leading killer in the United States. They account for almost 10 percent of all American deaths. Many of the people who die from a human error might have lived, had their doctors been equipped with electronic health records, mobile devices, and Siri. To put it plainly, information technology saves lives.

Pilots in aircraft are essential, but the technologies that monitor their flights and help make course corrections are more reliable. In fact, you'd refuse to board any plane without these technological safeguards, and rightly so. And yet most of us fail to see the danger of receiving medical care from a doctor who is unaided by modern information technology.

When doctors keep paper records, your medical information is un-available to anyone outside that office. On average, patients see nineteen different doctors in their lifetime. And if you are like most patients, that amounts to nineteen different physicians asking you about your allergies, medications, and past test results (tests they'll likely repeat if they them-selves didn't conduct or order them). That's annoying, inefficient, and dangerous. Only one of the doctors needs to get the information wrong to spell disaster. The bigger problem, however, is that when these medical offices are closed, so too is access to your complete medical history.

Imagine you get taken by ambulance to the nearest Emergency De-partment after hours and the ER physicians treating you can't access your records. Invariably, you will suffer delays in your care and may even expe-rience medical complications.

Those aren't the only risks involved when your physician relies on a paper medical record. A *Time* magazine story revealed that doctors' sloppy penmanship kills more than 7,000 people each year. Electronic order entry can prevent this error and save nearly all of those 7,000 lives.

Across the nation, patients overrate the dangers of privacy problems and digital errors, and they undervalue the safety and convenience inherent in computerized systems. But there are ways to reverse these perceptions.

Industry leaders have told me that one of the biggest challenges Uber faced in the beginning was the fear people had of getting into a normal car with a stranger, and that the company had worked hard to address this concern. Riders were used to taxi drivers and perceived the number atop the cab and the logo on the side of the car as indicators of safety. Of course, there was no reason for passengers to assume cabbies were any more trustworthy than Uber drivers. But every single one of us has been warned since childhood not to get into a car with a stranger. Four or five years ago, Uber drivers would have been the strangers. The company needed a way to assure passengers that they were safe.

So Uber decided to provide riders with each driver's name, headshot, and car make and model, along with GPS tracking of the car's location and the driver's rating from previous passengers—information it gave to riders before they ever set foot inside the vehicle. So, by the time the car arrived, the driver wasn't a stranger anymore.

Uber made this information available for a variety of business reasons, but perhaps none of them more important than establishing the rider's trust. By altering the context, Uber took fear out of the equation (or at least reduced it considerably). And now, people feel as safe (if not safer) in an Uber vehicle than when hailing a typical city cab. This important shift has made Uber a $62-billion company and, according to the *New York Times*, "the world's most valuable private start-up."

Since the dawn of medicine, the trust between patients and their physicians has been central to the delivery of health care. And in spite of all the problems with health care delivery today, surveys show people still trust their physicians.

The profession of doctor was founded on the willingness of certain individuals to put the health of others first. Back when plagues and disease were ravaging towns and villages, doctors did exactly that—they put the lives of their patients ahead of their own. During devastating epidemics, doctors went out in the streets and into people's homes to care for the sick.

This same selfless desire to heal exists in the twenty-first century, too. Each year, more than 40,000 students apply to our nation's medical schools, ready and willing to commit a decade of hard work toward improving and saving people's lives. This commitment and sense of purpose continues today as it always did. What has changed is the role of technology.

Telemedicine can serve as a bridge between our busy lives and the care we need, bringing the physician into the patient's home. It can bring the house call of yesteryear into the twenty-first century.

Recently, a cardiologist told me about a patient he is treating with heart failure. This patient had numerous hospital admissions over the years due to his cardiac problems. Time and again, the doctor had counselled the patient on proper diet and limiting salt intake. So, following discharge, the doctor scheduled a video visit with the patient in his home to see how he was doing. After a few minutes of talking, the doctor asked the patient to take him into the kitchen. When the physician saw the potato chips and pretzels on the shelves, he immediately recognized the difference between what his patient told him in the office and what was actually happening in his life. Convincing the patient to throw away the snacks helped reduce his need for further hospitalization.

As we think about the not-so-distant future of medicine, we may be inclined to perceive technology and the personal relationship between doctors and patients as conflicting. And for some physicians, installing a computer system in their office has created such a conflict. Doctors lament that completing the electronic health record has forced them to focus more on the computer screen than on the patient. Some have even hired scribes, either in-person or virtual ones to enter the information into the computer for them. It doesn't have to be this way. Technology and personalized medicine can be integrated. In the future, that will require improved medical technology, and better applications and training. Modern electronic health-record systems today are clunky, but they do save lives.

Telling Patients the Truth

When people put their lives in someone else's hands, trust is unquestionably essential. In my career, I have experienced the effects of death on others many times. I have helped families confront the reality that no matter what I did, their loved ones would die. And in my life, I have stood with my siblings at our father's hospital bed, each of us faced with an impossible choice: to hope for a miracle or to accept the inevitability of death.

American culture doesn't handle the reality of death well. As a result, most doctors are uncomfortable telling patients the truth about their medical problems and having honest conversations about what will happen to them.

Dr. George York, the neurologist you met in the preface of this book, has a deep understanding of how the subconscious brain responds in the context of fear and reward, which greatly aided my understanding of the subject. He is also a well-versed medical historian who, years ago, told me how physicians in the past would communicate the inevitability of death to other physicians.

Prior to the modern era of surgery and anesthesia, he said, cancer was a death sentence. As grim as that may sound, it was the reality of the time. The doctors, wanting to be respectful and supportive of their colleagues in delivering the diagnosis, introduced an elegant ritual. Carrying a silver tray with two glasses of fine champagne, the doctor would enter his colleague's room to deliver the truth with compassion rather than blurting out the details and leaving the patient to grieve alone. Together, the two doctors would discuss the sick physician's life, his accomplishments, and their friendship. This ritual communicated to the patient that the treating physician would be there in whatever way was needed. And yet it left no ambiguity as to the prognosis.

Physicians today aren't so direct or compassionate. Day after day, in hospitals and medical offices all across America, doctors hide from the reality of death and fill their patients with false hope. Doctors tell themselves they don't want their patients giving up, but the truth is they prefer to avoid the painful and time-consuming conversations that accompany the end of life.

Advanced cancer is one such situation. Save for rare circumstances, leukemia and lymphoma among them, chemotherapy doesn't produce a cure. Once the cancer spreads through the blood and lymph systems to the vital organs—the liver, lung, and brain—chemotherapy can't eradicate the disease. At most, it can relieve the symptoms or, in some cases, delay recurrence. And yet, published studies show that when patients with advanced cancer are asked about the purpose of their chemotherapy treatments, two-thirds believe the drugs are being administered to cure them.

Ask oncologists why they recommend continued courses of chemo to patients who are likely to die in the next month or two, and they'll assure you it's what their patients want. Research published in the *New England Journal of Medicine* demonstrates the opposite. Patients who are given palliative, supportive care instead of suffering through another round of chemotherapy report that their final days are less painful and more fulfilling. None of this seems surprising. What did surprise researchers, however, was that these patients also lived longer on average.

Knowing that death is near can be incredibly frightening and yet profoundly empowering. By understanding the hard truth of their situation, patients can make difficult but necessary end-of-life decisions. They have the opportunity to put their finances in order and make their last days fuller. They can have important conversations with loved ones and check items off their proverbial bucket list. When asked, over 80 percent of patients say they prefer the whole truth from their physicians. Almost all are glad when they receive it. Not enough patients do.

Are You Getting Excellent Care?

At the Stanford Graduate School of Business, I teach a seminar that attracts students with a deep interest in the business of health care. The first class of the semester is always interesting and eye-opening. I begin with this question: By show of hands, who believes they receive excellent medical care?

Like clockwork, about 90 percent of the students raise their hands. And what else would you expect? These are extremely smart students with a deep interest in health care. Of course they're getting excellent care. And then, with their hands still confidently aloft, I ask, "How do you know?"

Slowly, the hands come down and, for a few awkward seconds, the room is silent. As graduate students in the business school, these are skilled researchers with a deep appreciation for data. Yet it's in this moment they realize they have no objective information or data to explain the confidence they have just expressed.

These bright young minds would never make a financial decision without digging through spreadsheets and reports. They would laugh at someone who bought stocks solely because a friend or relative said it was a good investment. They would roll their eyes at a fellow student who accepted a job simply because the company was headquartered in an attractive building. But that's exactly what they've done with their health care choices.

Of course, students have a good excuse for not knowing how good their health care really is. After all, most are still in their twenties, some only go to the doctor for sports physicals, and few have experienced a serious medical problem. It stands to reason that they would be unable to rattle off the quality ratings for the top heart surgeons in the area. Student or not, the problem is that almost none of us can discern on our own whether we're getting great medical care.

When I get asked about "the best doctor" to treat a certain condition, I'm reminded how naïve I was during my medical school days. Back then, I assumed that once I finished my training, patients and other doctors would somehow be able to check my quality "statistics" as if they were printed on the back of a baseball card.

What I didn't know then was (1) how impossible that would be, and (2) how relatively useless that information would be in making personal decisions on health care. Quality outcomes today rarely reflect individual physician ability, but rather the performance of the entire team providing medical care. If we want to improve the health care choices we make in the future, we'll need to think differently about the quality question.

Organizations such as the Institute for Healthcare Improvement have demonstrated that in the twenty-first century, health care is a "team sport" and the system of care affects quality outcomes far more than does individual ability.

Sure, there are a few physicians of very poor quality, and everyone would be well advised to avoid them. But contrary to what we see on TV shows, there are no physicians who can best their peers through sheer brilliance or unparalleled dexterity. They don't exist in real life. The reason some physicians achieve superior outcomes has much more to do with whether they work in an integrated system or a fragmented one, and whether they have access to advanced (and connected) information technology. Success is determined much more by whether doctors are reimbursed for the quality of their outcomes or the quantity of the procedures they perform. This context shapes not just doctors' perceptions but also their clinical performance.

The Quality Conundrum

Even if we could obtain data on individual outcomes, we would have a hard time figuring out what it meant. Most physicians don't do enough of any one thing to reach a statistically reliable set of conclusions. And again, because most procedures today are relatively safe, it takes a lot of procedures to discern skill from luck.

Outside of cardiac surgery, with its higher complication rate and more limited scope of procedures, you'd need to look at a thousand cases before you could find valid data on most operations. As a result, regardless of the specialty or specific procedure, the best way to obtain statistically reliable outcome data is by looking at institutions, not at individual physicians. Only when patients compare outcomes by health system or hospital do the numbers become statistically significant for most medical problems. If you go to the National Committee for Quality Assurance (NCQA) website, you can find ratings for entire health systems, grouped on a five-point scale. The same is true for Medicare Advantage programs on the Centers for Medicare and Medicaid Services (CMS) website, which use a five-star evaluation system. These ratings are based on results from hundreds of thousands of patients or more. Statistically, that's very significant.

On the whole, high-performing organizations succeed in finding the best doctors and weeding out those whose performance does not match their standards. In general, colleagues are the people best equipped to judge the competence of others in their field. That's why peer evaluation is an essential function in all large medical groups. This is particularly true when the person doing the evaluating can observe the individual actually performing his or her job. And that's exactly what happens in most of the five-star programs.

Similar to the NCQA and CMS, the Leapfrog Group has done admirable work in singling out the best hospitals and health systems. Leapfrog got its start when several major employers realized their businesses were spending billions on health care coverage for employees with no real way of comparing the quality of doctors and hospitals in their networks. By joining forces, the group's founders figured they could improve the health of their employees, and of all American patients, by ranking hospitals and by rewarding those that achieved the highest levels of quality and safety.

Their independent survey compares more than 2,500 hospitals using common national standards, assigning a letter grade—A, B, C, D, and F—depending on each hospital's success in preventing errors, achieving superior quality, and avoiding infections. Although participation is voluntary, the hospitals likely to score well usually participate. Those that would not fare so well tend to abstain.

Statistically significant data points are available for those interested in gauging access and service records as well. J.D. Power and Associates publishes an annual rating of health systems by geography on both.

All of these rankings are a great place to start in the quest to separate anecdote from data. And by picking the best system (based on these reports), patients will be much better off than when they try to identify "the best" individual doctor for their problems.

Who and What Matters to Your Doctor?

I mentioned earlier that there are a few physicians everyone would be better off avoiding. Some are inadequately trained, and some others generate frequent complications. As we've seen, figuring out who these individuals are proves difficult outside of medical groups. In contrast, it's easy to determine whether a physician's clinical decisions are being inappropriately influenced by drug-company money.

ProPublica, an independent nonprofit newsroom, first built its impressive "Dollars for Docs" database in 2010 and has since tracked more than $4 billion in disclosed payments. The site will show you which doctors are the biggest recipients of drug-company money and how much they receive—with some individuals raking in millions of dollars.

Ask doctors why they appear in a pharmaceutical "open payments" register, and they'll likely deny any relationship between the perks they get and the drugs they prescribe. They'll naively talk about how they provide invaluable expertise that leads to better medical outcomes. You can be certain that's not how drug and medical-device companies view the relationship.

Pharmaceutical companies don't align with individual doctors because they provide superior care or medical expertise. They do it because these doctors prescribe more of their products, particularly the most expensive ones. As a result, they know they can count on these doctors to keep prescribing their products and recommend them to their colleagues.

The pharmaceutical world is brilliant at shaping perception through rewards that fatten wallets and stroke egos. Drug reps provide doctors with food, flattery, and friendship, while their companies lure physicians with offers of lavish trips, dinners, and the opportunity to participate in industry talks that come with a handsome honorarium for their trouble.

In most cases, the influence is subtle, not explicit, but the results are always the same. These relationships create conflicts of interest that cloud clinical judgment. For the drug company, the influence is calculated and measured in terms of "return on investment." It is estimated that for every $1 a pharmaceutical company invests in marketing, it earns $10 in return.

And although it is never overtly stated, doctors on the receiving end understand that these perks will disappear as soon as they begin to prescribe a competing product. Confront doctors on the inappropriateness of these relationships, and they'll tell you their independent judgment is never influenced. Look at their behavior, and you can see how financial rewards distort their perceptions.

In 2010, recognizing the danger to patients, Congress passed a piece of legislation known as the Sunshine Act. As a result, pharmaceutical and medical-device companies are now required by law to release details of their payments to doctors and US teaching hospitals. And by going online, you can find out whether your doctor is one of them.

The Psychology of Choice

When it comes to picking the best care for ourselves and our families, patients resist making alternative choices even when data demonstrate far better options are available. It's a confounding paradox that's rooted partly in anchoring bias and partly in fear. But there's also a third element at play, one that is well demonstrated by a series of psychological experiments performed a few years ago.

In one study, people were given one of two relatively similar-looking coffee mugs. They were then asked how much they would sell their mug for and how much they would pay for the other. You might imagine some individual preferences would exist and that any given person might rate one mug better than the other. But researchers found that these randomly selected subjects valued the mug they were given much more than the other, by as much as 50 percent. And when researchers let participants choose the mug, they valued it even more.

The same goes for health care. Pick your own doctor, and you are likely to rate his or her ability as excellent, regardless of what the objective data would indicate. Select a particular hospital or a health plan, and you'll deem it superior to the alternatives.

Insurers know that you have an option to select a new health-insurance policy every year, but that you will most likely make the same choice year over year. In fact, it's estimated that it takes a 15 percent price differential to get people to move from one program to another. Similarly, drug manufacturers know that once patients are prescribed a medication for chronic disease, they are likely to demand it in the future, even when a less-expensive generic comes on the market. Rarely are these important decisions based on objective data. More often, they are a result of our subconscious fears and what's called prior-decision bias, a corollary to the concept of anchoring bias. With prior-decision bias, we hold tight to our choices, valuing the things we chose (like a coffee mug) more than the other options available to us.

The Reality of Modern Medicine

American health care is filled with strange incongruities that result in poorer health, higher costs, and unnecessary deaths. As was highlighted already, many of these contradictions derive from how the brains of both doctors and patients have evolved over tens of thousands of years. As a result of our subconscious processes, we trust the recommendation of a friend over published clinical data. We overrate the excellence of our

doctors and hospitals, and we resist change. We overestimate the likelihood of success in some circumstances (as with the launch of a new drug
or radical procedure) and underestimate it in others (as when doctors
recommend approaches that demand more from us than taking a pill).

These conclusions aren't logical, and that's the point. In the unique
context of medical care, the normative rules of decision making cease
to exist. In the end, context matters greatly, and significantly more than
most of us ever realize.

The American health care system is the best in the world, in some
ways. The speed of diagnoses and the breadth of treatments available in
the United States outpace those of health care systems in other nations.
And many of the world's leading medical discoveries and innovations
came from American researchers and scientists.

But as we have seen, our nation lags behind other advanced nations
in most health measures. Health care's culture, the context of medical
practice, and the evolution of our brains all contribute to this problem.
Although the human mind allows us to solve some of the most complicated and complex problems that exist, it also distorts our perception.

Homo sapiens is the only species to understand the genesis of disease
and the inevitability of death. These threats have terrified us throughout
our existence and, in spite of the medical advances of the past seven decades, we remain as fearful of them as ever. As a result, we often make
poor choices for ourselves.

However, the problem isn't entirely of our own doing. The medical
care we receive and our perception of its quality are greatly affected by
others. In fact, the influence of some of health care's biggest players, from
insurance companies to drug manufacturers, contributes greatly to the
problem and has serious negative consequences for us as well.

Chapter Four

THE LEGACY PLAYERS

Stanford's business school campus imparts spectacular views. It's an atmosphere that inspires collaborative and creative thinking. The main quad, known as "Town Square," is bound by the library and classrooms on two sides, and cafés on the others. Benches and tables offer places to sit and interact with the next generation of business leaders. Signs posted throughout the space announce upcoming lectures. As I peruse the flyers, I always look for the sessions with other CEOs. They come from a diverse set of industries to interact with students and faculty for an hour or more. I always learn much from their experiences.

Six years ago, I attended one such presentation led by outgoing Walmart CEO Lee Scott. I had never met him and had no idea what to expect. Walmart is a retail behemoth with dozens of case studies and books written about its aggressive business model.

I expected Mr. Scott to outline Walmart's world-leading distribution channels, cutting-edge information technology systems, and plans for further global expansion. Instead, he spent most of the time talking about bath towels.

He started by painting a picture of the typical family that comes to Walmart each week to shop. As he spoke, I could envision the mom and dad, along with their three kids. They're an average, hardworking, lower-middle-class family. The husband works a full-time blue-collar job. The wife cares for the children and works during the holiday season so they can supplement their income and purchase a few special gifts for the family. Together, they bring home a combined income of $35,000 a year.

By the time they have paid their taxes, written a rent check, and bought groceries, a set of bath towels becomes a significant purchase, Lee told us. Their world is different than that of families that go to Macy's or even Target for bath towels. He explained that if "Walmart families" can purchase two sets at $20 to $30, they'll have enough money in their budget to take the kids out for pizza on Saturday night. But if these towels fall apart on the second washing, it'll set them back a couple of weeks, maybe a month.

He then described searching the world for quality products—towels among them—and bargaining hard on behalf of these families. In response to one student's question, Lee explained that what got him out of bed each morning was the opportunity to make the life of this family, and millions of other families, better. He closed his remarks with a quote from Walmart's founder, Sam Walton.

"If we work together, we'll lower the cost of living for everyone. We'll give the world an opportunity to see what it's like to save and have a better life." I had come to the talk expecting to be impressed by Walmart's efficient business model. I left feeling inspired by Lee and moved by his commitment to improving the lives of the people who came to his stores.

The next day, I attended a labor management partnership meeting in Oakland, California. At the meeting, I sat next to John August, then director of the Coalition of Kaiser Permanente Unions, which has more than 100,000 of our employees in its membership.

I know John as a principled individual with a forty-year career in labor. When I mentioned the lecture I had just attended, he went ballistic. He had just come from a national labor meeting and described what he perceived to be the horrific treatment of Walmart employees, pointing to inadequate wages, skimpy benefits, and cruel management. He described the steps the AFL-CIO was getting ready to take in order to expose the company's practices to the public, hoping to force Walmart executives to admit their wrongdoing and make amends.

Both Lee and John became controversial figures in later years, but based on my interactions with them, I am convinced both men are sincere individuals, caring fathers, and good leaders. Having talked with colleagues of theirs, I am also convinced they were highly respected by most of their peers. And yet their views of the same company were diametrically opposed. One described Walmart as the defender of the common man, and the other viewed it as the evil empire.

That's the power of perception. When it comes to large legacy players such as Walmart—organizations with massive size, media attention, and clout—few people have neutral opinions. Emotions run high.

But when you work for a company such as Walmart, the largest in the world, with more than 2 million associates, or even for the AFL-CIO, the largest federation of unions, with 12 million members across the country, your views are shaped by the context of your environment.

Legacy players are defined as industry leaders, usually in a position of dominance for decades. Each has its own perception of the world and its place in it. Each invests time and money in shifting the perceptions of others toward viewpoints that best serve its interests. And each has a very hard time seeing or accepting opposing viewpoints.

Theoretically, Lee and John could have objectively examined and resolved their primary areas of disagreement. Using publicly reported data and comparisons to competitors, they could have agreed to a framework for analysis, using it to (1) assess Walmart's wages and benefits, (2) discover opportunities for improvement, and (3) find a common ground. After all, Walmart wants excellent employees and the union wants Walmart to expand and create even more jobs.

But when you are that large and successful, you are convinced your viewpoint is truth no matter what. There's an old saying that I've seen attributed to Anaïs Nin, which reminds us, "We don't see things as they are; we see them as we are." The same is true for the legacy players in health care.

The Legacy Player's Perspective

The 2016 presidential race revealed that our nation's perspectives are divided on a range of issues. Health care is among the most powerful examples.

Many Americans were fed up with the health care system and demanded change. At the same time, others saw the traditional model of care delivery as working well. They preferred that it be preserved with little modification. In general, legacy players fall into this latter category.

To them, American health care might require some tweaks, but not dramatic shifts, and all of them should be accomplished with limited government interference. This preference, along with their antipathy toward President Obama's health care reform programs, can be traced back a full presidential term earlier.

Amid the furious 2012 debates surrounding US health care reform, then House Speaker John Boehner told CBS's *Face the Nation* that "Obamacare will bankrupt our country and ruin the best health care delivery system in the world."

There are a whole lot of claims and concepts packed into that sentence. First, as one would predict, it contains the GOP leader's negative view of the president's signature legislation, which subsequently underwent thirty-seven repeal attempts by Republicans leading up to the 2016 national elections. Layered on top of that is the former House Speaker's pessimism about the act's economic viability. Finally, it encompasses the belief, held widely across the health care continuum, that America has the best delivery system on the planet—or at least it did before the government intervened.

Regardless of your politics, what Boehner said in 2012 had some important economic truth to it. For decades, health care has consumed an ever-greater percentage of tax revenue each year, a trend that poses a serious risk to our nation's financial well-being. And it's true that expanding insurance coverage to tens of millions of Americans through the Affordable Care Act increased total spending, at least in the short term. This was predictable. The advocates accepted it as necessary in their quest to provide medical care to Americans who could not access it before. Today, more than 30 percent of all US government spending goes to health care—a combination of Medicare, Medicaid, veterans' care, marketplace subsidies, and medical research. Those costs will continue to rise rapidly as eligibility for Medicare climbs at an annual rate of 3.5 percent, while the growth of America's populace expands at just 1 percent each year. Legislators like the former House Speaker are rightly concerned about whether our country can generate the tax revenue necessary to fund the rising cost of health care in the future, at least without triggering negative consequences elsewhere in American society.

Of course, congressional politics is partisan. Just as Lee Scott zeroed in on the shopper and John August on the worker, Republicans like Boehner perceive health care reform (as enacted under Democratic leadership) to be an economic threat, whereas the Democrats see it as a solution for helping the millions of Americans who previously lacked insurance coverage. Politics aside, both points have validity. But health care is political and therefore biased. And so are the views of most legacy players.

Going back to the former House Speaker's remark about America boasting the world's best delivery system, there exists a fundamental divergence between his perspective and the objective data. American health care is the costliest system in the world, but its quality outcomes rank nowhere near the top, according to almost all independent global analyses.

In essence, American health care is analogous to paying several thousand dollars for a single bath towel that falls apart on the first wash, not the second.

In the latest Social Progress Index report on health and wellness, the United States ranked sixty-sixth, behind such countries as Canada, Japan, Brazil, Iceland, Sweden, and Israel, to name just a few. And in a biennial survey from the Commonwealth Fund, a private foundation promoting high performance in health care, the US system ranked dead last in several quality measures among eleven of the world's wealthiest countries (mostly in Western Europe, plus Canada, New Zealand, and Australia).

Contrary to John Boehner's belief, the American health care delivery system is mediocre at best. As a result, American adults don't live as long and our child mortality rate is higher when compared to people in almost all other industrialized countries.

Just about the only area in which the United States leads is in how much we spend. In that measure, we aren't just ahead of the rest of the world, we've lapped the field. In raw numbers, US health care accounts for 18 percent of every dollar Americans spend. That's $3 trillion all told. Americans spend more on health care than each of the world's 195 other nations (save for Germany, Japan, and China) spend on everything its citizens purchase or produce.

Our system is overpriced and under-delivering. And though that may be what the objective data demonstrate, that is not at all how health care's biggest players perceive the situation. The way they see it, America needs to keep the health care system it has and, if anything, expand on the traditional approaches they believe have worked for decades. They argue that Americans need more, not fewer, prescription drugs, medical devices, high-priced health insurance plans, and invasive procedures. And with their massive profits, media platforms, and lobbying influence, the views of legacy players have become our nation's collective reality. The numbers tell us that we're buying what they're selling.

As a legacy player, you want to preserve your dominance and position. To do that, you focus on appealing to those individuals who are most valuable to your organization. If you're the head of a drug or device company, for example, you court the doctors, nurses, and patients who prescribe or use your most expensive drugs and devices.

Elected officials share similar characteristics with health care's leading legacy players. If you're an elected official, you may care about all the people you serve, but you care the most about those who increase your chances of getting reelected.

That's not a comment on the politician's personal values or ethics. That's simply the mindset necessary to run for and stay in office. If you were in that same context, you would see that people who show up at the polls are seen as more important than those who don't. You would perceive those who can deliver entire voting blocs as more important still, and those who make the largest campaign contributions as most important of all. Citizens who do none of those things would likely get pushed to the periphery.

Seeing the world as legacy players do is the first step in understanding the types of decisions they make and the impact they have on American health. Ask politicians if they view some citizens as more important than others, and they'll assure you they don't. Look at their actions, and it is hard to come away with any other conclusion. This imbalance between words and actions results in the mistreatment of certain individuals. And as you're about to see, the result of this imbalance can be catastrophic.

Lead in the Water

Flint, Michigan, is the second-most-poverty-stricken city in the country and has long struggled with financial difficulties. In 2014, with the fear of bankruptcy looming, a newly appointed official pitched an idea to save the city $5 million by shifting its water source. Local legislators jumped at the opportunity.

From 1974 to 2014, the main conduits carrying water from Lake Huron into Flint were up to code and fairly lead-free, thanks to prior replacement efforts. But many of the pipes that carried water into people's homes had been installed long ago.

Although low levels of lead had been in the drinking water for some time, the amount of lead found in children through regular blood-lead levels (BLL) tests was relatively minimal. That all changed when the city shifted its main water source to the Flint River.

Lead (Pb), a naturally occurring heavy metal, is highly toxic to the body's organs, including the heart, kidneys, intestines, and bones. Its most serious impact, though, is on the developing brain, particularly in children under the age of six. Best estimates suggest elevated levels of lead in the body produce a five- to ten-point reduction in IQ. Increasing evidence now points to a link between these neurotoxins and the future development of mental-health problems.

That's why flipping the switch on a city's water supply was a big deal—a decision worthy of a detailed water-composition analysis that never took place. If it had, inspectors would have recognized the water's new source was more acidic than the old one, causing lead to leach out of the pipes and into the drinking water.

Not long after switching the water source, residents complained about the quality, citing the water's unusual color, taste, and smell—complaints that went ignored by city officials.

Dr. Mona Hanna-Attisha, a physician on staff at Flint's Hurley Medical Center, reported that lead levels had doubled in the most recent BLL tests of her pediatric patients. State officials ignored the data and accused her of overreacting. Dr. Hanna-Attisha refused to be intimidated. She knew her data were accurate. The water was more acidic, the lead concentrations had increased, and the risks to the children were real.

As city and state officials contemplated the serious financial implications of going back to the old water source, it is very difficult to imagine they would consciously choose to ignore the data and harm the children of their community. But it's not at all difficult to imagine that these politicians simply couldn't see what they were doing in the context of this developing financial crisis.

A month later, when Dr. Hanna-Attisha threatened to go to the press and involve representatives at the federal level, officials were caught up in a political crisis that was spiraling out of control. By then, they had no choice but to see and address the water problem.

Soon, Flint mayor Karen Weaver stressed to residents the importance of picking up lead-testing kits. A few days later, officers from the Michigan State Police started delivering cases of clean water to people's homes. In January 2016, then president Obama declared a state of emergency in the city and surrounding Genesee County, and at a news conference less than a month later, the mayor said the city would remove and replace all 15,000 water service lines that contained lead piping. Work was expected to begin at a cost of $55 million. What started as a desperate attempt to save $5 million in the city budget had turned into a national crisis with a price tag of over $50 million.

Flint's population is 57 percent black and 40 percent poor. The city's crime rate is nearly 50 percent higher than the national average, with an unemployment rate nearly double that of the average city. As stories began to emerge of undocumented residents in Flint being refused bottled water and medical care, residents began to wonder how politicians would have viewed the situation if a threefold increase in lead levels were detected among kindergarten-aged children in an upper-class, predominantly white community like Bloomfield Hills, Michigan. And it wasn't just the residents of Flint who wondered that.

"I'll tell you what, if the kids in a rich suburb of Detroit had been drinking contaminated water and being bathed in it, there would've been action," said Hillary Clinton in early 2016 at the end of a presidential debate, a sentiment believed by some but not all. The legacy players have unique perceptions of the world, often at odds with what they say. For elected officials, votes influence how they view the world and determine what is most important. For traditional legacy players, money is the most influential and important element.

Meet Health Care's Legacy Players

Legacy players in health care represent some of the biggest organizations in America—multibillion-dollar companies and associations that advocate on behalf of the most powerful industry sectors. Together they wield massive influence with market control that, in some cases, borders on monopolistic. Through their lobbying, advertising, and financial donations, they effectively shape the perceptions of doctors, patients, regulators, and legislators.

Their impact on the health care industry is widespread and dichotomous: they simultaneously account for major advances in medical care and yet create some of the biggest barriers to progress. As with Walmart, you can laud their contributions and accomplishments or criticize their abuses of power. But to truly understand the factors shaping American medicine, both now and in the future, you'll need to understand health care's legacy players better. Let's meet the four most important players in health care today.

1. Major insurers. Providing coverage to more than half of the US population, the five largest health-insurance companies have dominated for decades. The annual revenue for each of them currently exceeds $30 billion and is projected to exceed $100 billion per company if these powerhouses successfully consolidate down into three. When and if regulators approve these mergers and acquisitions, we can predict that each insurer will exert even more industry control and that their CEOs, who today earn tens of millions each year in salary, stock, and incentives, will be rewarded handsomely for completing the deals.
2. Hospitals. With nearly 6 million employees across the United States, community hospitals are the second-largest source of private-sector jobs. Their boards comprise CEOs and other business leaders. Similar to insurance company executives, hospital administrators are well compensated, often in proportion to the number of beds they fill and the profits they generate. Community hospitals account for more than 30 percent of all health care costs in the United States, driven in no small part by inefficiencies in the way they deliver care.
3. Physician specialty societies. Not all physician membership groups are created equal. There are about 200,000 primary-care physicians in the United States. That's a lot of doctors. But in the pecking and economic order of American medicine, they exert very little influence. By contrast, the American societies for cardiology, orthopedics, oncology, and other high-cost specialties have a huge impact. With their ties to drug and device companies, they have deep resources to lobby for their members and affect legislation.

4. Drug and device companies. These two prominent manufacturing sectors exert major influence over US politicians, doctors, and patients. As drug prices continue to increase at double-digit rates, these players account for much of health care's rapidly rising costs. Patent laws and restrictive regulations on prescription drugs in the United States protect drug-company profits more than they protect patients.

All four of these legacy players rose to power over many decades. They designed the system's current policies and practices, and they are likely to shape health care well into the future. They wrote the rules governing how health care is structured, reimbursed, and technologically supported. Each has contributed to the best aspects of our current system, but all have worked hard to tip the balance of power in their favor and resist true change. Today, the design and economics of the American health care system reflect their influence.

Playing Favorites

You've probably heard this story before. A father and his son are involved in a terrible car accident. The father dies on impact, but his son is rushed to the Emergency Room for surgery. The surgeon takes one look at the child and says, "I cannot operate on this boy. He's my son." How can that be?

It's a classic riddle on gender bias, with an important lesson for understanding the subconscious perceptions that affect our decisions and actions. Recently, a Boston University researcher ran this riddle by nearly two hundred psychology students and more than one hundred summer-camp kids, ages seven to seventeen. Only about 15 percent from each group guessed the surgeon could be the boy's mother. Some of the kids in the study got downright creative, suggesting the surgeon might be a robot or even a ghost. Most participants, however, couldn't get beyond their internal associations. In the context of their lives and experiences, they generally perceived surgeons as men.

Science has the ability to quantify this bias. The Implicit Association Test, or IAT, can be taken online by those interested in learning more about their own hidden biases relative to gender, race, sexuality, age, or physical appearance.

To complete the test, you sit in front of a computer and perform a series of rapid-fire labeling tasks. You might see the word "doctor" appear in the middle of the screen. You must then tap one of two keys to file the word either under the grouping of "female and career" on the left side of the screen or under "male and family" on the right. Clearly, since the words "doctor" and "career" are complementary, you'd want to tap the left key. The words in the middle of the screen change with each selection, from "doctor" to "wedding" to "child." A little later, the two options on the side of the screen change to "male and career" and "female and family."

As you make your picks, the IAT measures your reaction time in nano-seconds. Of course, if you were without bias, you would place doctor under "female and career" just as quickly as you did "male and career," but that's rarely what happens. Consistently, people are quicker to put professions under male and child-rearing activities under female.

Subconscious Bias Is Universal

All of us have subconscious biases. Some of them are embedded in our brains through evolution, and some reflect the culture in which we are raised. Some are taught to us by our parents and friends, and some result from the conscious efforts of advertisers and prominent cultural influencers.

In the interest of full disclosure, I need to acknowledge that in some ways I am a legacy player and see the world differently than others. I teach at a large academic institution, belong to several national specialty societies, and lead two large medical groups, serving as CEO for the "Permanente" side of Kaiser Permanente.

At the same time, Kaiser Permanente is a not-for-profit, and the medical groups I lead are not publicly traded. My involvement in the Stanford Business and Medical Schools is unpaid. And even in the national societies, I have focused on educating the members rather than taking a leadership role.

In writing this book, I have tried to remain aware that I, too, am vulnerable to subconscious biases, no different than anyone else. As much as possible, I have relied on published, objective information from others to support the contents of *Mistreated*. And by being exposed to the many different sides of American health care, I hope that I can offer a more balanced assessment of the current system, its successes and failures, and the role of legacy players in shaping it.

To better explore the context and the perceptions of these legacy players, I will examine each of the four in greater detail, "zooming out" to offer a broader, more global look at their respective industries before "zooming in" to analyze the factors that influence how each American legacy player operates.

1. Insurers

Zooming Out: Is Health Care a Human Right or a Privilege?
Regardless of the issue at hand, those who clearly see one reality find it difficult to acknowledge the perceptions of others. A story from a few years ago demonstrates this precept well.

If you were on the Internet in February 2015, you doubtless remember the controversy that surrounded a particular dress. When someone on the social media site Tumblr asked her friends to settle a dispute about whether the dress in the photo she had posted was black and blue or white and gold, an Internet frenzy erupted. Every single person who looked at the dress saw it one way or the other. And just about everybody was baffled as to why others couldn't see it their way.

Experts such as Arthur Shapiro, an American University professor specializing in visual perception, provided the scientific explanation: "Color is our perception—our interpretation of the light that's in the world. Individual wavelengths don't have color, it's how our brains interpret the wavelengths that create color."

After 20 million views and a seemingly endless debate on social media, the dressmaker gave us all the answer we were waiting for. On Twitter, British clothier Roman Originals wrote: "We can confirm #TheDress is blue and black!"

That may have resolved the scientific and fashion industry dispute, but it didn't end the debate. Even when people were exposed to the objectively measured truth, those who saw it as white and gold refused to accept the perceptions of those who saw it as black and blue.

In certain situations, everyone sees things the same and their view aligns with the objective reality. But, for a variety of reasons, there are times when what we see differs from what's commonly accepted.

As with the dress, it's not a question of what we think, believe, or decide, but what we actually experience. Even when presented with a scientifically accurate conclusion, it's not enough to change people's perception.

This same variation in perception exists in the way people in different countries view the issue of government-sponsored universal health care coverage.

In the countries that provide health care coverage for all, an overwhelming percentage of their citizens perceive health care as a fundamental human right. In countries that don't, particularly in the United States, coverage is seen as something earned, by virtue of a job or old age, or as a result of economic hardship.

Starting half a century ago, governments across Europe, Canada, and Australia began planning and building centralized health care systems. Today, they continue to provide universal coverage and have built into their tax structure the means to fund it. In some nations, such as England and Canada, the government controls both the financing and certain aspects of health care delivery. In others, including Australia, Sweden, and Germany, medical care is publicly funded, though in large part it is privately delivered.

In the United States, our health care approach and beliefs have evolved quite differently. Until the 1960s, few Americans had government or employer-provided comprehensive coverage. A variety of social and political events at the time caused Congress to expand insurance coverage to millions more at the urging of President Lyndon Johnson. As part of the president's Great Society agenda, the House and Senate enacted legislation that provided Medicare to those over sixty-five and Medicaid to those with extremely low incomes.

Interestingly, organized medicine and the specialty organizations of that era predicted such a move would undermine the excellence of American health care and lead to socialized medicine. But when the expansion in coverage brought them new patients and added income, their perceptions changed and they warmed up to the idea.

Parallel to these expansions of public coverage, private companies hoping to take advantage of favorable tax treatments began expanding coverage for their employees, as well. As unions negotiated and ratified contracts for the steel and auto workers, health care benefits boomed throughout America.

Fast-forward some fifty years and the United States now offers health care coverage through a staggering array of channels. The government continues to provide public health services for our seniors while state-based programs cover individuals with limited resources. We have commercial health care, offered through employer-sponsored insurance plans, along with the online health-insurance exchanges and private brokers who help individuals find coverage. And, of course, with the election of Donald Trump as the forty-fifth president of the United States, new options have been discussed and many of the current programs may change. In Chapter 6, I'll analyze some of the possibilities.

Regardless of what the current president and Congress do, this potpourri of alternatives—some publicly funded, and some private—fits our nation's preference for individual freedom and choice.

Travel the world and you'll meet people with totally different perspectives on how best to provide health care, each opinion held as firmly as the opinions of those who viewed the much-disputed dress.

I have observed these differences in perspective in my own travels. During my training years at Stanford, I spent six months in Calgary, Canada, working in a university hospital. And for over a decade, we at Kaiser Permanente have collaborated with the British National Health System in search of best practices for both outpatient and hospital care. More recently, I traveled to Sweden and Australia, where I had the opportunity to discuss their health care systems with citizens and local experts.

In each location, I spoke with dozens of people covered through their respective national programs. Overwhelmingly, they appreciated the financial security of government-provided health care coverage. In exchange, they were willing to tolerate limitations in their choice of doctors and frequent delays for routine care. Although the details of each system varied slightly one from another, the locals were largely appreciative for what they had and how their systems were run. And in the Commonwealth Fund report, all of these countries rank ahead of the United States in quality outcomes and overall population health.

Given all the problems with US health care, you might predict that its design would have changed decades ago. But that's the problem with perception. In the United States, our culture views the trade-offs of universal coverage rather negatively. We value individual choice over a single, uniform approach. As the 2016 US elections demonstrated, we are leery of the government's ability to operate efficiently. And as a huge, diverse nation, we are less focused on those without coverage than are citizens who live in smaller, more homogeneous nations.

To Americans, the shortcomings of the British or Canadian systems, with their restrictions and delays, are seen as extremely problematic. And we assume their citizens must feel that way as well. But when surveyed, residents of the United Kingdom, Canada, Sweden, and Australia report satisfaction levels with their national health systems at around 85 to 90 percent, significantly higher than Americans rank their own system.

Zooming In: US Legacy Insurers and Payers

As the 2016 election process demonstrated, Americans span the spectrum in how they believe health care coverage should be provided. For Bernie Sanders, the Independent senator from Vermont, and for many of his millennial followers, a single-payer system run by the government would be best. For Secretary Clinton, a traditional Democrat, expanding the Affordable Care Act, particularly Medicaid and the online insurance marketplace, was the best next step. And for the new president, the most popular refrain was "repeal and replace," which offered up a medley of free-market options.

But the biggest issue for our nation isn't who funds it. In reality, it doesn't make much of a difference whether the funding is paid directly through employers or via government taxes. The iceberg that awaits is the total cost of providing care. Over time, if health care inflation continues at the current rate, all the choices will be bad. The only options will be: (1) charge people more, (2) cut benefits, or (3) ration care for those who can't afford it. Regardless, health outcomes will suffer.

To reverse the escalation of cost in American health care, we need to improve the performance (efficiency and effectiveness) of the care we provide. You might think that with their power and market clout, insurance companies would be able to restructure US health care delivery. However, historically, these "payers" have had very little influence over the provision of care. It's not that they don't want to improve performance at the care-delivery level. They just don't know how. And when they've tried in the past, the results have been dismal. There's an old adage that says when the only tool you have is a hammer, everything looks like a nail. To insurers, money and financial incentives are the solution to every problem.

An example from a few years back was the concept of "pay for performance." It makes logical sense in theory: pay doctors increments of money to achieve higher levels of preventive screening (mammograms and colonoscopies), and you'll increase your health plan's performance and improve patient health.

The problem with using money to change physician behavior isn't that it fails to work. The problem is that it works too well.

Remember that doctors get accepted into medical schools by doing well on tests. Pay for performance is just another test. The outcomes of this financial-incentive experiment reminded me of a research effort that happened overseas many years ago.

Wanting to isolate a hormone called human chorionic gonadotropin (hCG), scientists in the 1960s traveled to a remote village in Papua New Guinea with a high fertility rate. They offered pregnant women there a modest payment for every liter of their urine, a source of this protein. Everything went well for the first week. But over the next few weeks, scientists noticed the urine had become less concentrated and the hormone harder to extract. They wondered what was happening with the population's biology. Soon, they realized the women weren't the only ones participating in the research. They were asking their husbands, children, and non-pregnant friends to pee in the container as well.

And that's basically what happened with the doctors in the pay-for-performance system. Rather than focusing on the proper indications for the screening tests (that is, which patients would benefit from them), doctors started ordering them for everyone, in order to collect the financial reward. The program did increase the rate of screening, but not necessarily for the patients who needed the studies the most. And in parallel, the doctors stopped focusing on the important preventive interventions that weren't being rewarded. As a result, most insurers have eliminated these types of programs or cut them back significantly.

Pains and Claims

Observing the decisions of legacy players from afar, the economics of their world often appear upside down. The medical loss ratio, or MLR, is a good example. MLR is the percent of an insurer's premium spent on direct patient care and quality improvement, as opposed to administrative overhead and profit. In health care, you would assume companies that exist to insure people should want to maximize the medical care they reimburse.

If that were true, the higher the MLR, the better. You might assume that a 90 or 95 percent MLR would signal great success, as it would mean more money was going toward improvements in quality and patient health. But insurance company executives are rewarded and their stock prices rise the fastest when their ratio is as low as possible.

Prior to the passage of the Affordable Care Act, many for-profit insurance companies were achieving MLRs in the 70 to 75 percent range. The problem got so bad that the federal government mandated through ACA legislation that insurance companies had to spend at least 85 percent of the premiums they collected from medium and large businesses on direct medical care.

And that's not the only practice the ACA prohibited. It also did away with what insurers called "cherry-picking" and "lemon-dropping." These were cute names for insurance tricks that had very real consequences for patients and working people. The goal for insurers was to maximize profits by (1) encouraging relatively healthy people (cherries) to join a health plan, and (2) discouraging relatively sick people (lemons) from seeking coverage under the company's plan. Insurers accomplished this by denying coverage to individuals with preexisting conditions and by denying reimbursement for as many health care services as possible, including maternity care.

When confronted with the ACA's prohibitions, commercial health insurers switched tactics in 2014 and began offering subscribers "narrow networks." These new coverage options offer lower premiums in exchange for a reduced choice of care providers, anywhere from 30 to 70 percent fewer in-network physicians. This makes sense in circumstances where insurers limit the choices to only the doctors and health systems with the highest-quality measures and lowest prices. But that wasn't the criteria they used. Instead, they looked at claims data and selected the least expensive providers, regardless of their clinical outcomes.

Even this choice might have been acceptable to some policyholders if they could have figured out who was included in these narrow networks and who wasn't. At least then patients and employers could have assessed the quality of the providers available and figured out how much extra they were willing to pay for broader choice.

But amid the frequent adding, dropping, and replacing of physicians, the in-network lists were rarely up-to-date or accurate. Some patients who sought care learned the hard way just how narrow their network had become. In some states, patients faced with unexpected medical bills for newly out-of-network doctors sued the insurance companies that failed to let them know.

The latest health-insurance-industry solution to address financial woes: mergers and acquisitions. Through regulatory approval, the "big five" had hoped to clear the legal hurdles and become the even-bigger three. Anthem wanted to merge with Cigna, Aetna with Humana. Even United-Healthcare, already the biggest fish in the sea, expanded its influence through Optum, its data analytics arm. Already, however, the Aetna merger with Humana has been blocked, and the Anthem-Cigna union is being opposed by the Department of Justice.

It's hard to predict exactly where all this focus on consolidation and increased market clout will lead. Theoretically, insurers could use this added influence to obtain concessions from doctors and hospitals that lead to greater savings for policyholders. More likely, they will try to use the reduced competition to charge higher premiums for businesses and individuals. Industry observers have been watching closely to see what President Trump and Congress will do. Will they continue to oppose these mergers as aggressively as the Obama administration or will they change course and let insurers sell their products across state lines? If so, we could see insurance companies with even greater market clout introducing even narrower plans.

Through the lens of the major insurance companies, their job is to calculate risk and price plans accordingly. And from their perspective, the rising cost of health care is hardly their fault. Blame the hospitals, doctors, and drug companies for that. And when you see the world in this way, you perceive consolidation not as anticompetitive but as an important tool in the battle to maximize your market power. But even without that increased power, insurers are still doing just fine financially. UnitedHealthcare has seen its share price increase 375 percent since 2010. In parallel, every one of the big five has watched its shares reach record highs in recent years. When insurance companies earn huge profits and when executive take-home salaries exceed $15 million a year, they don't see the current health care system as broken. The same is true for the politicians who received $152 million in annual campaign contributions from the insurance industry during the most recent election cycle.

To the rest of the world, our system makes no sense. Earning a profit by selling health care coverage seems inappropriate to people in other countries. They believe that allowing insurance companies to become so dominant through merger and acquisition is not in the public's interest. And the thought of people having to declare bankruptcy because of high medical bills feels unconscionable.

When you perceive health insurance as a right, you embrace the compromises needed for the government to cover all of its citizens. Delays in routine care and higher taxes are seen as a small price to pay. In contrast, when you see health care as a privilege, not a right, you dismiss the financial challenges of those without coverage, deride universal systems, and scoff at how long it takes citizens in other countries to obtain routine procedures and tests.

Like the way we see the dress, the issue is not whether one perception is right and the other is wrong. It's a matter of how we see that world. And when we see the world of health care one way, we can't possibly see it any other way.

2. Hospitals

Zooming Out: The Swedish Formula

A few years ago, I spent a week visiting the main hospital in Jönköping, a lakeside town in southern Sweden. Health care experts around the world regard this hospital as the crown jewel of clinical outcomes. As I observed the hospital's remarkable efficiency and highly coordinated care, it became quickly clear how perception and culture affect clinical quality. These forces combine for the benefit of Swedish patients in a nation that, overall, ranks third globally in the Commonwealth Fund report.

In Sweden's medical culture, physicians and hospital administrators view health care as a public service. To them, providing medical care is an honor. The ideals of collaboration, not competition, power their day-to-day practices as Swedish health care professionals work together as a team on behalf of the entire population. It's a mindset that contrasts vividly with American medical culture, which elevates and celebrates the contributions of individuals.

This difference in cultures shouldn't be surprising. The citizens of Sweden are overwhelmingly Scandinavian, reflecting a common culture and national values. They're appalled when one of their own suffers or hurts another, which explains why the nation has some of the strictest drunk driving laws in the world.

And because most of Sweden's citizens embody a shared history and ethnicity, Swedes embrace a strong sense of familial kinship. As in most families, the greater good trumps the desire for personal freedom and individual accomplishment. Cooperation and concern for the well-being of others makes for a powerful societal norm, which in turn has made the Swedish health care system both high performing and incredibly safe for patients.

The facility I visited was built decades ago and would be considered dated by American standards. The hospital, however, was medically outstanding. The hospital team generates world-class clinical outcomes for every problem the doctors treat. Working together, physicians, nurses, and hospital leaders analyze data on clinical outcomes to determine the best approaches for all patients. They translate these practices into consistent pathways that all physicians follow, scrutinizing them down to the smallest detail.

For each medical problem a patient may experience, physician leaders in the hospital and the associated outpatient facilities identify the best set of steps for treatment and get agreement from all to use them. Everyone, from the most senior to the newest physicians, follows these clinical protocols. Tell this to American doctors and patients, and they'd be skeptical. How could a consensus-building medical culture be better or more efficient than ours? The answer is simple. By elevating the performance of every doctor to match the best, the entire hospital achieves superior outcomes at lower costs.

For example, by agreeing on a single type of orthopedic implant, everyone on the operative team learns how to use it, thereby reducing the risk of medical error. And rather than having to stock a variety of implant types in all different sizes simply to match the preferences of individual surgeons, the Swedes figure which is actually the best, and they purchase it in higher volumes at reduced prices. The esprit de corps and level of fulfillment I observed among the doctors and nurses in this hospital were nothing short of inspiring.

Zooming In: The Inconsistencies of US Hospitals

In American medical culture, doctors in hospitals perceive variation in practice as a positive, not a problem.

It's yet another paradox of American medical practice. Our doctors spend hours each month reading the latest medical journals and insist that research studies should be scientifically controlled and subject to statistical analysis. Then when it comes to their own practices, they resist the idea that there is a best approach and that every doctor should adhere to specific evidence-based best practices.

To understand the impact of this paradox on patient care, let's start with the following question: If you knew you were going to be admitted to the hospital for a serious and unexpected medical problem, on which day of the week would you want it to happen?

If you said Monday or Tuesday, you'd be correct. Those are the best days to get sick if you need immediate hospital care. If you said Friday or Saturday, guess again. If you're admitted on a weekend, treatment for your non-life-threatening problem will be delayed. You'll spend a day longer in the hospital on average. And that extra day may prove very hazardous to your health.

Most people think of hospitals as the safest place to be. They are not. Bacteria abound. Hospital-acquired infections affect more than 700,000 people in acute care facilities and prove deadly for 10 percent of them.

Hospitals on weekends are worse for one basic reason: they are under-staffed compared to weekdays. Not by necessity, but by choice.

Doctors and nurses defend the current staffing approach. They assume that seven-day coverage would require as many people on Saturday and Sunday as they currently have Monday through Friday, thereby raising costs excessively. They will reassure you that in case of a life-threatening emergency, the on-call staff is available. What they can't see is how the delay from Saturday to Monday ushers in the risk of infection, the anxiety of waiting, and the added cost to our nation's health care system. There is a solution. Spread the elective work over all seven days, providing enough staff every day while avoiding overtime and on-call pay during weekends. But that would mean doctors would need to work more Saturdays and Sundays than they prefer. And in the context of their personal life, they don't see that as an optimal solution. When it's your weekend and you want to spend time with your family, you don't notice the impact on patients.

Today's wait-and-see approach leads to predictable and problematic outcomes. A 2008 *Journal of the American Medical Association* (*JAMA*) study found that hospitalized patients who suffered a cardiac arrest over the weekend were less likely to survive than those admitted on a weekday. It doesn't have to be this way.

Imagine if hospitals had to post signs in their lobby detailing the average time delay for patients awaiting care on weekends. Or imagine if they were prohibited from billing insurance companies for the extra day. It would be the right thing for the patient. But don't expect this type of transparency anytime soon in a hospital near you.

3. Physician Specialty Societies

Zooming Out: Protecting Your Turf

Every major medical specialty has a national society looking out for the interests of its physicians, from the American Society of Cardiology to the American Association of Orthopedic Surgeons and the American Society of Clinical Oncology. Each is dedicated to two objectives: advancing clinical practice and advancing the financial success of its members. Often, these two objectives conflict.

For example, it's commonly assumed that early prostate cancer detection saves lives. But two large clinical trials show no overall benefit from mass screening. A positive prostate-specific antigen (PSA) test is typically followed with a biopsy to confirm the presence of cancer. But even when the test rightly identifies a patient with cancer, aggressive radiation and surgical treatment have virtually no effect on the person's life or longevity. In fact, a recent study in the *New England Journal of Medicine* showed that aggressive treatment of early stage prostate cancer was no better than an observational approach known as "watchful waiting." Of the 1,600 men observed in this study over ten years, only seventeen (1 percent) died of prostate cancer. And yet urologists still recommend the aggressive approach, so many of their patients choose this treatment, too.

Many US primary-care organizations recommend men without symptoms skip the PSA test. Some even point out the many ways the test leads to more harm than good, including higher risks of infection, impotence, and incontinence from the resulting surgery.

That's not what urologists who do the surgical resection want to hear or what their specialty society recommends. This may sound like a standard disagreement among physicians over which approach is best, but it's more than that. For primary-care physicians, it's a question of observing the scientific literature and seeing that surgery is no better than monitoring low-risk patients over time. For the urologists, they simply don't understand how you can argue against operating on cancer, despite what the published clinical trials may indicate. For them, it's a question of income.

A similar perceptual conflict exists with the most commonly performed orthopedic procedure in the United States: meniscus surgery, an operation to repair a tear in the cartilage of the knee that about 400,000 people undergo each year. Several large studies have shown that the operation, plus physical therapy, is no better than physical therapy alone.

Specifically, researchers found the surgery to be "a highly questionable practice without supporting evidence of even moderate quality." Much of the research proving the futility of this surgery was conducted through one of the world's best academic orthopedic programs. Of interest, this program was in Canada, not the United States. The Canadian faculty members attend the same conferences as their colleagues south of the border. They read the same peer-reviewed journals. And yet, their perceptions of the same operation turned out to be extremely different. Once again, this is the influence of context on human perception.

When asked to identify the five biggest opportunities to reduce health care costs without compromising quality, the American Association of Orthopedic Surgeons made no mention of eliminating meniscus surgery. Compared to what they actually recommended, rethinking meniscus surgery would have had one hundred times the impact. Through the lens of people who are paid to maximize the income of orthopedic surgeons, the specialty association leaders simply couldn't see what other experts in their field were able to identify so easily. As is the case with many legacy players, the line between conscious choice and subconscious perception is blurred. After all, it's not as though the AAOS decided to continue performing meniscus surgery out of greed. It's that it couldn't see the value in doing away with it, even though it was so obvious to others.

In the United States, physician specialty societies advocate not only for a higher volume of procedures for their members, but also for higher reimbursement per procedure. For American medical culture, that may seem appropriate. Medical leaders elsewhere in the world see the situation differently.

At the Jönköping hospital in Sweden, I was surprised to learn how narrow the salary gap was between primary-care physicians and surgical specialists. In the United States, surgeons and medical subspecialists who do procedures stand at the top of the income pyramid. Orthopedic surgeons and cardiologists in the United States earn two to three times more on average than a family-medicine doctor or pediatrician.

It's hard to know which came first for specialty physicians—the money or the status. But in practice, one simply reinforces the other.

When a patient suffering from a heart attack is brought back to life in the Emergency Room, the cardiologist who unclogs the artery is labeled a hero. There are kudos from colleagues and thank-you cards from grateful family members. The fee schedule (a complete list of fees used to pay doctors/hospitals) aligns with this hero status, reinforcing the perception that intervening during a crisis is more difficult and more valuable than preventing one.

Compare the surgeon's experience to that of a primary-care physician. Through prevention and aggressive management of chronic conditions, the typical primary-care physician saves a comparable number of lives. But unlike the cardiologist, primary-care physicians can't name the specific patients whose deaths they prevented. So, for the preventive-care specialist, there are far fewer cheers and thank-you notes.

This difference in context has a huge impact on American health and the provision of health care. It leads us to overvalue the impact of doctors who operate on people and undervalue the physicians who keep us off the operating table in the first place. Consequently, the United States ranks first in the world in the proportion of specialists to generalists, and there's not a close second. This imbalance is becoming worse, not better.

Across the nation, there is a growing physician shortage in primary care, but counterintuitively, there are not enough residency positions for the number of medical students graduating. Over the past fifteen years, the number of newly trained doctors has gone up 30 percent, but the number of US resident slots has held relatively flat. This past year, 1,000 graduating medical students failed to find a residency match, and most of the recently created positions have been designated for training additional specialists, not more primary-care physicians. This trend is the opposite of what our nation needs if we're going to match the quality outcomes of other countries.

The reasons for this rift are largely economic. Since the 1960s, residency programs have been federally subsidized through Medicare, with few additional investments coming from elsewhere. And in the United States, hospitals receive the same financial reimbursement from the government whether they train primary-care physicians or orthopedic surgeons.

Administrators know that having more orthopedic residents will encourage attending surgeons to operate in their facilities rather than at competing hospitals. Residents help take care of the patients, so that attending physicians are bothered less at night with questions or problems. Admitting physicians appreciate this service.

With more orthopedic residents (and more community doctors wanting to operate in places with these residents), these hospitals will do more total joint replacements, particularly those that require complex surgical procedures and generate more-lucrative reimbursements. To a hospital administrator, training a resident in a surgical specialty is almost certain to positively affect the hospital's bottom line, whereas the financial impact of adding another primary-care resident will be minimal.

Ask health care leaders about primary care and all will agree: we have a national shortage and should train more. They're right. But when they have the opportunity to hire and train more of them, that's usually not what they choose to do.

Zooming In: Heart Surgeries and Hysterectomies

Silicon Valley houses the headquarters of many tech-industry icons: Google, Apple, and Facebook among them. Along the valley's stretch of Highway 101, between San Francisco and San Jose, you will pass ten community hospitals that offer cardiac surgery. Three of these facilities perform less than one surgery per day on average, which means on some days they do a couple and on other days none. Now, try to imagine a technology manufacturing plant that would pay a full shift of skilled laborers to stand around for an entire day and not produce any new widgets.

In the manufacturing world, this would not be tolerated, and the solution would be simple: combine the three low-volume centers into one to maximize expertise, boost quality, and lower cost. And in most industries, these three inefficient businesses would either merge or go bankrupt. Easy choice. But in this respect, health care defies the usual rules of business and logic. Any hospital executive who decides to consolidate and send his or her facility's heart-surgery patients five miles up the road would be fired for undermining the medical center's brand. It would be the right move for the patients and the community, but it would be a career-ender for the CEO.

Contrast that logic with the practices in Switzerland, which ranks second in the world for health care quality based on the Commonwealth Fund report. There, about a dozen surgeons perform all total joint surgeries for the nation's 8 million residents. These surgeons are some of the top orthopedic specialists in the world. That's partly because they possess about five to ten times the experience (and expertise) of their US counterparts. The United States is about forty times the size of Switzerland and has approximately 5,000 surgeons who perform this procedure. If we tried to match Switzerland's clinical success, we'd need to limit that number to 500 or so. That is not something the national orthopedic societies are likely to encourage, even when data on the relationship between volume and quality outcomes indicate it would be better for patient care.

The math is straightforward: do an operation infrequently and you will have less expertise and more complications than when you perform it often. Ask any surgeon if he or she would be willing to undergo an operation performed by a colleague who does that procedure rarely, and the answer will be no. Then compare the number of surgeons in America with the number of procedures performed, and you'll see the double standard that exists. This kind of math problem isn't just confined to total joint surgeries.

There was a time when the hysterectomy, a procedure to remove a woman's uterus, was a very common operation in the United States. Surgeons saw performing the procedure as something that would benefit most women once they reached a certain age, like getting your wisdom teeth or tonsils removed. That's no longer the case.

With a better understanding of the indications (knowing when and whether to do the procedure) and the emergence of less-invasive alternative treatments, the rate of hysterectomy procedures has dropped dramatically.

Still, the majority of OB-GYN physicians in community practice continue to do the procedure, even as the total number of hysterectomies performed each year declines. Currently, there are two different approaches available. There's the newer, less invasive approach that can be completed through a laparoscope and on an outpatient basis. And then there's the old way, in which the OB-GYN physician makes a long incision in the patient's abdomen, requiring the woman to spend several nights in the hospital and weeks in recovery. The new way, using the telescope-like device, leads to faster healing and a much shorter hospital stay. But there's a catch for doctors when making the shift from a large incision to a small one. Laparoscopy is much more technically demanding. And with fewer hysterectomies being performed, many physicians lack expertise with the new approach, causing higher rates of complication.

No female surgeon would ever agree to undergo a hysterectomy performed by a doctor who does fewer than a dozen a year. But last year, half of the doctors performing the procedure did not reach even *that* threshold.

More Is Not Better

If you calculated the number of procedures performed per 1,000 people living in different parts of the country, you'd see a huge variation from one location to the next. Your first assumption might be that the numbers reflect the rate of disease, illness, or injury in the area. But that's not what is happening. Strange as it may sound, the best predictor for higher volumes of surgery in a given geography isn't the rate of disease but the number of surgeons practicing there.

Simply put: Oversupply a city with spine surgeons and the number of back surgeries will grow in proportion. Oversupply a town with high-tech testing machines, and you'll see more studies ordered.

According to the authors of the Dartmouth Atlas Project who document variations in how medical resources are distributed and used in the United States: "In regions where there are relatively fewer medical resources, patients get less care; however, there is no evidence that these patients are worse off than their counterparts in high-resourced, high-spending regions. Patients do not experience improved survival or better quality of life if they live in regions with more care. In fact, the care they receive appears to be worse."

It's important to emphasize the last point, "the care they receive appears to be worse." In places oversupplied by surgeons, more procedures actually worsen clinical outcomes. The reason is simple. Operate on people with minimal indications, and the complications will exceed the benefits. Based on the independent data available to us, we don't need more surgeons. We need to shift more dollars from specialty to primary care. Of course, that's not how the specialty societies and their members perceive the situation.

4. Drug and Device Companies

Zooming Out: A Global Prescription

Pharmaceutical manufacturing and sales is a profitable venture the world over. According to one recent report, it may be the most profitable industry that exists. Here in the United States, drug companies benefit from long-term patent protections and regulations that prohibit the federal government from negotiating favorable pricing for Medicare patients.

Recently, the International Federation of Health Plans issued a report on prescription medication costs in the United States versus countries such as Canada, Spain, the United Kingdom, and the Netherlands. In it, unit pricing for various drugs (ranging from HIV/AIDS and pain medications to pills for depression and arthritis) was displayed on a chart side by side, nation by nation. From top to bottom, the United States registered the highest price for every medication, on the list, and it wasn't even close.

Take Nexium, a moderately priced and popular acid-reflux medication. It costs $30 a month in Canada, $42 in the United Kingdom, $58 in Spain, and $23 in the Netherlands. Here in the United States, a month's supply will cost you $305. On the other end of the pricing spectrum, the drug Gleevec, which treats a particular type of leukemia, is available for $989 per month in New Zealand and $1,141 in Canada. The average US health plan, however, prices the same drug at around $8,500 per month.

In the past six years, the average price for the most widely used brand-name drugs in the United States has increased 128 percent. And though prescription-drug coverage blinds most Americans to these astronomical fees, insurers pass along the costs to patients through higher premiums, deductibles, and copayments.

Americans wrongly perceive much of their health care to be free. In fact, because of the rapid rise in health care costs, hourly wages for US workers have remained relatively flat over the past two decades.

Because our government is legislatively prohibited from negotiating or regulating prescription prices and because such countries as Canada, Spain, the United Kingdom, and the Netherlands have government agencies that do, US payers and patients contribute to a disproportionately higher share of drug-company profits.

Although some elected officials (and all drug-company lobbyists) will tell you the safety of patients is their primary concern, that's not the reason Americans are legally prohibited from buying medications from pharmacies in Canada. Tainted drugs are no more a problem north of the border than here in the United States. Rather, the law reflects the economic power of the pharmaceutical industry, its lobbying efforts, and the shifts in political perception that accompany large campaign donations.

It doesn't have to be this way. During his presidential campaign, candidate Trump talked about easing this restriction as well as allowing Medicare to negotiate for lower prices, as is done in other countries. How aggressively he will pursue these options as president, and whether Congress will legislate the necessary changes, given the power of the pharmaceutical lobby, remains to be seen.

Zooming In: US Drugs, Devices, and Destiny

For more than a decade, pharmaceutical and medical-device manufacturers have been criticized for their role in driving up US health care costs. In spite of public reproach, the pace of drug-cost inflation in the United States is accelerating rapidly. The industry is well aware that most patients have no choice but to pay the asking price. They take advantage of this with every opportunity they see.

Mylan manufactures a product called an EpiPen. The device allows parents to safely inject epinephrine in children who are experiencing dangerous allergic responses. The drug is safe and costs little to produce. And because epinephrine is a naturally occurring chemical in the human body, it can't be patented.

The injection device itself, however, is under patent, even though it was developed by a NASA engineer for the federal government thirty-four years before Mylan bought the rights. For a while, the cost for a two-pen set was approximately $100, an affordable price for most families.

From 2007 to 2015, the price Mylan charged for their EpiPens increased by 600 percent, despite the company not investing a single dollar in research and development. Over that same time frame, the compensation for Mylan's CEO rose 671 percent, from $2.5 million to $18.9 million a year.

When the story made front-page headlines in 2016, the company offered to provide uninsured patients with a rebate coupon, a gesture the
company knew would have little impact on the total product revenue.
And when that move was ridiculed as insignificant and self-serving, the
company said it would release a generic version of the same product for
$300, a seemingly nonsensical solution, given all they had to do was drop
the price of the EpiPen itself.

But there was more strategy here than meets the eye. Mylan's executives knew that if doctors wrote out a prescription for "EpiPen," phar-
macists would be legally required to sell the patient the expensive name
brand, not the new generic. And as a result of legislation, which Mylan
played a role in passing, schools in most states had to purchase EpiPen,
not the generic alternative.

In spite of condemnation by numerous members of Congress and polls
showing that 65 percent of Americans favor steps to control drug prices,
little has changed in the pharmaceutical industry. Drug companies can
still purchase the rights to long-established products, invest no additional
dollars in them, and raise their prices excessively. No legislation has been
passed to limit the abuses of existing patent protections. Lobbying and
campaign donations from "Big Pharma" helped create this context.

Patent laws are designed to encourage research and development and to
reward companies that take risks. Increasingly in the drug world, they do
neither. Instead, these companies are allowed to engage in price gouging.
There is no other way to objectively describe their recent actions. For a
variety of medications, there is only one manufacturer. The companies
know that patients have no alternative but to buy their products. And
they are confident that when they announce price increases, no one will
or can stop them.

That brings us to Sofosbuvir, a hepatitis C medication sold by Gilead
Sciences under the brand name Sovaldi. The medication is effective in
ridding the body of the virus that causes the infection. For that reason,
the manufacturer could have appropriately justified a relatively high price.

Instead, Gilead went sky high. What makes the company's actions
so egregious is that Gilead didn't research or develop Sovaldi. Rather, it
simply bought the rights to it from another drug company for $11 billion,
with absolute certainty that a handsome profit was in store.

Pharmasset, the company that did the R&D, had planned to sell the drug at a total cost of treatment for around $30,000. But when Gilead realized it could charge whatever it wanted, the company affixed a price tag of $1,000 a pill, approximately $84,000 for a course of treatment. It has been estimated that Gilead recouped its total investment in less than eighteen months, with revenues projected to reach $269 billion over the drug's life span. That's a 2,500 percent return on investment, essentially guaranteed and relatively risk free.

Pharmasset and Gilead represent two diverging sides of the legacy drug companies. On the one hand, Pharmasset radically changed the prognosis for patients with chronic hepatitis. On the other hand, Gilead used its size, power, and patent protection to extract exorbitant profits from insurers and patients. As a nation, drug spending through Medicare increased by $17 billion from 2013 to 2014. Almost 20 percent of that was because of Sovaldi.

Gilead's decision to jack up its hepatitis C drug price signaled to the industry that patients, insurance companies, and even the federal government were in no position to say no to predatory pricing.

Enter Martin Shkreli, a hedge-fund manager who studied Gilead and realized that successful drug companies didn't have to conduct any R&D or even create new products, for that matter. He concluded that you don't even need to know much about drugs or health care to become a pharmaceutical CEO. So, he granted himself the title, purchased the rights to an essential drug that had been around for more than half a century, and marked it up. In fact, he marked it way up: 5,000 percent, to be exact.

Shkreli didn't write the playbook. He just executed it like no one else had before: (1) Find a drug that's relatively low in cost and essential, (2) buy the rights, (3) jack up the price, and (4) raise it again every few months.

His purchase, an anti-parasitic medication given to patients with compromised immune systems, is a must-have medication for anyone living with AIDS. Shkreli knew these patients had no choice but to purchase this life-saving medication, regardless of the price. The magnitude of his greed, combined with his lack of compassion, brought intense congressional scrutiny. His perception of himself as untouchable extended to his testimony, during which he showed disdain for Congress, both in his words and defiant body language. More than a year later, he continues to defend his actions as appropriate.

How drug companies are perceived is complicated and depends a lot on the eye of the beholder, as proves true for so many legacy players. Visit one of their corporate headquarters and you'll see the walls are covered with pictures of patients cured of life-threatening diseases. Read their mission statement, and you might even be inspired by how they talk about their purpose and dedication to improving lives.

Learn about the free samples they give away and the price reductions they offer for those who can't pay, and you may perceive these pharmaceutical companies as angelic. Watch patients become "brand loyalists" as a result, and you will conclude it was all a scam, a calculated marketing ploy.

Drug companies and their executives want to develop life-saving medications for patients. And there's no reason to believe that the people who work there aren't motivated by a righteous mission. But over the past decade, there has been a fundamental shift in the drug industry. Rather than focus on major R&D investments to address the most severe problems patients face, they are using acquisition, patent protection, and price escalation to fatten their balance sheets. And central to their marketing efforts is shaping perception through persuasive advertising messages.

In print publications and TV commercials, on the Internet and radio, drug companies spend millions on marketing and use celebrities with vast social networks to tout their products and drive up demand. A couple of decades ago, they recognized it would be much easier and more effective to change the perceptions of patients with a medical problem, rather than their doctors. So the drug companies went heavy on direct-to-patient advertising. It was a calculated maneuver. They knew that most of the time when patients request a new brand-name medication from their doctor, they get it.

Increasingly, drug companies are using famous people, including TV and social-media personalities such as the Kardashians, to hype their products. It's an interesting choice. Why not pay a reputable gynecologist, cardiologist, or oncologist to tout your product? The reason they prefer a celebrity endorsement brings us back, once again, to brain neurophysiology.

We may think that TV ads with famous people don't influence our buying habits, but marketing firms know better. We have already seen how powerful a friend's recommendation is when it comes to selecting a doctor or health plan. And even though very few of us know a celebrity personally, we follow their lives on TV and in social media and feel like we can relate to them. This perceived intimacy, combined with the equity of fame, significantly elevates the value of the products they recommend. One research experiment demonstrated how the perceived value of "premium goods" is wired into our brains.

The Illusion of Quality

In 2008, Stanford researchers asked paid volunteers to evaluate the taste of wine. Participants were hooked up to brain scanners measuring the flow of blood to different parts of the brain. Researchers then poured wine from two bottles with fake price tags attached, one for $5 and the other for $45. The trick was that each bottle contained the same wine. As participants noted the difference in price, they reported the more expensive wine as the better of the two. That part was predictable. But what truly surprised researchers wasn't the conscious choice people made but the activity demonstrated on their brain scans. As the tasters sipped the seemingly more expensive wine, the pleasure centers of their brains became stimulated, even though their taste and olfactory nerves experienced the identical chemicals in both.

When drugs are advertised on TV and endorsed by famous celebrities, patients are likely to request them, even though generics are identical in chemical structure and efficacy. And when a drug is covered by prescription insurance, the price differential becomes even less relevant.

Drug companies are not the only health care manufacturers to have figured out how to game perception. Medical-device manufacturers understand this scheme, too. Take, for example, the promise and hype surrounding the "surgical robot."

Mention the use of a "robot" in the context of health care and people will automatically associate it with the most advanced technology available and, therefore, assume they're in for a better clinical outcome. Published outcome data do not validate this perception.

The surgical robot was first approved by the Food and Drug Administration in 2000. As noted earlier, resecting prostate cancer is fraught with severe complications, ranging from impotence to having to wear a diaper for the rest of your life due to urinary incontinence.

Using a robot sounds sexy and, intuitively, its use in prostate surgery makes sense. After all, the robot has steady hands and can work through a smaller incision. But the results, in terms of both cancer eradication and surgical complications, are similar to more traditional alternatives. And for most surgeons, the robot-assisted procedure takes longer.

The price of this device totals more than $1 million. However, the "up-sell" feature is not the machine itself, but rather the robot's disposable arms. Each arm has a built-in obsolescence factor that forces hospitals to replace them after ten uses. The requirement to replace them every week or two has little to do with safety. It's about profit. The manufacturer could have built a robot that could complete one hundred procedures. In fact, there's little evidence that using them more than ten times poses any risk to patients. However, once the manufacturer slapped a warning label on the device, no hospital in America would risk using the arms eleven times. But here is a question worth asking: Why did hospitals purchase surgical robots in the first place, especially when there were alternatives that cost less and delivered similar outcomes?

Like so many legacy players, the company that developed the robot understood the power of perception. It put up billboards along the highway advertising the hospitals that had bought these robots, communicating to passersby that these institutions were cutting-edge. Of course, there was no evidence those who bought these machines were any more advanced technologically or achieved better results than their competitors. But that's the power of perception. Once a few hospitals jumped on board, others had no choice but to follow or lose patients.

As in the drug world, device manufacturers understand that most patients are relatively insulated from the total cost of these procedures. But even if patients had to foot the entire bill themselves, they would still have relatively limited control when it comes to the cost of their medical care.

Consumers can choose to pay more for an Apple computer than a comparably functioning Windows PC. Or they can go with an off-label computer or none of the above. Similarly, consumers can opt to pay twice as much to stay at a Ritz Carlton or get an equivalent night's sleep at the Marriott down the street. Whether it's a computer or hotel accommodations, branding makes a big difference in the choices people make. But it's their choice and their wallet.

Medical drugs and devices are different. People don't have the same options. Doctors decide what devices they'll use, and hospitals get to decide how much extra to bill for the technology. And in general, insurance companies pay up, then raise their prices the next year to compensate.

Our Prescription Addiction

Profit motives have driven up prices across the drug and device industries. They also have cost hundreds of thousands of patients their lives.

When we think about people dying from drug overdoses, our minds conjure up stereotypes of individuals from the wrong side of the tracks. We assume the pushers are gang-related dealers forcing innocent civilians into the clutches of addiction. What few realize is that the most successful pushers in history are drug companies and doctors.

Every year, 40,000 people die from drug overdoses in the United States. Up to 60 percent of these deaths come from prescription medications. That number is climbing. Between 1990 and 2012, the frequency of patients dying from a drug overdose increased more than 100 percent. This didn't happen by chance. It was the result of a deliberate effort by some drug manufacturers to shift doctors' perception in favor of prescribing more of these dangerous medications.

Opioid use is now the most common cause of death from injury in the United States. And today, three in four drug-overdose deaths involve an "opioid analgesic" painkiller such as oxycodone, hydrocodone, or methadone. Opioids exact an enormous toll on human lives in the United States and cost employers a fortune in missed work and additional health care expenses, upward of $53 billion a year.

But the story of painkillers is complex. Opioids are essential to modern medicine. Used properly, they are some of the most important medications available. After surgery or acute trauma, opioids provide patients with essential pain relief, offering improved sleep, rest, and recovery.

Here in the United States, figuring out the best balance to get the positive therapeutic outcomes without the complications of addiction has taken American medicine on a roller-coaster trajectory.

In the 1960s, the United States saw a sharp increase in the use of both prescription and illicit drugs. In response, the federal government began a crackdown on prescription medications as Congress tightened restrictions to limit counterfeits. In parallel, there was a cultural shift underway within the field of medicine. Watching the consequences of addiction take a toll, physicians became more cautious and decreased the frequency of opiate prescription, hoping to curtail abuses.

These developments drove down the quantity of opioids prescribed for pain. As is so often the case in medical practice, a directionally appropriate response was taken too far, and the pendulum needed to swing back the other way. Studies conducted in the late 1980s and early 1990s confirmed that health care providers were, in some cases, undertreating pain.

So, pain management experts (many found and funded by the manufacturers of these powerful medications) began assuring doctors through continuing-medical-education programs and meetings that dependence and addiction would not occur in the face of genuine pain. Many taught doctors that their patients would become immune to the life-threatening consequences of high-dose administration over time. Therefore, there was no limit to how high the dosages could go. They encouraged the use of these medications for treatment of any pain, not only pain from surgery, trauma, or cancer. This all but guaranteed users for life. Nearly all of these assertions about the protection from addiction and resistance to overdose have been proven wrong since then.

We now recognize that as patients take narcotics in ever-greater doses, the euphoric side effects increase the desire for more and spur addiction. And as the dosages increase, the associated depression of the breathing center in the brain causes a growing number of patients never to wake up.

Prescribing an opioid to a patient with vague pain and no obvious diagnosis is much less time-consuming for doctors than explaining that they can't find a medical cause for the problem. Drug manufacturers know this and use it to their advantage.

Today, the United States consumes over 80 percent of the world's most addictive oral pain pills and 99 percent of its hydrocodone, a highly addictive compound found in Vicodin. From the perspective of the companies that sell these opioids, overdoses and addiction have become unavoidable "collateral damage."

Health Care as a Cultural Imperative

In many ways, legacy players are like nations. They speak their own language. They have unique cultures. And the perceptions of the people in them are shaped by contextual forces.

It would be almost impossible to confuse Italy's culture with Germany's. Similarly, any new employee who walks through the doors of a drug or device manufacturer learns almost immediately what beliefs are valued, what actions are encouraged, and how to differentiate the organization and its products when communicating with others.

Join a pharmaceutical giant, and you will quickly perceive the products sold as exceptional, the prices appropriate, and the company's mission worthwhile. When you are hired as a drug representative, you will be trained for several weeks. Part of the training educates you on the specific medications. Much of the training, however, is designed to inculcate you into the culture and teach you how to influence the prescribing habits of doctors and their office staff.

The laws of our nation and the unique culture of our health care system make the impact of the legacy players far greater in the United States than in the rest of the world. Elsewhere, governments constrain their power and influence by providing citizens with health coverage, by regulating drug prices, and by influencing the number of doctors trained in each specialty.

In contrast, America was born in revolution, an experience that is embedded into our nation's psyche and our unique approach to health care. It's not right or wrong. It's the context that exists. And it's extremely powerful.

As a country, we value the individual over the group, freedom over restriction. Our history celebrates people who overcame huge odds to achieve massive success. We see this as a virtue, one that made us a global leader in science and technology. It has helped Americans win more Nobel Prizes in medicine, physics, and chemistry than any other nation's scientists.

But the same characteristics that drive innovation and the free market have also driven the costs of medical care to excessive and unaffordable levels. They have led our nation to undervalue prevention and, as we'll soon examine, ignore disparities in medical outcomes by race and socioeconomic status.

Our belief in individual autonomy has produced a health care system that tolerates major variation in practice, the insufficient surgical expertise of many doctors, and frequent medical errors. In total, the culture of American medicine has produced below-average quality outcomes, despite $3 trillion in health care expenditures.

It should be no surprise that the large legacy players have greater influence in the United States than in other countries. And it should be obvious that if our nation seeks to address the economic difficulties that health care spending creates, the legacy players will do their best to stop it. This is the unwritten law of health care economics.

In the year 2000, the United States spent $4,878 per person on health care. Ten years later, we were spending $8,402 on average. In 2016, it surpassed $10,000. For perspective, that's 30 percent more than Norway, the second-highest per capita health care spender.

Hypothetically, if we had transformed care delivery fifteen years ago and, over that time, limited health care inflation even slightly (let's say $1,000 less per person), we would still be spending more than twice the average of other developed countries. But as a nation, we would have an additional $300 billion a year to invest in education, infrastructure, the arts, or anything else that might have advanced our society.

For most Americans, this would have been a great improvement and a welcome outcome. For the legacy players, it would have been a disaster. Individuals and companies can decide to make the health care system more efficient, or they can use its existing inefficiencies to drive their profits ever higher. Rarely can they do both.

It is in the financial interest of legacy players to resist change, even when the change imperative is obvious to health-policy experts. Looking forward, the health care legacy players are likely to be successful in their resistance for some time. A lesson from history provides a powerful example as to why.

Scurvy is a disease we rarely see or hear much about today, but it was once a brutal killer. In the eighteenth century, it took out more British sailors than enemy combat.

Indeed, back when ships transported the majority of the world's goods, scurvy proved incredibly problematic during long voyages. While sailing between England and India, around the southern tip of the African continent, more than 40 percent of every crew would die from the disease.

In 1601, four ships set sail under the command of Captain James Lancaster. Three were stocked with the typical provisions, and the death toll on these boats was as expected. One ship, however, for reasons still unknown, carried lemon juice, a potent source of vitamin C. No one on that ship died of scurvy. It doesn't take a statistical expert to realize that something important had happened, something that could save a tremendous number of lives. But for more than a century, nothing changed.

In 1747, a physician named James Lind embarked on a scientific trial. On six ships heading out to sea, Dr. Lind varied the diets of each crew. Two of them carried citrus fruits, while others dined on traditional rations. When the ships carrying the fruit returned all their sailors alive, Lind had scientific, controlled proof that vitamin C prevented the deadly disease. Yet it would take another forty-eight years for citrus to become a seafaring standard aboard British naval ships, and another seventy years more until it was required.

In all, 264 years elapsed between a clear medical finding and broad, systemic change. The reason for the delay in progress was the same then as it is today: the power of perception. Meat and bread served as staples on long voyages out to sea, but captains perceived fruit—with its relatively high weight and cost—as a "luxury." As a result, they refused to stock it, even when it would have saved the lives of hundreds of crew members.

In many ways, the American health care system resembles the British navy of yesteryear. We have seen the economic threats for decades and done little to change the rate of health care inflation. We have known about opportunities to prevent heart attacks, strokes, and some cancers for years, and yet we failed to embrace the opportunities to correct course. And for close to twenty years, we have talked about patient safety and ways to reduce medical error. Yet the number of unnecessary deaths remains about the same every year.

As previous chapters have confirmed, our resistance to change comes in part from patients and doctors. But much of the blame for our current health care problems can be placed squarely on the shoulders of the legacy players. Of course, that's not the way they see it. From their perspective, our health care system is the best in the world, and they would be happy if it stayed unchanged forever.

Chapter Five

WHAT YOU GET ISN'T WHAT YOU SEE

In the early 1970s, a high school biology teacher named David Werner led a small group of American students along a series of trails in the foothills of western Mexico's Sierra Madre Occidental. They had traveled from California to study the flora and fauna of the lush mountain range. Along the way, they discovered a tragic situation affecting the lives of local villagers.

The people of Ajoya, most of them poor, subsisted on three basic food sources. They grew their own vegetables, they bought flour and made tortillas, and they trapped animals for meat.

On the morning that David and his students set out to gaze upon the birds and the plants of the area, a teenage girl from Ajoya went exploring in the mountains alone. On her journey, the young girl fell into a well-disguised trapping pit, a man-made hole in the ground about three feet deep. The pit was covered with twigs and leaves, and filled with corrosive lye. This common hunting technique was effective in catching and killing small prey—as the creatures fell through the camouflage brush, they succumbed to the powerful chemicals below. Unfortunately, the traps also worked on unsuspecting villagers. All who fell into the lye were burned from their feet to their thighs. Most died a slow and painful death from infection.

David arrived on the scene just after the villagers. Although he wasn't a doctor, his background in biology and general first-aid knowledge came in handy. He immediately washed the lye off the girl's legs and accompanied her back to the village. He explained to her family how to keep the wounds clean, making sure the water they used was properly boiled. He instructed them to change her wound dressings several times a day. Thanks to the diligence of her parents and David's know-how, the girl survived.

As word of her recovery spread, the villagers began to embrace David as a healer. Each time he returned to Ajoya, they sought his help for ever-more-complicated problems. To better provide assistance, he began reading books on basic medical treatment. Over time, he expanded his clinical knowledge. But the more he learned about the villagers' health problems, the more concerned he became about one problem in particular: the extremely high incidence of deaths among babies in Ajoya.

As he would later calculate, infant mortality in the village exceeded 30 percent at a time when the death rate for American babies was less than 1 percent.

As he studied the problem, he kept hearing the same story from grieving mothers. Young children, usually under the age of two, would become sick and develop severe diarrhea. As the babies grew increasingly ill, they would get progressively more lethargic. Their skin would lose its normal color and elasticity.

Soon, most of these babies would develop an ominous symptom, one that was well recognized in the village as a sign of impending death. On the heads of these very young children, the soft spots (what doctors call the "fontanelles") would begin to sink inward and collapse. Once the fontanelles began to cave in, local healers would be summoned to provide treatment. Relying on the traditions of their elders, the healers administered herbs before putting their fingers inside the mouths of the infants and pushing up on the palate.

For some babies, the treatment worked and the fontanelles expanded, much to the relief of the parents. They knew then that their child was more likely to survive than if the collapse had persisted.

Their prognostic observations were accurate, but what they didn't understand was that they were confusing cause and effect. In all infants, crying increases intracranial pressure, which pushes the fontanelles outward. Pushing up on the palate was simply a mechanism to induce discomfort and crying. Infants did not survive because of this maneuver or the resulting expansion of their fontanelles. Instead, the babies who lived were the ones suffering the least amount of dehydration. In other words, these children still had enough fluid in their bodies. For them, crying was sufficient to elevate the soft spots. The others were simply too far gone.

Back in the states, David told this story to physicians. They immediately recognized what was happening. The underlying problem was intestinal infection, causing massive diarrhea and life-threatening dehydration. They recommended David administer large volumes of fluids for treatment.

So the next time David returned to Ajoya, he instructed mothers in the village to boil water. He taught them how to calculate the amount of fluid required to restore and maintain adequate hydration. Once the infants drank enough liquids, the effects of dehydration reversed and most lived. David's reputation as a healer spread even further.

Hearing this story for the first time, Americans might shake their heads at the ignorance of the villagers. After all, even without a medical degree, most of us would correctly diagnose the problem as diarrhea, fluid loss, and death from dehydration. We would instantly recognize that trying to manually elevate the soft spot in the skull makes no sense, a classic example of confusing cause and effect. But to assume that such a mistake is relegated to certain cultures and regions would be, in itself, a mistake.

What We Can Stomach

If you saw my dad and his older brother, Herb, standing together, you wouldn't think they were related. My father was tall, thin, and athletic. Herb was shorter and heavier, a studious type. My dad was outgoing and took on a variety of leadership roles in his community, whereas Herb, more the introvert, would probably be labeled a nerd today.

Although my uncle was reserved in most aspects of his life, when it came to his surgical practice, he positively lit up. It was his passion for medicine that inspired me to follow in his professional footsteps. He was a skilled general surgeon who loved his practice and his patients. His joy was infectious, and I quickly caught the disease.

The first time I scrubbed into a surgical procedure was with him. I was a first-year medical student, home for the holidays, and had asked my uncle Herb if I could tag along and shadow him for the day. After a morning in the office, he asked me if I wanted to go with him into the Operating Room. He didn't have to ask twice. The patient was a woman in her forties with pain in the upper-right side of her abdomen, and he would be removing her gallbladder. I remember the procedure well and, perhaps, with the kind of fervor not everyone would share. If you're squeamish, skip ahead two paragraphs.

With the first incision, well-oxygenated blood seeped from the wound margins. Expeditiously, my uncle called for a sponge, suction, clamp, and suture as if he were on the set of *General Hospital*. As he cut down deeper into the cavity of the woman's abdomen, her peritoneum (the lining around the intestines) glistened under the Operating Room lights. Once inside the peritoneal cavity, her internal organs pulsed with life, quite the opposite of the cadaver dissections I'd recently completed in medical school.

Dissecting through the tissues, he deftly exposed the gallbladder, filled with green bile and lined with pebble-like stones. As his hands moved with speed and grace, my uncle separated the duct that drains the gallbladder from that which drains the liver. These adjacent structures are easily confused and, like a spy diffusing a bomb with two red wires, my uncle told me that tying off the wrong one would spell certain disaster and likely death. With the woman's gallbladder sac now removed, my uncle made sure there were no stones left in the passageways before closing up the tissue in layers.

The whole operation lasted maybe forty-five minutes, but decades later, I can still picture it clearly. My uncle, so uncomfortable in social situations, was always at home in the Operating Room. The same qualities that made him bookish also made him an excellent surgeon.

Herb was a content man until, in his fifties, he began developing pain in his upper abdomen, just below his ribs in an area called the epigastrium. He ignored it at first, but the pain got worse and worse.

His doctors diagnosed him with a peptic ulcer, blaming it on a combination of stress and the spicy foods my aunt loved to cook. When the problem worsened, physicians removed most of his stomach. They didn't need to. Like the healers in Ajoya, my uncle's doctors had confused cause and effect.

The medical community has long known that when we eat, the glands in our stomach secrete hydrochloric acid to aid with digestion. In fact, our bodies produce more than a liter of the stuff each day. As you can imagine, our gastrointestinal tract has a way of protecting itself from this powerful, corrosive acid. Naturally occurring mucus works perfectly to coat the lining of our stomachs. That is, until the lining is damaged. When that happens, the acid penetrates below the surface and destroys the underlying tissues, producing the kind of pain my uncle experienced.

At the time, American physicians were taught in medical school that spicy foods caused this stomach erosion. It was just as logical as believing that the collapsed fontanelles caused infant mortality, and it was equally wrong.

Spicy foods do lead to acid production, but no more so than in patients without an ulcer. And were it not for two physicians working on the other side of the world, doctors in the United States would still be blaming ulcerous patients for eating spicy foods and living stressful lives. And they'd still be recommending a major resection of the stomach as treatment.

In the early 1980s, an internal medicine doctor in Australia named Barry Marshall became obsessed with studying ulceration of the stomach. By 1982, he and his collaborator, a pathologist named Robin Warren, had made a remarkable discovery. They realized that *Helicobacter pylori* (a bacterium more commonly called *H. pylori*) was present in 80 percent of all stomach ulcers and 90 percent of ulcers originating in the first part of the small intestine, the duodenum. Dr. Marshall believed this bacterium, not stress or spicy food, was the cause of peptic ulcers in nearly all patients.

But when he and Dr. Warren presented this idea at scientific meetings, their hypothesis was met with broad skepticism.

"Everyone was against me," Marshall recalled in a later interview, "but I knew I was right."

So, three years after developing his hypothesis, and out of complete frustration, Dr. Marshall decided to experiment on himself. First, he passed an endoscope into his stomach. This long and flexible tube with a light and camera attached showed his stomach had no ulceration. Next, he obtained a biopsy to prove his stomach didn't harbor *H. pylori*, the bacterium he and his associate had identified so commonly in patients with ulcers.

He then collected bacteria from a patient with stomach ulceration, put the material in a petri dish and let the organisms multiply for several days. Can you guess what Dr. Marshall did next? He downed the whole thing. With the bacteria now festering inside him, the doctor reexamined his stomach with the endoscope, confirming a serious *H. pylori* infection with destruction of mucous membrane. Finally, he took a course of antibiotics, cured himself completely, and disproved decades of conventional wisdom about stomach ulcers. It was a remarkable discovery.

Three things in particular stand out about this story. One, Dr. Marshall had gone to such lengths and put himself at great personal risk to educate physicians and change medical practice. Two, Dr. Marshall had followed, to an exacting degree, a century-old scientific process to definitively prove his hypothesis. Three, in spite of everything he did, medical practice didn't change.

He published his research in the peer-reviewed *Medical Journal of Australia* in 1985 and expected his findings would rapidly transform medical practice. But for over a decade, doctors continued to blame spicy foods and stress instead of the real cause: infection. By 1997, research showed that three-fourths of all patients continued to be treated for peptic ulcers as in the past.

In fact, little progress was made until 2005, when Drs. Marshall and Warren shocked the world by winning the Nobel Prize in Medicine, an honor almost always reserved for PhD scientists. To date, more than 25,000 articles have been published on ulcers. The findings of Marshall and Warren have been confirmed every time.

The Problem with Conventional Wisdom

There's a quote from Mark Twain at the start of the movie *The Big Short* that reads, "It ain't what you don't know that gets you into trouble. It's what you know for sure that just ain't so."

It's an insightful truism about the dangerous assumptions we make and about how incorrect ideas get repeated again and again until everyone believes them. Quite a few movie reviewers cited the quote as central to the film's theme. But what's most interesting is that there's no evidence Twain ever wrote or said it.

That's the problem with conventional wisdom. Something that sounds as if it could be true gets repeated often enough that everyone assumes it's true, even when there's no basis for it.

This phenomenon applies to cultures the world over, from Ajoya to America, in small villages and powerhouse nations alike. Be it the curative effect of elevating the fontanelles or the belief that spicy foods produce gastric ulcers, people comfortably buy into conventional wisdom that, it turns out, isn't all that accurate or all that wise.

Even in a scientific discipline such as medicine, erroneous beliefs and conclusions persist long after someone discovers the truth.

In the nineteenth century, Hungarian doctor Ignaz Semmelweis postulated that obstetricians who failed to wash their hands between patients were transmitting living organisms that led to infection and higher mortality rates. His theory was rejected, and he was ridiculed for this concern. After all, how could something unseen be so destructive? It wasn't until years after his death in an asylum that Semmelweis's theory started gaining acceptance. French chemist and microbiologist Louis Pasteur, who himself had lost three daughters to infectious disease, was finally able to persuade scientists of the time that the germ theory of disease could be proven through rigorous experimentation.

Today, the field of science continues to evolve with new evidence disproving commonly accepted theories. What seems logical is, to an increasing extent, being proven wrong.

Human immunodeficiency virus (HIV) is a retrovirus that slowly replicates and weakens the immune system. Those infected become highly vulnerable to disease. Scientists recognize that HIV attacks and destroys what are called "CD4+ T helper cells." These T cells are essential in helping fight off various infections.

Once a person's T-cell count drops below two hundred, the diagnosis advances from HIV to AIDS, and the risk of a life-threatening infection escalates. Until recently, clinicians and scientists believed the human body attacked and killed the "helper cells" that were most infected by the virus. Logically, they assumed, this was the body's way of trying to limit the disease. It was a reasoned conclusion, but wrong nonetheless.

An immunologist in San Francisco named Warner Greene discovered that 95 percent of the time, the body destroys the less infected "resting cells," rather than those actively fighting the virus. Researchers don't know why, exactly, but they were able to show that as the immune system kills these relatively healthy cells, the body releases chemicals that attract more of them to the scene. The more resting cells present, the faster the T-cell count drops.

Although contrary to logic and common knowledge, this finding allowed the scientists to identify a specific protein that contributes to this process. And with this new information, researchers recognized that an existing drug could be used to block this part of the sequence, thus maintaining T-cell counts and preventing the infection from progressing to AIDS. Ultimately, this discovery may provide new insights in the fight against a variety of other infectious diseases, potentially even cancer.

Commonly accepted beliefs are common, naturally, and therefore in great supply. Most of them seem logical. To the villagers, it seemed logical that pushing up on the palate and expanding the soft spots would help save the lives of children whose fontanelles had collapsed. To American doctors, it seemed logical that stress and spicy foods would lead to gastric ulcers, and that the body would destroy the most infected cells in patients with HIV.

These assumptions weren't frivolous or completely without merit. Each conclusion was based on some level of observation, practical application, and prior success. But as these assumptions evolved into absolute certainties, and as their merits went unquestioned, it became all the more difficult to prove the experts wrong. And when it comes to the greatest threats facing our health, it just goes to show that much of what we know for sure "just ain't so."

Social Determinants of Health

You might assume that what happens inside the walls of America's health care institutions would have the greatest impact on American health. After all, clinics, oncology suites, and hospitals are the kinds of places people go when they're sick and need to get better. And as a corollary, you might assume that if we wanted to improve the health of Americans, that's precisely where we should start looking for answers and making investments. Neither assumption is accurate.

What happens outside of traditional medical practice shapes our health and life expectancy much more than what takes place inside American care facilities. In fact, the conditions of our daily lives influence our health to a far greater degree than traditional medicine ever could.

As an example, improving heart and cancer surgery outcomes might save a few thousand lives. But proactively addressing the causes of heart disease and cancer through preventive screening, diet, and exercise has the potential to save hundreds of thousands of lives each year.

It's a lesson David Werner embraced when he moved to Ajoya, established a medical clinic, and invited physicians like me to visit. Once he had his treatment center up and running, David quickly figured out why so many children in the village were experiencing intestinal diarrhea and dehydration in the first place.

The streams of Ajoya supplied the village's drinking water. These same streams ran through cow pastures where the water was being contaminated by feces. And because the village itself had no sanitary facilities for the disposal of human waste, the very ground where children played was being contaminated as well.

David understood that addressing the source of the problem was better than treating it afterward. But the village could not afford to pay a construction company to modernize the village's infrastructure. David could have applied for grants to fund the project, but that would have been chancy and, even if successful, could have taken years. So he took a different path.

He began by establishing an innovative fee schedule at his clinic, creating two payment options. Villagers could either pay $50 for a year's worth of visits or they could volunteer two hours of their time after receiving medical services and recovering from their diseases.

Most rural villages in Mexico have a few wealthy individuals who own nearly all of the arable land and farm it at a great profit. Ajoya had three such landowners. These individuals chose to pay the fee and cover each person in their family, thereby funding the entire clinic on an annual basis. Everyone else volunteered their time.

So, with the volunteer labor, David had villagers install pipes to carry water from high in the hills, above the cows, to the land down below. And when that project was finished, the villagers constructed latrines with similar pipes to carry away human waste.

Almost immediately, the childhood mortality rate in the village plummeted into the single digits. David realized that maximizing health takes more than treating people's acute medical problems. It demands that people recognize and address underlying social and public-health issues, a reality that holds as true in the United States today as it did in the mountains of Mexico back in the 1970s.

If you asked Americans to explain which factors contribute most to their health care outcomes, the first three items on the list most likely would include doctors, hospitals, and medications, maybe along with diet or exercise. Almost no one would mention the zip code in which a person is born, a factor that alone can lengthen or shorten a person's life by seven years. Few would cite race or family income, two factors that account for at least 20 percent of a person's health status.

In effect, the quality of your local hospital or your choice of a doctor wouldn't even crack the top ten. Rather, some of the greatest determinants of our overall health and life expectancy are environmental factors: where we're born and raised; where we work, play, and socialize.

Health institutes like the Centers for Disease Control (CDC) and the World Health Organization (WHO) have done extensive research to understand and quantify the impact these "social determinants of health" have on our well-being.

These organizations have studied the deterioration in health that occurs when communities lack balanced food options, safe places to play, and community programs that encourage healthy behaviors. They have quantified the impact of high crime rates, unemployment, polluted air, and contaminated drinking water on life expectancy.

In fact, based on analysis of nearly fifty studies, researchers have found that such social dynamics as education, racial segregation, social support systems, and poverty account for more than one-third of all American deaths in any given year.

Overall, social settings are two times more likely to determine a person's risk of premature death than the places in which he or she receives medical care.

By cleaning up the drinking water in Ajoya, David Werner and the local villagers reduced child mortality by two-thirds. That outcome wouldn't surprise most Americans, who would quickly associate these types of sanitary and environmental issues with the diseases found in the mountainous regions of Mexico. Yet we as Americans overlook many of the social factors compromising the health of people in our own communities.

Smoking in America

Decades before the US surgeon general identified smoking as a cancer-causing habit, the research was perfectly clear. The chemicals in tobacco smoke were found to have a toxic impact not just on the throat and lungs but on just about every organ in the human body, from the heart and brain to the kidneys and blood vessels of the feet.

Cigarette companies hid the information for years, killing tens of thousands in the process. Today, that information is public and is being used to fuel educational campaigns intended to reverse smoking trends in America. And after decades of public outreach, we might expect that smoking would be all but stamped out by now. It's not. One in six American adults continues to light up regularly. As a result, cigarettes account for 20 percent of all deaths in the United States. If we cut that percentage in half, we'd save 250,000 lives a year.

It certainly feels a bit foolish, writing about smoking as a health hazard in 2017. We've all seen the warnings and we understand the risks.

But in spite of everything we know, smoking remains a deadly addiction that starts early in life. That's by design. Over the years, tobacco companies have funded billions of dollars in cigarette promotions, many of them devised to entice teenagers and young adults into becoming life-long customers. Their efforts are effective. Each day more than 3,200 teens smoke their very first cigarette.

But that's usually where the health experts leave us: with one finger aimed at addiction and another pointed at the tobacco companies. Often left out of this discussion is the fact that smoking has just as much to do with the effects of social context. This is a crucial cog, one that can give us a better grasp of why smoking persists despite our almost universal understanding of the consequences.

Educational programs and medical statistics have a minimal impact on smokers. We know that because if we quizzed a hundred smokers on the dangers and risks involved, ninety or more would get all the answers correct, and yet they still smoke. The reason they do speaks to the powerful relationship between context and perception.

If you don't smoke, you see cigarettes as a disgusting habit and a leading cause of death. The statistics confirm your viewpoint. In round numbers, a smoker is twenty times more likely to die from lung cancer than you are. You don't understand why people would consciously increase their risk of dying. As a nonsmoker, it's likely you support smoking prohibitions in restaurants and perhaps even favor banning their sale altogether. From your perspective, smoking is a dirty, life-threatening choice.

But smokers see cigarettes rather differently. If you smoke, you perceive your chances of dying from lung cancer as relatively low. After all, many of your relatives and friends smoke. Few if any of them have been hospitalized for smoking-related illnesses. The reality is that only about 14 percent of smokers die from lung cancer caused by cigarettes. As such, smokers see the low overall risk as reassuring.

Phrased differently, nonsmokers see the dramatically higher *relative* risk. Smokers, by contrast, focus on the *absolute* risk. The odds are that the majority of smokers will die from something else. They may not know the exact statistics, but they recognize that their probability of developing lung cancer is relatively low. Besides, they tell themselves they can always quit if it becomes a problem.

At a societal level, perceptions of smoking also involve probabilistic math. Americans are generally aware that the annual death toll from smoking is high, but they underestimate the impact it has on our nation's overall health, and more important, they don't hold the manufacturers of cigarettes directly accountable. It's contrary to the facts and figures, but so is the nature of perception.

Imagine if a man put arsenic in a commonly sold product and killed seven hundred people. We'd prosecute him as a mass murderer, every media outlet would cover the story for weeks, and our nation would mourn the tragedy. When cigarettes kill exactly that many people each day, tobacco companies are allowed to continue selling these toxic substances. Their actions don't make front-page news.

That's because our brains make a point of differentiating direct and indirect causality. In the (hypothetical) case of the arsenic, everyone who consumed the product died and the consequences were immediate. In the (real) case of cigarettes, the victims are measured in probabilities. We can't be absolutely sure who died directly from smoking. As a result, one is a felony and the other is a source of tax revenue.

This same probabilistic logic applies to how we perceive medical prevention. When doctors fail to screen for colon cancer, statistics tell us that about 26,500 people will die each year (that is, half of all people who die from colon cancer annually). But we can't be sure who is in which half, so we tolerate the failure. Just as we do with cigarettes.

Kill a patient from a dirty colonoscope, and a host of regulators will be in your office the next day. Kill a patient by failing to schedule a colon-cancer screening, and no one gets blamed. One is malpractice. The other is mistreatment.

Each victim of malpractice has a face and a name. When a patient dies from malpractice, the grieving family knows who caused it, or at least who they can blame, and they frequently sue on the victim's behalf.

Victims of mistreatment, however, are statistical and faceless. We can't be sure whether a person will die if *not* screened for cancer any more than we can be sure that someone would have lived even if screened. But make no mistake, this kind of mistreatment is lethal. It kills hundreds of times more people than malpractice.

What our brains perceive and how we estimate the odds of dying from a problem are distorted by context. When we develop a medical problem, we overrate the impact of intervention. But when we're not yet sick, we fail to take the steps necessary to prevent the problem from happening in the first place.

If you were to tell people who have colon cancer that there's a machine somewhere in the world that will increase their chances of being cured by 5 percent, they would hop on a plane the next day. But guess what happens when you tell people who are at risk of colon cancer that there's a safe, painless, once-a-year fecal immunochemical test (or FIT) that (1) can reliably detect cancer, (2) takes only five minutes to complete, (3) can be done in the privacy of their own bathroom, and (4) reduces their odds of dying by 50 percent? What happens is that people pay very little attention, nearly half ignore the recommendation, and tens of thousands of Americans die unnecessarily.

Rarely do these calculations occur in our brains at a conscious level. Most of the odds and likelihoods that drive our behaviors are sorted out subconsciously. All are heavily influenced by our personal circumstances, and each is affected by social context.

Smoking serves as a great case study for understanding this problem. Depending on (1) where you live, (2) the policies that govern your state, and (3) the social structure in place, your likelihood of being a smoker will vary by upward of 15 percent.

In Kentucky, for example, about 30 percent of all residents still reach for a pack regularly. Some conclude that the habit is culturally ingrained in a state where tobacco was once the "King of Kentucky crops" and where smoking has brought farming families together since the 1800s. Others, including health experts, point to the absence of a statewide ban on smoking in workplaces, restaurants, and bars. Regardless of which social influence you point to, smoking accounts for about 40 percent of all cancer-related deaths in Kentucky.

Now, compare Kentucky with Utah, which boasts the lowest rate of cigarette smokers in the land (about 12 percent). Utah has had a statewide ban on smoking in indoor spaces since 1998. These strict government ordinances combine with other environmental factors, such as the state's high religious composition, to help stamp out smoking in homes and workplaces and at social gatherings.

What you have in Utah is the antithesis of Kentucky: positive, not negative, determinants of health.

Nonsmokers and public-health advocates judge smoking as a "bad habit" and smokers as bad decision makers. But these are value-laden judgments that ignore the influence of a person's environment. Context is value-neutral. Place one teenager in Kentucky and another in Utah. The teen in Kentucky will have a three times higher probability of developing chronic obstructive lung disease and dying from cancer. It's simply a fact.

When it comes to the factors that influence our health, context matters immensely. And when we accept that context matters a great deal in shaping our perceptions and decisions, we're able to identify a wide range of medical problems that are societally based. More important, we can develop new and better ideas for solving them.

Obesity and Chronic Illness in America

As dangerous as smoking is, obesity in the United States is even more problematic. Obesity costs our nation an estimated $190 billion in medical spending each year. It's the number-one cause of diabetes and prediabetes, conditions that combine to impact one-third of all Americans.

These days, people use the word "epidemic" loosely. But it's hard to find a better word for America's weight problem. According to CDC data, America's obesity rate held between 13 and 15 percent between 1960 and 1980. The latest projections now indicate that 42 percent of all Americans will be obese by the year 2030.

Anyone who has tried losing weight knows it's difficult. It requires eating fewer calories and engaging in more activity each day. Neither alone is sufficient, and both together are vexing, especially for those carrying excess weight.

Still, just fifteen minutes of exercise a day could reduce a person's mortality risk by 14 percent and increase life expectancy by three years. And according to findings published in the *Journal of the American Heart Association*, thirty minutes of exercise five days a week will save the average American $2,500 a year in medical expenses.

Indeed, exercise has innumerable benefits. It can reduce premature death from heart attacks and stroke, lower the risk of diabetes, control blood pressure, prevent osteoporosis, and alleviate symptoms of depression and anxiety. Combined with a healthy diet, it improves quality of sleep, increases confidence, and facilitates weight loss without any negative side effects.

As with the findings on smoking, we all know it is important to exercise and avoid excess weight. But once again, knowing something and doing something about it are two very different things.

The epidemic of obesity has many possible causes, almost all of them linked to fairly recent changes in American culture and daily practices. Dietitians point to higher intakes of sugary sodas and the overflowing portion sizes found on fast-food menus. Health experts connect the problem, in part, to dips in exercise and even the sedentary nature of America's workforce, noting that American jobs that involve intense physical activity have declined from 50 percent in 1960 to less than 20 percent in recent years. Physical activity is estimated to cause up to 10 percent of premature deaths, a mortality level on par with smoking. Psychologists point to weight, diet, and exercise as "contagious." If your friends are overweight with excessive food intake and inadequate exercise, your chances of "catching" the problems are much higher than if your social circle is healthier.

So, if those are the causes, the question becomes, what can any of us do about it? Once again, the answer depends on whom you ask.

Travel to Boston and talk with Clayton Christensen, the celebrated Harvard business scholar who coined the term "disruptive innovation," and he'll offer you a financial solution. He begins by pointing out that businesses shoulder most of their employees' health care costs and that they're no doubt invested in trying to find a solution. But he thinks US companies are approaching the problem all wrong. Christensen notes that employers currently spend thousands each year on employee "wellness programs" with little to show for their efforts.

"We're pushing the wrong levers," he says.

Wellness programs are nice-to-haves. But Christensen thinks the better solution would be to create financial incentives for employees to exercise, manage their weight, and get the preventive screenings they need.

"In that way, their businesses can reduce the burden of chronic illness in their companies and flatten the rate of health care inflation."

In his mind, the shift could save lives, while saving employers millions in health care costs. So, that's one solution.

Now, hop a train to New York City and speak with Malcolm Gladwell, the noted journalist, social scientist, and author of such best-selling books as *The Tipping Point* and *Outliers*.

He'll tell you, "We aren't, as human beings, very good at acting in our best interest."

That's why Gladwell is a fan of nudging change through small, incremental improvements, a concept promulgated by Richard Thaler and Cass Sunstein in their book *Nudge*. Citing the auto industry as an example of what is possible through a series of small steps over many years, Gladwell said, "In the '60s, legislators started nudging car makers to improve safety by requiring them to equip all cars with seatbelts. Then in the '70s, they set standards for fuel economy. Having been nudged in both of these areas, car makers started innovating on their own, developing airbags and perfecting hybrids."

The result has been cleaner and safer cars with a future that now holds the possibility of fully automated, driverless vehicles.

Advances in the auto industry show us how a combination of aggressive and smart regulation can move people and companies in a direction that is best for our nation. Applying this concept to health, Gladwell questions why we can't find more opportunities to encourage healthier behaviors, particularly around exercise.

"When I go to my health club and it's in the basement, I have to take the elevator down. This drives me crazy. Why can't there be a stairway? At least make it as easy to exercise as it is to not exercise. It's in society's interest for me to take the stairs."

Ultimately, Gladwell believes human beings need a little help to get started. "As a society we have to push people, nudge them in the right direction."

Finally, fly to Northern California and talk to Chip Heath, who, along with his brother, Dan, coauthored the best sellers *Switch* and *Made to Stick*. They'll offer you a psychological solution like the one they used to improve upon the US Department of Agriculture's perplexing food pyramid.

The problem with the pyramid? Only a nutritionist could look at it and determine what any one person should be eating, Chip recalls. So, the Heath brothers helped the USDA come up with the concept of "MyPlate."

Chip notes, "The brilliance of MyPlate is that you look at the picture and half the plate is filled with fruits and vegetables. Now you know exactly what is expected if you're trying to improve your diet. Just make sure your plate looks like the picture on the diagram."

Simple, actionable advice is something Chip believes can have a profound impact on American health. "I think exercise is particularly hard because we have a cultural picture of it that's just unrealistic. We think the only way to exercise is by dressing up in black spandex and going to a gym and glistening attractively."

If our goal is to help people get out and exercise 150 minutes a week, we need to help them accomplish this feat in a more sustainable way, he says. Instead of running out and buying a gym membership to get our fitness fill, "What if we broke that down into five-minute stretches of exercise, five or six times a day? Imagine walking up the stairs for five minutes or parking five minutes from your destination. When we simplify what a person needs to do, suddenly we can picture exercise in a way that doesn't seem so overwhelming."

So, there you have it. Three of the nation's leading thinkers on behavioral change, each with a different approach to solving America's obesity epidemic. One offers financial incentives, the second thinks nudges can create momentum, and the third focuses on shrinking the change and reinforcing the sense of achievement.

The challenge in solving the obesity epidemic in the United States is a bit like the challenge of solving the sepsis crisis in hospitals. Many people are responsible for the solution, and yet it's no one's biggest priority. Being obese will affect nearly every aspect of a person's medical care, and yet none of the doctors caring for that patient are likely to invest the time to make a major difference.

As David Werner learned, fixing Ajoya's health problems literally took a village. And even with the help of the village, David still needed a clear vision and a detailed plan to implement it. In many ways, David's approach combined the best thinking of Clay, Malcolm, and Chip. David offered free medical care in exchange for two hours of work (financial incentives). He didn't try to solve all the childhood mortality problems in a single step. Instead, he focused on one opportunity: cleaning up the water (a nudge). And finally, David gave moms with sick infants a set of clear and simple instructions. Boil the water and give babies a large but specific amount every few hours (shrink the change).

Unfortunately, David's vision was ahead of its time and as a result, Ajoya's story didn't come with a fairytale ending. Once David had addressed the bacteria that led to diarrhea, he introduced another nudge. He offered vaccines to further reduce childhood mortality. And then he offered another, focusing on bolstering the village's education.

Soon, as the villagers grew more aware of the social and historical context in which they lived, they started questioning the privilege of the wealthy landowners. Why should they have so much when everyone else had so little? A revolt erupted over land reform, and when the authorities heard about it, they came into the town, put down the unrest, and killed many villagers in the process. After that, the health care experiment was drained of its energy.

David returned home to complete a book of his learnings, *Donde No Hay Doctor* (Where There Is No Doctor). The book has since been reprinted in seventy languages and is recommended by the World Health Organization and UNICEF for care workers.

Stress, Depression, and Anxiety in America

When it comes to social determinants of health, one problem often creates or compounds another. The intersections of stress, anxiety, and physical disease provide a noteworthy example.

Like obesity, stress and anxiety are becoming ever more prevalent and now are endemic in America. One in five adults today reports extremely high levels of what clinicians call "everyday psychological distress."

People who experience high stress and elevated anxiety levels—most commonly originating from their jobs, financial pressures, family responsibilities, relationships, and personal health concerns—are less likely to exercise, eat well, get enough sleep, or moderate their alcohol consumption.

And though the positive associations between physical activity and reduced stress are well established, we're beginning to realize the opposite is true. That is, individuals who make poor health and lifestyle choices experience increased stress that leads to a variety of serious health problems, such as clinical depression, cardiovascular disease, and more frequent colds. It's a vicious cycle.

Studies show stress also affects our nation's work productivity and overall health care system. One-third of all US workers report feeling very stressed at work. This job-related stress costs American industry an estimated $300 billion a year in absenteeism, turnover, diminished productivity, and on-the-job accidents. In addition, health care expenditures are nearly 50 percent greater for workers who report high levels of stress.

The negative consequences of stress increase dramatically when the problem becomes more severe. Depression and severe anxiety affect 20 to 25 percent of adults in a given year, with devastating effects on physical health.

Just as with stress, the connection between psychological disorders and medical issues cuts both ways. Chronic health problems such as diabetes, heart disease, and arthritis lead to various psychological disorders, including depression, which alone doubles the risk of cardiovascular disease and more than doubles the risk of a person becoming sick enough to require hospitalization. This compounding effect of the physical and the psychological can send lives spiraling out of control, ruining families and careers.

Every year, depression results in 200 million lost workdays, costing employers up to $44 billion. In total, the calculated impact of depression and anxiety disorders on the workplace exceeds the cost of diabetes and heart disease.

None of these associations are surprising to scientists who study the intersection of the mind and body. For over a century, physicians have recognized that pain and discomfort stem from our brains, regardless of whether the sensation originated in a distant organ or in the mind itself. But only recently have doctors begun to understand the magnitude of the connection. Nearly seven in ten people with a major psychological disorder suffer from at least one medical condition. And 29 percent of those with a medical condition have a "co-morbid" (associated) psychological disorder.

The bottom line: depression and anxiety disorders are very common and deeply entwined with chronic disease. If either the psychological or the physical issue isn't recognized and effectively treated, patients are more likely to develop both down the road.

According to an American Psychological Association report, 33 percent of patients have never discussed managing their stress with a health care professional and only 22 percent say that their health care provider supports them in managing stress. Doctors do a poor job of spotting these symptoms. Although nearly all physicians agree it's important to counsel patients about these conditions, nearly half admit to "rarely" or "never" bringing it up with their patients.

Childhood Trauma: America's Silent Killer

Sometimes stress, anxiety, and depression result from factors that arise in a person's current situation (what's happening now). But we are just starting to recognize how often these problems date back to childhood.

Researchers are now uncovering the startling frequency with which American children suffer from abuse, neglect, and trauma, though the magnitude is still grossly underreported. In some cases, children suffer publicly recognized tragedies such as the loss of a parent. Too often, however, the source of the problem is a deep, dark secret: the result of growing up in a home with domestic violence, mental illness, or addiction. These physical and emotional traumas damage the lives of children in ways that linger throughout adulthood.

In the United States, we talk freely about the bodily harm that household chemicals, pollution, and secondhand smoke can inflict on children. Yet we rarely talk about childhood trauma, an even more potent killer.

The troubling cause-and-effect relationship between early and later life events is well documented. But as a society, we do little to break this cycle or even openly acknowledge it. Unless physicians explicitly ask about childhood trauma, patients rarely volunteer the information. People who are abused in childhood learn not to trust any authority figure.

Researchers found that those who have had an adverse childhood experience (ACE) face a much higher risk of illness and premature death than those who haven't. In adulthood, they report more frequent problems with job performance and significantly lower incomes. They experience poorer health and worse quality of life. As teenagers, they are more likely to smoke, overeat, and abuse alcohol or drugs, or both, compounding the negative impact of the adverse childhood experience on the development of their body and brain.

For this reason, the CDC has identified adverse childhood experience as one of the nation's leading causes of poor health.

The degree of trauma can be calculated through a ten-question survey. For each type of trauma experienced, you add a point. Respondents who have experienced four different adverse childhood experiences are twelve times more likely to commit suicide and seven times more likely to become an alcoholic. The correlation between a traumatic social environment and lifelong health issues is clear.

As much as some might like to believe that these childhood traumas happen only in families with lower incomes or less education or among those living in less-desirable neighborhoods, it's simply not true. When clinicians screen for ACE, they find that adverse childhood experiences are common, regardless of race, ethnicity, or socioeconomic status.

When clinicians treat childhood trauma like any other traumatic injury, they reduce the risk of long-term consequences and lessen the potential for that person to one day harm others through domestic abuse, another sad and silent killer in America.

Intimate Partner Violence in America

Historically, domestic violence has been viewed as a criminal issue, categorized as physical battery inflicted on a spouse, most often the wife. According to police records, nearly one in three female homicide victims is killed by an intimate partner. But these cases are just the tip of the iceberg. The number of unreported attacks, both physical and psychological, dwarfs the number of crimes investigated.

We are slowly beginning to understand domestic violence as a major social issue with serious health implications.

Facial bruising and broken bones are the well-recognized signs of domestic abuse. In the United States, 24 percent of adult women and 14 percent of adult men have been physically assaulted by a partner at some point in their lives. It is the most common cause of injury for women ages eighteen to forty-four. But physical signs make up only one piece of the puzzle.

The symptoms of abuse are usually much more subtle: a woman complains to her doctor of depression or insomnia, a coworker stays late in the office every night. Usually, these subtle warning signs of abuse go unnoticed.

Some American businesses have taken action and seen results. Companies such as Verizon, Allstate, Prudential, Avon, Mary Kay, Macy's, and Home Depot have trained their employee assistance teams to screen for signs of abuse. They've provided necessary information to their staffs, and as a result, they've seen the rate of identification increase significantly.

But until the medical profession begins to recognize the symptoms of domestic violence more consistently, the majority of victims won't receive the help they need to reduce the long-term consequences.

The Affordable Care Act identified domestic-violence screening as a national health priority. And studies show that when women talk with their physicians about domestic violence, they are four times more likely to get the services they need to end the abusive relationship.

Although there are significant differences in the roles that colleagues, health care professionals, and friends can play, the secret nature of domestic violence requires vigilance from everyone. The good news is that regardless of who helps identify the problem or provides the care needed, the majority of individuals who end a violent relationship do not experience another one.

Social Inequities in America

Although incidences of childhood trauma and domestic abuse occur across all social classes, some medical problems are more prevalent among specific races and socioeconomic groups. It's a discomfiting reality, but major health care disparities exist among minority groups throughout the United States, and they dramatically reduce life expectancy.

In the United States, health and status maintain a symbiotic relationship. The lower the income, the shorter one's life expectancy. The fewer years of education completed, the more likely a person is to die prematurely. These problems go beyond the individual, too.

Sadly, these social factors impact the health of children just as much as their parents, creating a ripple effect within families that can last for generations. Some disparities in health can be attributed to specific genetic patterns associated with certain racial and ethnic groups. For example, high blood pressure is most prevalent among African Americans. Approximately 42 percent of black Americans experience hypertension, compared to only 29 percent of people nationwide.

Although genetics plays a major role in disease prevalence, failure on the part of health care providers to offer appropriate and aggressive treatment leads to preventable deaths. Fortunately, with heightened attention and awareness, success is possible. For example, some large medical groups have made addressing hypertension among African Americans a priority and have dramatically reduced, and in some cases completely eliminated, this disparity in clinical outcomes.

Unfortunately, the disparities don't end with blood pressure. Health experts continue to observe variations in screening for a variety of conditions. For instance, black patients are less likely to be screened for high cholesterol than white Americans. This failure, combined with poorer blood-pressure control, results in dramatically higher rates of heart failure and strokes for African Americans.

Similarly, the death rate from breast cancer for African American women is significantly higher than for white women, a result of lower rates of screening and difficulties accessing medical care. African Americans aren't the only minority group affected by disparities in health outcomes. Latino populations have a higher incidence of diabetes compared to other ethnic groups. Women of Southeast Asian descent experience more heart attacks than others in the same communities. And certain cancers are more prevalent in people of Chinese descent.

Among health care experts and public officials, there's broad agreement that inequities exist. Historically, a major contributor to these inequities was the higher rate of African Americans and Latinos without health insurance. The expansion of coverage through the Affordable Care Act was designed to close the gap and, to date, the ACA has helped increase coverage for these populations.

Parallel to those changes happening at the federal level, creative solutions have come from local government and grassroots organizations as well. The city of Baltimore offers one example.

Solving Social Problems

At age eight, Leana Wen came to the United States from China with her parents. She graduated from college at eighteen, trained at the Washington University School of Medicine, and served as president of the American Medical Student Association. Along the way, she earned two master's degrees, one in modern Chinese studies and the other in economic and social history from the University of Oxford in England. She was a Rhodes scholar and worked on the faculty of both the Harvard Medical School and George Washington School of Medicine.

So what is Dr. Wen doing today? In 2015, she was selected as health commissioner for the city of Baltimore, Maryland, and was retained under mayor-elect Catherine Pugh the following year.

Under any administration, this is no small assignment. In the short amount of time that she has served in this role, she has had to address a series of major crises, from a rash of gun violence to the rise of opioid overdoses. Baltimore is the city that put to rest Freddie Gray, the twenty-five-year-old black man who died in police custody and under circumstances that remain unclear. His funeral was followed by rioting and looting in the downtown area. Baltimore is also a city that has seen the number of drug overdose deaths double since 2010. It's the place one *Washington Post* reporter described as "a combustible mix of poverty, crime, and hopelessness."

On day one in her new role, Dr. Wen recognized that if she wanted to improve the health of the community, she would need to address disparities in health outcomes, particularly when it came to child mortality. At the start of her tenure, the infant death rate for African Americans was five times that of whites.

She could have tried a traditional medical solution, but instead she began by tackling a few of the underlying social determinants. She convened a citywide meeting for public and private partners, including hospitals, clinics, foundations, sororities, and churches.

Together, they established a coalition of committed individuals and groups that founded the program "B'more for Healthy Babies." Their approach was multipronged and included educational programs for new parents to reduce infant deaths during sleep, home visits from nurses to evaluate the health of babies, and universal triage and preventive services for all pregnant women on Medicaid.

The approach is working. Dr. Wen's coalition has reduced the infant mortality rate by 28 percent. They've halved the frequency with which babies die during sleep. And they've closed the gap between black and white infant deaths by 40 percent.

Keeping Our Focus

Addressing social determinants of health is important to improve the well-being of our nation and extend the life expectancy of our citizens.

That's easier said than done. How we view these problems, and whether we see closing the gaps as important, is a matter of context.

Specifically, those who have never experienced domestic violence or major childhood trauma will view these events and their consequences differently than those who have been directly affected by them. Those who don't smoke scoff at those who do and wonder why they're consciously deciding to kill themselves. When a socially determined problem does not affect us or those around us, we're more likely to blame the individual, fail to factor in the social context, and underestimate the magnitude of its consequences.

All That Glitters

The nature of human perception leads us to overlook powerful forces that impact our health. We focus instead on approaches that sound attractive, often overestimating their ability to cure our bodies and improve American health care.

As Americans, we are constantly distracted by what's shiny and new. The explanation for this error in perception is neurobiological. The reward and pleasure centers of our brain light up when we see things that are fresh and exciting, be they in the realms of fashion, entertainment, technology, or even health care.

Like a moth to a flame, American patients are drawn to the health care products and practices that "glitter."

The Twenty-First-Century Gold Rush

Since the 1840s, California has attracted wide-eyed entrepreneurs hoping to strike it rich. And though most of California's gold was harvested over a century ago, the promise of fantastic wealth remains in the land they call the Golden State.

Every year, budding entrepreneurs flock to Silicon Valley to make their mark on the world. Some begin by taking classes at the Stanford Graduate School of Business, with its impressive course titles such as "Entrepreneurship: Formation of New Ventures" and "Managing Growing Enterprises." Others rent a garage, purchase computer services, and begin working sixteen hours a day to launch the next multibillion-dollar tech company. All of them have big dreams and revolutionary ideas. And increasingly, they're setting their sights on the $3 trillion industry that is American health care.

Although these eager entrepreneurs come armed with data, degrees, and start-up dollars, most fail—largely because their approaches follow a faulty and predictable pattern.

They begin with a new product or service that they've invented or defined. As entrepreneurs, they then reach out to venture-capital firms and convince them to invest based on growth assumptions that, on a chart, most closely resemble a hockey stick. The investors, armed with similarly big dreams, value these companies in the billions, often before these young businesses even have a viable product to sell. In fact, there's a name for these heavily capitalized but money-draining ventures. They are "unicorns," start-ups without a track record but with a stock-market valuation of more than $1 billion. Create such an animal (and keep it alive long enough), and you will be financially set for life.

Unfortunately, as many investors in the health care sector learn the hard way, all that glitters isn't gold.

The Young Bloods of Health Care

Elizabeth Holmes, a former Stanford enrollee, established a start-up called Real-Time Cures in Palo Alto before changing its name to Theranos, a clever fusion of "therapy" and "diagnosis." The big idea was to offer low-cost blood tests with only a small amount of blood obtained through a finger stick rather than a big, scary needle.

Holmes sold her investors and customers on a story about how she feared having blood drawn. She promised her company's technology would help millions like her overcome that fear, and that, better yet, her tests would cost only half as much as tests done in a traditional laboratory.

The idea was popular. Holmes and her cofounders raised $700 million on their way to a $9 billion company valuation. The business community and media hailed her as health care's next great entrepreneur. Holmes was able to generate all of this investor and media frenzy before anyone in the medical community had even tested the breakthrough device she had code-named "Edison." There wasn't a single published article about it in a peer-reviewed journal. It is hard to imagine a medical advance physicians would accept without this type of scientific review, but when you're hunting for a unicorn, your expectations and beliefs have to defy the laws of nature.

Holmes's idea glittered, a lot, and it helped make her Wall Street royalty, a crown she wore for several years. That was until it was discovered that Theranos's glitter was nothing more than fool's gold.

The *Wall Street Journal*, after months of investigating Theranos, revealed that the company's patented blood-testing technology was a ruse. Of the many kinds of tests the company promised, there was really only one available, and its substance didn't match the hype. Soon after, regulators determined the test results were suspect, and in response, the start-up's founders scrambled to cover their tracks. Six months earlier, Holmes's personal wealth was estimated at $4.5 billion. After Medicare withdrew payments for Theranos's services, that number plunged to zero.

In the aftermath, a *Wired.com* article pointed to "a deeper problem with the way Silicon Valley tries to spin hype into start-up gold." Although the problem isn't confined to Silicon Valley, many of the promises made by health care start-ups prove to be more alchemic than authentic.

In practice, few new medical breakthroughs match their hype. That's because the biology of human disease blunts their impact. When an idea that sounds great is tested on people, the results may be statistically significant, but the impact on life expectancy is often insignificant. In cancer, for example, tumors mutate and change their biology, rendering the efficacy of most new cancer drugs short-lived. Often, these very expensive and highly publicized new treatments extend life by days or, at most, weeks—rarely months and almost never years.

The 5 Percent Solution

Over the past decade, policy experts looking to solve the economic challenges of health care have searched diligently for opportunities hiding among the 5 percent of patients who account for 50 percent of all health care costs each year. On paper, they draw out scenarios in which even a relatively small degree of improvement produces hundreds of billions of dollars in savings. Reality, it turns out, is much more complex. The 5 percent is a heterogeneous group. About one-third of them are on the list because of a one-time event like a major car wreck or the birth of a very premature child. They're unlikely to suffer the same difficulties the following year. At the other extreme, about one-third of these high-cost patients are in the top 5 percent as a result of being so sick that no matter what doctors do, their medical problems will continue to worsen, rendering efforts to reduce the expenses futile. And even for the remaining one-third, reducing their health care expenditures requires major investments, often canceling out the savings. I'll explain this problem with a comparison.

In the field of information technology, innovations drive huge returns on investment. That's because the cost of creating an application may be expensive, but the cost of offering it to millions of people is relatively cheap. In health care, by contrast, a solution that helps twice as many patients often requires twice as many doctors and nurses. Programs designed to help the sickest 5 percent are important, but identifying cost-saving opportunities among them has been elusive.

What's more, in the technology world, innovators such as Steve Jobs and Mark Zuckerberg were able to create tools and applications with an almost exact knowledge of how they would affect our daily lives and to what degree. In health care, most ideas and approaches aimed at the 5 percent end up being less effective than their creators hoped or promised. Human biology simply lessens the impact.

The Future of Genomics Isn't Now (Yet)

Call it what you will: personalized medicine, predictive medicine, targeted medicine, or genomic medicine. Whatever you call it, the promise has so far yet to match the reality.

The field of genomics isn't new. DNA, the very foundation of genomics, was first discovered in the 1860s, almost a century before James Watson and Francis Crick demonstrated that the DNA molecule was, in fact, a three-dimensional double helix.

Fast-forward to 2000 when Bill Clinton and Tony Blair, the leaders of the Western world, stood side by side at the White House to announce the sequencing of the human genome was nearing completion. The information would soon be released to all, they said. They reported that the project took more than a decade and cost over $1 billion. Since then, scientists have found progressively less expensive ways to sequence the human genome of individuals and, today, offer the service for less than $2,000.

The set of genes we inherit from our parents determines much of who we are. Although there are a few dozen diseases for which medicine understands the precise genetic basis, including cystic fibrosis and sickle cell anemia, most problems, including heart disease, schizophrenia, and cancer, are far more complex. Specific genetic abnormalities don't exist among them.

Somewhere in between these two extremes lies another set of genetic mutations that have high association rates with particular diseases, most often cancer. Two of them are specific to breast cancer.

The clinical importance of these genes drew mass-media headlines in 2015 when noted actress Angelina Jolie was found to have one of these abnormalities and decided to undergo a double mastectomy and subsequent breast reconstruction.

The actress tested positive for a rare mutation in a gene (BRCA1) that assists in the repair of DNA. Mutations of the BRCA1 gene place people at significantly greater risk for developing breast and ovarian cancer. In her case, Jolie's family history demonstrated a much higher frequency of breast cancer than usual, and an inheritance pattern that led her doctors to order the test. It was the right decision for her—with an emphasis on "for her."

Only 5 to 10 percent of women with breast cancer have this particular abnormality. That's why this type of testing fails to provide any actionable information for the overwhelming majority of women and is therefore not routinely recommended by cancer experts.

It's logical to assume that if we fully understood the approximately 24,000 genes in our bodies, we would be able to predict our future health and better understand the basis of disease. But in spite of genetic sequencing data pulled from hundreds of thousands of patients, diagnostic answers are incredibly scarce. So far, genomics has produced many more correlations than demonstrated causalities. That means some genetic patterns are found more commonly in people with certain medical problems, but it doesn't mean these specific genes cause a higher incidence of problems or poorer health outcomes. The associations are simply more frequent, but far from universal.

Show patients a genomics test that demonstrates a 20 percent correlation with heart disease, rather than 12 percent, and they are unlikely to modify what they eat or exercise more often. Showing those same statistics to a doctor wouldn't change the course of care or recommendations provided, either. Make it a 100 percent correlation, and that would be a different story. We are many years away from that possibility.

For close to a decade, genomics companies and even some drug manufacturers have promised to deliver tests that could identify which patients
will or won't respond to a particular chemotherapy agent. Once again,
scientists have identified a few genetic markers that could make a difference and not much more.

Jolie's story raises our hopes for genomic testing while underscoring
the problem with things that glitter. Unlike the Theranos case, in which
there was no technology behind the curtain, genomic technology is elegant, accurate, and exciting. But when it comes to the human body,
knowing more about it doesn't directly improve medical care. As a result,
the industry's projections for applying genomics to human disease and
improving health remain heavy in hype and light on proof.

Simply put, the amount of data and information we have accumulated
year after year grows exponentially, but the impact of human DNA testing increases minimally.

In contrast, the medical community has learned a lot about the genomics of cancer cells themselves over the past fifteen years. So much so
that, one day, we will no longer refer to cancers by organ (lung or breast)
but by their specific genetic markers. Unfortunately, that day remains far
in the future.

For now, regardless of what genomic or genetic testing may indicate,
everyone would be better off eating healthier foods, exercising regularly,
and getting the appropriate prevention screenings based on their age, sex,
and medical history. In spite of our vast and complex genomes, when it
comes to our health, most humans have roughly the same basic needs
and risks.

"Revolutionizing" Health Insurance

Consumers take roughly sixteen times longer to choose a computer than
a new health plan. We shouldn't be surprised by this. For decades, health
plans have differed greatly in terms of marketing strategies but only
slightly in terms of the doctors and hospitals they make available.

And if the available care was essentially the same from insurer to insurer—with similarities in clinical quality, access, and service experience—it would make sense that it should only take you a few minutes to
decide which price, plan design, or company logo you liked most. That

may change in the future as insurance networks become narrower and the provider options grow more diverse.

In health insurance, you'll often hear that quality "is a given," or "table stakes." That couldn't be further from the truth. In the past, consumers have had no easy way of quantifying the differences in clinical outcomes from health plan to health plan, but that too is changing in the era of health care reform.

As the most recent data demonstrate, we now know that the old "quality-is-a-given" claim isn't just false, it's dangerous. Depending on (1) the health plan you select, and (2) the in-network care providers available to you, the quality of clinical outcomes you'll get (and your chances of dying of certain diseases) varies by 20 percent or more.

As will be detailed more fully in the next chapter, the Affordable Care Act expanded the insurance pool and stirred up competition among insurance companies. And by lowering the barrier to entry through the new online exchanges, new companies entered the picture.

Oscar Health, which made its debut on the New York health insurance exchange in 2014, seized the opportunity. Rather than sneaking up on traditional insurers, the company bragged on its website, "We're revolutionizing health insurance through technology, data, and design." Oscar was ready to take on the competition.

We expect new technologies and drugs to be doused in glitter, but this was the first insurance company to go that route.

Oscar sees itself as a technology company. Its website, the first point of contact for many consumers, is "cool." It offers user-friendly information on doctors in the neighborhood, along with easily clickable icons that take members to any of Oscar's five different social-media platforms. What's more, patients can learn how much money different providers will charge to treat their problem and how other patients have rated their experiences.

Patients preferring modern technology to an in-person office visit can connect virtually with doctors and find alternative treatments for their problem. Oscar even offers enrollees a free, wearable tracking device, along with rewards for members who use it to monitor their steps and exercise more often.

In the years since it launched, Oscar has grown its footprint and now sells insurance in New Jersey, California, and Texas. A recent investment from mutual-fund giant Fidelity to the tune of $400 million means that Oscar is now valued at an eye-popping $2.7 billion.

But the sparkle of this newish company appears to have outshone its true value. Despite all the excitement, the company has continued to lose millions of dollars year after year. In 2015, Oscar took a hit of $105 million and posted a loss of $52 million more in the first half of 2016. As *Fast Company* pointed out, "Many health experts agree that where Oscar excels isn't in its plan benefit design, but in the way that it markets these offerings to its members."

Although Oscar amassed a total of 150,000 new members since hitting the exchanges, that's less than 1 percent of the enrollment of the largest insurance companies and significantly below industry expectations. In addition, if Congress votes to reduce subsidies through the exchanges, the impact on Oscar and exchange-based newcomers like it will be massive: currently, 86 percent of participants receive financial assistance from the government to help pay their premiums.

Meanwhile, Oscar remains a small fish in a tank of sharks. And in health care insurance, where marketing budgets and economies of scale matter, the sharks are trying to team up through mergers and acquisitions. And if they succeed, Oscar's competitors will be able to negotiate lower prices with providers while creating networks the likes of which Oscar can't replicate.

After several years of claiming to be different, Oscar is now being forced to use the same cost-cutting approaches as the other guys. The company has shrunk its network of available doctors, transferred more of the cost onto the patient, and pulled out of overly competitive markets. At the same time, other insurance programs have modernized their websites and begun to offer the same patient conveniences that once helped Oscar stand apart.

Without excelling in the basics of insurance or being able to build a more efficient delivery-system model, Oscar will likely be devoured or, at any rate, sold to one of its larger competitors. This may in fact be the company's long-term strategy.

Nevertheless, Oscar maintains its enthusiasm and hope. But rather than living up to its billing as a powerful market disrupter, the heavily hyped insurer is looking more and more like a smaller version of the same old thing.

The Wrist of the Story

Every year, scores of Americans make resolutions to lose weight and get fit. And to ensure this year is really the year, many rely on technology for a boost.

They purchase and proudly display the hottest health wearables, for instance, the FitBit, the Misfit, and the Apple Watch. They sign onto their social channels and #humblebrag about their workouts. This health-tech frenzy has made the wearable device industry a Wall Street favorite. And so far, these investments have proven financially remunerative. But if we're looking to these wearables to significantly improve American health, we're better off looking elsewhere.

For all of the enthusiasm and hype these devices drum up, they essentially provide us with data on only two basic functions: sleep and exercise. Most of us already know whether we slept well. And even if the wearable informs us that we tossed and turned last night, what can we do about it? The wrist monitor quantifies our steps, calculates the distance we covered, and even estimates the calories we burned. But most of that information can be obtained through the smartphone we already own (and carry with us everywhere) or by clipping a $5 pedometer to our shorts.

Wearable devices do motivate some people to begin an exercise program or increase weekly mileage. But their impact on American health has been limited. For most people, the hope for greater health doesn't align with the results, because, in reality, attractive wristbands can't roll you out of bed or put your walking shoes on for you.

A recent study published in the *Journal of the American Medical Association* found that people who wore fitness trackers actually had a tougher time losing weight than people who logged their activity on a website.

Not surprisingly then, one-third of all consumers abandon their smart wearables within six months. And so, if they don't increase exercise for most individuals, and if most people can acquire the same information at minimal or no added cost, how are so many getting sold in the first place?

In short, fitness wearables solve the "December Dilemma." The holidays are coming and you're looking to buy a cool present for someone you love. Your budget is around $200 and you want the present to communicate how much you care. Voilà! The FitBit/Misfit/Apple Watch fits the bill.

The December Dilemma has been around for quite some time. In the 1990s, Americans solved it with inline skates. These shiny plastic boots with their wheels all in a row were beautiful to look at and trendy to own. But for one-third of all recipients, that morning in late December was the last time they put them on.

In health care, "home monitoring devices" have become the hot new thing. These wearables can measure core vital functions and would seem helpful for patients with chronic conditions. These wireless trackers range from blood-pressure monitors and pulse counters to blood-oxygen calcu-lators and blood-sugar evaluators. They can capture and send thousands of electrocardiogram (EKG) tracings, blood-sugar levels, or other bodily statistics directly to the computers of health care professionals.

However, except in the rarest cases, no doctor benefits from this stream of information. For 98 percent of patients, one, two, or three EKGs are useful. One hundred or 1,000 additional rhythm strips don't add value. Doctors don't want all of that information clogging up their electronic health records, particularly when the additional data don't help their patients.

Home monitoring devices are also seen as a potentially helpful way to reduce the number of patients idling in hospitals. If we could send people home earlier in their recovery and monitor their vital signs from afar, it could theoretically reduce health care costs. But that's not what happens in practice. When physicians are that concerned about a person's vital signs, they usually want to keep the patient in the hospital.

Knowing that a patient's blood pressure is dangerously low is better than not knowing, but what doctors really want is to be able to adminis-ter fluids and raise the patient's blood pressure back into the normal range within minutes. Home monitoring devices can't do that. Only doctors and nurses can. Of course, there are a few patients who would benefit from home monitoring, and a small number of people who could be dis-charged a day earlier, but not nearly enough of them to justify the billion-dollar valuations for the companies that manufacture them.

Why Big Ideas Lose Their Luster

Across the country, from Boston to San Francisco, new medical tech-nology ("med-tech") conferences sprout up each year. If you sat in the audience of one, you'd think the practice of medicine was undergoing a revolution. And if you sat in the audience of the same conference twelve months later, you'd realize that all the talks sound just like they did the previous year.

Browse the exhibition hall during the breaks and you'll meet excited sales and marketing reps hawking all sorts of sleek and shiny new gadgets. But few physicians are recommending them, and fewer insurance companies are paying for them. Why is that?

1. Many Big Ideas Don't Address the Real Problem

First, as we now know, tech entrepreneurs usually take a backward approach to innovation. They start by discovering a nifty technology. Next, they try to figure out how people can use the product. Finally, they focus on how to monetize it. It's a recipe for failure.

In practice, developing the monitor is the easy part. Figuring out how it will raise the quality of health or lower health care costs is the tricky part. And figuring out how to get someone to pay for it is almost impossible.

If you could connect your new blood-sugar monitor to a device that immediately administered insulin, the product would be equivalent to an artificial pancreas. That would most certainly be of interest to doctors. But a device that simply monitors a patient's blood sugar hundreds of times a day offers minimal utility and proves to be only slightly better than asking the patient to keep track of the numbers manually.

Sometimes, existing tech-enabled solutions can be used in new and innovative ways within a medical setting. For example, we know patients in the Intensive Care Unit often lose strength and become deconditioned as they lie in bed all day. Getting them out of bed and ambulating them several times a day contributes to speedier recovery and reduces the likelihood of readmission. Getting nurses to walk patients who are intubated proves difficult. That's why physicians in some of Kaiser Permanente's hospitals started giving their ICU patients an exercise tracker to ensure they got their necessary steps. Although the results are preliminary, more patients are getting up and out of bed. And thanks to the tracker, everyone is aware when they aren't.

The hope is that the trackers will motivate patients and nurses to accomplish a little more together each day. If it works, recovery times will speed up. But for the tech companies that make them, the number of new devices sold will be minimal compared to whatever business plan they showed their investors.

2. Tech Companies Don't Want the Malpractice Risk

Doctors don't want an hour's worth of EKG tracings from a monitor. But there's one technological opportunity that would prove incredibly useful to both doctors and patients. Physicians would love a home monitoring tool that informs patients when they are at risk and in need of medical intervention. For example, imagine a device that would alert patients immediately when the number of abnormal heartbeats exceeded a predetermined frequency. These patients could then call their doctor and transmit the recorded information to the physician's office.

Because most of the medical decisions physicians make are algorithmic, this information could prove useful. But there is a catch (for the manufacturers). A tool that could separate the "signal from the noise" for patients, telling them when they're at risk and when not to worry, would expose device makers to legal action and malpractice suits, should patients suffer a major complication. That's why tech manufacturers have chosen the simpler path: they transmit all of the data to the doctor, which almost no doctor wants.

3. No One Wants to Pay for New Technologies

Creating an innovative tool or app that can help doctors and patients isn't enough. These products must also be monetized, particularly the more expensive monitors designed to be used by patients with complex chronic illnesses, and for those being discharged from the hospital.

Even when patients, physicians, hospitals, and insurance companies all want these gadgets, each of these sectors believes that someone else should pay. Patients believe the doctor's office should provide it and that their insurance should pay for it. The physician believes the gadget is not part of the treatment and that the patient should contact the insurance company. The health plan says this technology, like most personal devices, is excluded from medical coverage and that the patient should pay.

Until our payment model moves from fee-for-service to "pay-for-value," some of the most effective technological solutions imaginable will be hard to sell.

4. Many Physicians See Technology as Impersonal

For millennials, technology is personal, helpful, and central to their identities. But few physicians in the later stages of their careers share those same perceptions.

For some physicians, the thought of Siri doling out advice—or, rather, looking over their shoulders and watching for mistakes—terrifies them. And the idea that patients could use technology to make their own health care decisions is also scary, but for different reasons. Some doctors fear it will devalue their years of training and erode the traditions of medical culture.

Increasingly, doctors find themselves frustrated at technologies that require them to spend more time staring at a computer screen than looking the patient in the eye. They worry that technology will force them to be on call 24/7 or that it will serve as a constant distraction in their day-to-day practice.

But for a growing number of patients, the absence of technology in a doctor's office proves equally impersonal, inconvenient, and frustrating.

Patients want to be able to schedule their appointments online, but doctors insist they call during business hours. Many individuals with routine questions and problems would prefer to use video chat or e-mail to consult a physician, but doctors are unwilling to provide the service, even when this means their patients have to miss work or school. Patients are concerned about high out-of-pocket payments for in-office visits, but doctors are more worried that insurance companies won't pay them unless the care is provided in the flesh.

In spite of all the lofty promises of new technical innovations, only a small fraction has succeeded in improving health care's quality while reducing its costs. Ironically, the health care innovations that have achieved both aims are ones few people would label as "breakthroughs."

Gold in Health Care Rarely Glitters

We've all heard the adage "seat belts save lives." Indeed they do and, as *Freakonomics* authors Stephen J. Dubner and Steven Levitt once pointed out, they're one of the few life-saving innovations of the past fifty years that have actually been cost effective.

The first modern seat belt, the kind used in most consumer vehicles today, was patented by American inventors Roger Griswold and Hugh DeHaven in 1955, the year actor James Dean was killed in a two-vehicle crash along a quiet stretch of California highway. That was also around the time that Volvo, a brand now synonymous with safety, became the first car company to offer seat belts as standard equipment, citing the rapid rise in fatal car accidents throughout Sweden.

However, it wasn't until nearly a decade later that US legislators would finally enact standards for seat belts, so that "passenger injuries in motor vehicle accidents can be kept to a minimum."

Today, car crashes remain a leading cause of death for people under the age of fifty-five. But according to the CDC, seat belts reduce serious crash-related injuries and deaths by about one-half. As a result, seat belts save more than 15,000 lives each year in the United States.

Unlike some of the cars they occupy, seat belts don't glitter. Their popularity is muted. Search for "seat belt" on Facebook and you'll find an interest page with just over 1,000 likes. That's less than one-tenth the number of Facebook users who like *The Seatbelts*, a Japanese band that entertains audiences with something called "space jazz." But what automotive seat belts lack in glitter, they more than make up for in value. That's something most new products can't claim.

Throughout the health care arena, there remains a huge gap between what many people think of as the most important innovations and what data show them to be.

The Value of Vaccines

Losing a child to an infectious disease was commonplace in the first half of the twentieth century. As I noted at the outset of the book, when my father was a child, his sister, Mary, died of measles. Today, we have safe and effective vaccines that can prevent measles and a slew of other infectious diseases.

Given that progress, scientists of a generation ago predicted that measles and mumps would someday be relegated to the history books. Yet in many of our wealthiest communities, we've seen a resurgence of these highly communicable viruses.

The concept of vaccination was pioneered by Edward Jenner more than two centuries ago. In the late 1700s, he discovered that milkmaids who had previously contracted cowpox, a disease with very mild effects on humans, were at little risk for becoming ill with smallpox, a disfiguring and often fatal disease.

He concluded that inoculating children with cowpox would prevent them from acquiring smallpox. From that observation, the first vaccine was born. Since Jenner's discovery, dozens of other vaccines have been developed, refined, and introduced into clinical medicine.

Many vaccines—like those for measles, polio, and tetanus—are mandated for children beginning school. But the impact of modern vaccines now extends far beyond the typical childhood illness.

A recent study found that 31,000 cancer deaths, including those of the cervix in women and in the oropharynx of both sexes, could be prevented each year through a safe vaccine now recommended for all against the human papillomavirus, or HPV.

Compared to most of the medical advances we herald today, the global impact of vaccines has been many times greater. We have seen the near elimination of vaccine-preventable diseases in the United States and the complete eradication of smallpox worldwide. Thanks to the efforts of such groups as the Bill and Melinda Gates Foundation, polio and its horrific consequences have been nearly eliminated around the world.

Through the Decades of Vaccines Collaboration, two hundred countries endorsed a shared world vision in which all individuals and communities enjoy lives free from vaccine-preventable diseases. Extending the full benefits of immunization to every person worldwide by 2020 would prevent an estimated 20 million deaths—mostly in children—and untold suffering from blindness, paralysis, and deafness for millions more.

In the United States, the days of school closures for measles and pertussis outbreaks have become relics of the past. Parents no longer have to keep their children home or away from public swimming pools to avoid exposure to polio.

Yet despite the virtues of vaccines, a growing number of children aren't getting them. Misleading science, outdated anecdotes, and fearmongering have exacted an unhealthy toll on American perceptions. In recent years, we have witnessed the scientifically ignorant (and sometimes deadly) impact of the anti-vaccine movement. Despite dozens of studies proving the safety and efficacy of these vaccines, there are those who continue to repeat false claims and resist universal vaccination.

When laboratory-produced vaccines were first introduced over fifty years ago, there were legitimate concerns about their safety. Many vaccines in their older forms were associated with the risk of rare but dangerous reactions. The vaccines we use today have minuscule risks, an extremely safe track record, and near-universal effectiveness in large-scale clinical trials. As a result, most pediatricians go through their entire practice without seeing a single major complication from the vaccines themselves or a patient death from any of the diseases against which they protect.

The misinformation and false alarms began in 1998 when a British physician published a study in the *Lancet* medical journal that falsely linked autism with the combined measles-mumps-rubella vaccine.

An investigation into the work revealed that the research was filled with fraudulent data and conflicts of interest. In 2010, the author's paper was fully retracted from the *Lancet*, an almost unheard of action in the world of peer-reviewed journals. Still, the damage was done. Vaccination rates in the United Kingdom plummeted, and reported cases of measles soared.

And as the trend crossed the pond, so did the threat. In the United States, if the already reduced vaccination rates in some communities were to drop much further, we would have another potential epidemic on our hands.

For the last two decades, fearmongers associated with the anti-vaccine movement in the United States and other developed countries have convinced thousands of parents to refuse vaccinations for their kids, citing concerns that the vaccines could cause autism in children. This overreaction results from a particular type of error in perception. We see problems that are common as far more dangerous than those we hardly ever encounter. Many people know someone who has a child with autism. Very few people know anyone whose son or daughter has developed measles.

When parents hear information that associates a vaccine with a problem that is familiar to them, they overrate the risks to their child. What they don't realize is that measles vaccination has prevented approximately 17 million deaths over the past fourteen years, "making [the] measles vaccine one of the best buys in public health," according to the World Health Organization.

The Boring Power of Prevention

When we hear the word "prevention," we tend to tune out. It has become the seat belt of medical practice: we all know we're safer with it than without it, but it remains an afterthought. After all, how tough could prevention be to accomplish? All the physician needs to do is order a test and prescribe a few pills. Surprisingly, the answer is very difficult.

Although Americans minimize its importance, the lack of prevention in our health care system helps explain why our quality scores pale in comparison with most other industrialized nations. Here at home, the inconsistency of our medical prevention efforts is evidenced by the massive variation in results from one group of physicians to the next.

Depending on the specific measure studied, health care providers who make prevention a priority are able to lower hypertensive disease, stroke, and heart attack rates anywhere from 10 to 30 percent below national averages. In fact, if every insured American received care from these higher performers, as many as 200,000 heart attacks and strokes could be prevented each year.

What is most baffling is that even though information on prevention outcomes is readily available—and even though the value of prevention is undeniable—people don't perceive it as important. As a result, they rarely make insurance decisions based on it, and almost never choose their doctors using the publicly reported data on performance.

The media reinforce this misperception, focusing on the glittery and gory. Headlines grab attention with the promise of unimaginable medical breakthroughs and the evildoings of medicine's villains. In news outlets, there's very little real estate dedicated to rigorously tested solutions that succeed through constant effort and hard work.

But suppose news outlets were to get creative. Instead of reporting the percentage of stroke, heart attack, or cancer deaths that could be *prevented*—or the number of lives that could be *saved*—what if they decided to reverse the language? Imagine coming across this salacious headline in your morning newsfeed: *200,000+ People Killed by Physicians Last Year.*

When a doctor harms a few specific individuals, everyone pays attention. Press outlets assign multiple reporters to cover the story, medical institutions assign blame, and patients insist on swift justice and immediate change. But when hundreds of thousands of nameless individuals die unnecessarily each year, our nation shrugs its shoulders. The press can and most likely will continue to ignore it, but 200,000 avoidable deaths each year represents the pinnacle of mistreatment.

Solutions in Context

The first half of the book analyzed the effects of context on doctors, patients, and large, lucrative organizations. Through the work of researchers like Philip Zimbardo, we now understand the psychology behind (and reasons for) much of the poor treatment patients endure in American health care today.

The remaining chapters of this book focus on the fixes. Many of them don't glitter, but all of them have the potential to shift the context of health care for the better, changing perceptions and altering behaviors in ways that would improve the quality of our care. When we obsess over what's shiny and new, we miss out on solutions that can have a far greater impact on our health. My belief is that if researchers like Zimbardo and Milgram have the power to affect human perception in negative and destructive ways, then we have the power to do the opposite. We can modify the structure, financing, and technology of medical practice in ways that lead to superior medical outcomes for patients and that create a professionally uplifting experience for doctors.

Along the way, it will be important to identify the specific changes necessary in health care, particularly those that differ from conventional wisdom. Doing so will require a focus on the massive gap between what we know about improving health care and how we currently go about it. Specifically, the following chapters will (1) examine the impact of the Affordable Care Act as a first step in what will be a long road to true health care reform and delivery-system improvement, (2) spell out a specific set of solutions that have the potential to address the root economic causes of our dysfunctional system and change the environment of medical practice for the better, and (3) present a potential road map for the future that begins and ends with what patients want.

Chapter Six

THE AFFORDABLE CARE ACT IN HINDSIGHT

On the evening of November 8, 2016, the talking heads on American news networks gasped in collective astonishment. As the polls closed and election results poured in, Donald J. Trump's lead in the presidential race grew insurmountable. It was a stunning upset. More than 60 million Americans voted for Trump, fewer than voted for Hillary Clinton but more than enough to secure an Electoral College victory for the candidate who campaigned on making America great again.

The results confirmed that pollsters and pundits had miscalculated, by a relatively large margin, the true feelings of a divided country. For many Trump supporters, making America great again meant, in part, pivoting away from the ineffectiveness of past administrations. Their fears, disappointments, and desires for political shake-up were foreseen in a survey conducted in the summer of 2016. The Pew Research Center polled registered voters, who ranked their most important issues as (1) the economy, (2) terrorism, and—not far behind those—(3) American health care.

Trump blasted the Affordable Care Act throughout his campaign, calling it "amazingly destructive." His political rival, Clinton, on the other hand, promised "to build on the progress we've made" with President Obama's health care plan. Looking back, the world that Hillary Clinton described contrasted vividly with the one Donald Trump portrayed. The contentious election of 2016 demonstrated, powerfully, the importance of context in shaping public and personal perceptions. Trump's supporters, many of whom felt left behind by society and government, saw the world very differently than those who voted for Secretary Clinton.

And as you're about to see, context was equally key in the creation, and now uncertain future, of the Affordable Care Act.

What We See

Students are brought into a room and asked to estimate the likelihood that an English word, selected at random, either begins with the letter "r" or contains "r" as its third letter. This isn't some kind of intensive Scrabble preparation. Rather, it's a test about how our minds call upon information.

What the researchers behind this study discovered is that we "judge words that begin with a given consonant to be more numerous than words in which the same consonant appears in the third position." And we do this incorrectly. Throughout the English lexicon, the letter "r" appears more than twice as frequently in the third position as in the first.

Daniel Kahneman, the same researcher behind the hypothetical outbreak of disease that was cited in Chapter 2, believes he knows why his research subjects got the answer to this alphabetical question wrong so often. It has to do with "availability bias," a concept he first explored with his collaborator, Amos Tversky, in their 1974 article, "Judgment Under Uncertainty: Heuristics and Biases."

The duo noted that "people approach this problem by recalling words that begin with r (road) and words that have r in the third position (car) and assess the relative frequency by the ease with which words of the two types come to mind." And unless you're a human dictionary, it's much easier for you to recall words by their first letter. They're the ones most available to us when we search our memory. And because it's easier for us to recall and recite words that begin with "r," we assume there must be more of them.

Think of availability bias as a mental shortcut that our brains use for estimating the likelihood of an event or particular frequency of occurrence. Take this example from Kahneman and Tversky: "It is a common experience that the subjective probability of traffic accidents rises temporarily when one sees a car overturned by the side of the road." Having just seen an accident, we begin to assume they're more a common occurrence than objective data would indicate.

This concept also applies to what we read, see on TV, and therefore have on our mind at any given moment. To give the theory of availability bias a more contemporary application, look at a 2014 poll conducted by the research group Ipsos MORI, which the firm titled, "Perceptions are not reality: Things the world gets wrong."

When asked to estimate the nation's Muslim population, Americans guessed, on average, 15 percent. That's not even close to being close. The Pew Research Center confirms that less than 1 percent of Americans are Muslim (0.6 percent, to be more precise). The discrepancy reflects the nation's lingering fear of terrorism and the Middle East, which has dominated the news for some time now. Meanwhile, amid the nation's ongoing job recovery and economic concerns, survey respondents also overshot the US unemployment rate by about 24 percent. Once again, this error in perception reflects what's on our minds and in the news. Context is extremely powerful in this equation.

What's especially interesting about availability bias is that the reverse of the theory also holds true. That is, events and figures that we know about but don't often encounter get pushed down into our subconscious, rarely entering our thought process. We might think of this as "unavailability bias." You'll find perhaps no better example of it than in US health care.

Unavailability Bias in US Health Care

For quite some time, the rate of uninsured in the United States hovered between 16 and 18 percent. In other words, about 50 million Americans (one in six) were living without health insurance.

About one-third of the 50 million were relatively poor (but not poor enough to qualify for Medicaid), one-third were lower to middle class (but not wealthy enough to buy private insurance), and the final one-third had preexisting conditions that made health insurance too exorbitant to purchase.

In any context, 50 million is a significant number. But if you weren't one of the uninsured, you probably didn't notice the problem—or at least you underestimated its magnitude. If you've always had health insurance and don't know people without it, you likely saw the uninsured population as relatively few in number, if you saw them at all. And if that was the case, you didn't perceive the lack of health coverage as a major problem for the country.

That's simply how our brains work. We filter out events and information that don't directly affect us to make room for the events and information that do.

So when Barack Obama stepped forward as the newly elected president of the United States in 2008, he set about a long and arduous journey to address the huge disparities he saw in access and clinical outcomes.

Through his own personal experience, Obama had witnessed the deteriorating health of low-income Americans living without health insurance. He had seen the discriminatory practices of health insurers and the difficulties they caused people with preexisting medical conditions. He had observed, firsthand, the reduced quality of care that poor patients received.

But he also knew he couldn't solve these problems until the American people noticed them, too. He needed to make the "unavailable" more readily apparent. So his first step was to help his fellow Americans see the issue.

Running Toward the Problem

Georgetown is a charming neighborhood in Washington, DC, a combination tourist stop, college town, and shopping extravaganza. As the CEO of The Mid-Atlantic Permanente Medical Group, I often stay there and look forward to my early morning runs. I usually start along the Potomac River and head down through Foggy Bottom to marvel at the majesty of the Lincoln Memorial, before venturing east toward the Washington Monument and, a few miles later, the US Capitol Dome.

But occasionally, I'll run alternative routes. From Georgetown, I sometimes head along Virginia Avenue toward Pennsylvania Avenue, passing the Western Presbyterian Church on my left. When I do, I often see an orderly line of people along the sidewalk out front.

Travel to DC in the context of a business trip or a vacation and you'll return home with great memories of the attractions, symbols of our democracy and the upbeat energy of a district that helps shape our national politics. Run along Virginia Avenue around 6:30 in the morning, and you're likely to see a line forming—men and women, cold and hungry, seeking food and shelter. Once you do, you can't un-see the people in it. It becomes difficult to ignore the problem.

To Have Not

Those familiar with the expression "to have and have not" may know it as the title of an Ernest Hemingway novel, written during the Great Depression. The book centers on a poor fishing-boat captain, an honest man, whose financial plight compels him to do illegal deeds to support his family. It's an insightful narrative, articulating how context alters mindset, sometimes blurring the lines between right and wrong, perception and reality. Our context—more than our convictions or values or conscious decisions—determines what we see and how we react to it. The presidential election of 2016 pivoted on that reality.

Throughout my career, I've treated millionaires and operated on those who struggle to make ends meet. My patients have included Nobel Prize winners and those without a roof over their head.

When you have enough to eat and a warm place to sleep, you often fail to notice those who don't. When you have health insurance, you also don't notice the one in six people without it. But once you've had to personally go without, you can't get that experience out of your head.

A few years ago, religious leaders in my community recruited people willing to try living on a typical food-stamp budget. The idea behind this "food-stamp challenge" was to help professionals understand what being poor is really like, what it means to have not. Along with about one hundred others, I was asked to limit my food intake for the week to what I could purchase for $31.50, less than $5 a day.

I never imagined how difficult it would be to experience the relative scarcity that millions of Americans find normal. The week felt interminable. I was constantly hungry. On less than $5 a day, a typical meal consisted of bread and peanut butter or a dry grain boiled in water. Apples and oranges were a treat. A cantaloupe was out of the question.

Going in, I knew full well this brief exercise in empathy and understanding would not fully capture the challenges of those living near the poverty line. But it took me almost no time at all to realize how absurd

I must have sounded when counseling my poorer patients on the importance of eating a healthy, balanced diet with fresh fruits and vegetables.

I also recognized that if you can't feed your family, buying medical insurance is not one of your top priorities. People don't go without insurance because they choose to. They go without insurance because they have no choice.

Sociologists and everyday Americans disagree about the origins of poverty in our country and the factors leading to the lack of proper food, shelter, and medical care. They disagree even more about the solutions. But everyone understands that the first step toward solving a problem is recognizing that it exists.

The story of the Affordable Care Act begins by understanding how Barack Obama, the forty-fourth president of the United Sates, came to see the nation's health care problem and the role government could play in solving it.

Seven years after its passage, and three years after broad implementation, Obama's signature legislation remains as controversial and incomplete as ever. At the same time, it represents the most significant change to American health care in over half of a century.

The Dawn of Health Care Reform

On the South Side of Chicago in 1985, a self-described "skinny kid with a funny name" accepted a job as a community organizer, a role subsidized by prominent members of the city's Jewish and Catholic communities. His assignment was to organize the nearly 5,000 residents of Altgeld Gardens Homes and convince them to push city hall for improved living conditions inside their run-down public-housing project. It was a clear objective with anything but a clear path.

To find a solution, Obama needed to connect with the projects' residents. To do that, he needed to gain credibility—this, according to biographer David Mendell. So he began by joining the well-known Trinity United Church of Christ under the leadership of its outspoken pastor, Reverend Jeremiah Wright.

Through the church, Obama met with families living in and around the projects and came face-to-face with the realities of their situation. This was new territory for the young man who had grown up in Hawaii and attended private school on Oahu. Although he had lived as a student in both Los Angeles and New York City, we can only imagine his first thoughts as he looked upon the dilapidated housing and impoverished neighborhoods of Chicago's South Side as a problem he was tasked to solve.

Obama witnessed firsthand the deprivation that infiltrated some of Chicago's roughest neighborhoods and saw how the conditions wreaked havoc on its residents. He came to understand how the lack of food, education, and medical care in the area precipitated high rates of crime, violence, and death.

He was overwhelmed and distressed by the realities he encountered, understandably. But he found encouragement in two of the community's most influential figures. The first was Jeremiah Wright, his church's spiritual leader, a gifted orator capable of galvanizing an entire congregation with his words and community outreach.

The second was Harold Washington, Chicago's first black mayor. Obama marveled at Washington's abilities as an influencer. He saw how a strong, black politician with a law degree could move the members of city hall into action and change people's lives for the better. It was Mayor Washington's example that helped the future president realize that if he truly wanted to make change happen in Chicago, he would need to earn a law degree.

Obama enrolled in Harvard Law School in 1988, where he became the first African American president of the *Harvard Law Review*. He would go on to graduate magna cum laude.

Law was the right choice for his intellect and personality. When Obama returned to Illinois, degree in hand, he became an effective force in the community. He taught constitutional law at the University of Chicago and helped lead a massive voter-registration drive. In 1996, Obama gained a seat in the state legislature, where he lobbied to fight racial profiling and expand health care coverage for children in need.

He had also become a skilled orator, telling impassioned stories of the South Side families he met during his days as a community organizer. As his political influence grew, so too did his aptitude for shaping and passing legislation.

Studying his later legislative efforts as US president, you can see how greatly he was influenced by his time in Chicago. Without that experience, he might have stayed blind to the lives and health care needs of tens of millions of Americans. He might have overlooked the massive gaps in medical care they experienced. Phrased differently, without his years as a community organizer, he might never have developed the health care "availability bias" he carried into his presidency. But having seen the problem with his own eyes, and having interacted directly with people in need, his focus sharpened.

Obama wasn't the first US president seeking to overhaul American medicine. He also wasn't the first to bring the context of his own life experience to the fore of his legislative efforts. If history is the best teacher, President Barack Obama was well informed by studying the efforts, and the failures, of his predecessors.

Lessons from the Past

Health care takes place in a professional setting, but it is undeniably personal—maybe the most personal of professions. When I meet with newly hired physicians, I ask them why they wanted to become doctors. Most of them describe powerful moments from their past, specific points in time when life and medicine intersected. For some, it was a significant childhood event, perhaps the death of a parent or sibling. For others, it was a positive memory, a particular physician who saved their life or the life of someone very close to them.

If you could ask American presidents throughout history why they pursued health care reform, you would hear the same kinds of stories. Absent that opportunity, one need only scan the archives of the presidential libraries. There, you'll uncover the deeply personal health care motivations of our nation's former leaders.

Take Franklin D. Roosevelt, who contracted polio at age thirty-nine, rendering him unable to stand or walk without assistance. With encouragement from his supporters, FDR formed the organization that would eventually become the March of Dimes, a nonprofit that helped raise millions of dollars in the fight against polio. Fortunately for children across the country, some of those funds went to American medical researcher and virologist Jonas Salk, the man who discovered and later developed the first successful polio vaccine.

Roosevelt's successor, Harry S. Truman, was a farmer from Missouri. He had grown up watching the common man struggle to get a fair shake in life. Small wonder this unlikely president opted to spend much of his time in office endorsing equal health-insurance coverage for all Americans. He saw it as one of the most important acts of his presidency. History, however, didn't give Truman a fair shake in return. Serving during a time dominated by fears of communism, President Truman could not overcome repeated attacks from the powerful American Medical Association (AMA), a group that labeled his federal health-insurance bill "socialized medicine." His plan died in congressional committee.

John F. Kennedy followed in FDR's footsteps to increase funding and federal support for people with disabilities. JFK's younger sister, Rosemary, was born with an intellectual disability, a health care problem long underfunded by the government and widely neglected by scientists of the time. Within the first year of his inauguration, Kennedy set about creating "a panel of outstanding scientists, doctors, and others to prescribe a plan of action in the field of mental retardation," leading in 1963 to legislation addressing intellectual and developmental disabilities.

Fast-forward to the early 1990s, when former Arkansas governor Bill Clinton found his own motives for passing health care reform legislation. Two years prior to his induction, Clinton's mother, Virginia, underwent a mastectomy. She was a nurse anesthetist by profession and extremely close with her son. Through her battle with breast cancer, President Clinton's passion for improving health care strengthened, elevating it to the top of his agenda.

Once elected, Clinton wasted little time announcing a White House task force to steer a massive reform effort. It was an ill-fated proposal from the start. Ultimately, three forces led him to abandon his cause and much of the political momentum that came with his new presidency.

First, rather than casting a wide net or conducting a rigorous search for a task-force leader, he called upon then first lady Hillary Clinton. A poll at the time reported that 44 percent of Americans thought there were better candidates for the job. Politically unripe, Mrs. Clinton relied on a tight inner circle of policy experts for input, in turn alienating a large swath of potential allies. Health care leaders, many of whom felt they were overlooked for the role, blamed the Clinton administration for ignoring the acumen of doctors and other health care experts in shaping the proposal.

The tanking economy of the early 1990s was President Clinton's second major headwind. The recession forced Clinton to abandon any approach that would increase government spending or expand the federal deficit. Third, as a result of the economic travails, Democrats lost the House during the midterm elections of 1994, a final and fatal dagger that put an end to his health care reform plan.

This brings us to President Obama, who, like those before him, brought a litany of personal and political motivations to his health care reform efforts, experiences that were very different from his successors'. He understood the devastating consequences afflicting the people he met and lived among in Chicago. He had urged the Illinois legislature to help them, and he helped write legislation to close some of the gaps. Once elected, he focused much of the first two years of his presidency on the challenges of Americans without health insurance, those constrained by the financial pressures of obtaining health care.

Making the Case

A little over a year into his first term in office, standing at a lectern in a downtown Chicago hotel, President Obama addressed the nation's most powerful constituency of US physicians, the American Medical Association, the same group that decades earlier had shot down Truman's reform efforts. Here, Obama spoke with passion about the economic stresses confronting the American people:

> Make no mistake, the cost of our health care is a threat to our economy. It is an escalating burden on our families and businesses. It is a ticking time-bomb for the federal budget. And it is unsustainable for the United States of America. It is unsustainable for Americans like Laura Klitzka, a young mother I met in Wisconsin last week, who has learned that the breast cancer she thought she'd beaten had spread to her bones; who is now being forced to spend time worrying about how to cover the $50,000 in medical debts she has already accumulated, when all she wants to do is spend time with

her two children and focus on getting well. These are not worries a
woman like Laura should have to face in a nation as wealthy as ours.

All of the physicians assembled at the AMA conference that day knew
a Laura from their own practices. They had all taken care of a patient who
couldn't afford treatment for a disease like cancer. They knew people with
chronic illnesses who had to choose between their care and their family's
financial well-being.

Barack Obama, surveying the massive hill he'd need to climb to effect
meaningful change, started his ascent by putting a human face on the
imperative to expand health care coverage and restrain its escalating costs.

His speech to the AMA didn't change every mind in the room that
day. And as he repeated his message both privately and in public, he didn't
alter the perceptions of every person in Congress, either. But the effect
of his words, his ability to make people see the problem, was the catalyst
needed to kick-start radical change in America's health care system.

A Policy Born of Political Reality

The immediate future of health care policy is nothing if not uncertain.
But we can infer a lot about what might happen by understanding the
congressional mathematics of the past. President Obama entered the
White House in 2009 with a veto-proof Congress, comprising fifty-eight
Democrats and two Democratic-leaning Independents in the Senate.
That, along with a solid majority in the House of Representatives, meant
the president had just enough votes to advance health care reform over
GOP objections. It was the last time until this most recent election that
a political party controlled the Senate, the House, and the presidency.

Still, Obama recognized his journey was fraught with barriers and that
he didn't have a single vote to spare. So out of a combination of political
necessity and personal style, the president embraced a different strategy
than his predecessors.

Specifically, Obama was cautious from the start. He knew that opposing lobbyists needed to flip only one of his Senate supporters. And if they
succeeded, the Republicans would surely "talk his bill to death" through
filibuster.

That's why he announced that the nation's health care reform plan would be handled openly and transparently from the outset. We can assume that Obama, as the head of the Democratic Party, was involved in all key decisions, but we know he wasn't alone in the decision-making process. In fact, he even offered to work hand in hand with Republican leaders, remembering well the expensive advertising campaigns and lobbying avalanches that buried the past reform bills.

As a student of political history, having closely analyzed the Clinton health care proposal, Obama concluded that it would be unproductive to send Congress a well-baked yet poorly backed plan. Instead, he took a hands-off approach in the early stages, asking lawmakers to sketch out a first draft, preferring consensus over personal preference.

And to the surprise of many, rather than painting the legacy players as villains or obstructionists, the president included them in the discussions, too. He invited representatives from Big Pharma, community hospitals, and for-profit health plans to the White House for a "health summit" in March 2009.

As a national health care CEO and the leader of the country's largest medical group, I was there to help provide a physician's perspective on the challenges facing patients and doctors. It was an incredibly exciting time in health care's storied history. As you might imagine, with $3 trillion of health care spending in play, the environment was one of constant frenzy. Every organization wanted its voice heard. From community leaders to insurers to drug companies, the nation's most powerful health care players lobbied the White House and Congress hard, often into the wee hours of the morning.

For my part, I focused on opportunities to increase coverage and improve the effectiveness of clinical outcomes, arguing that all Americans were entitled to high-quality medical care. I explained that rewarding physicians for superior results through a "pay for value" rather than a fee-for-service reimbursement model would improve the nation's health and benefit everyone in the long run. Some of this thinking ended up in the final bill. Although, with hundreds of voices flooding the debate and many arguing for similar things, it's impossible to pinpoint the contributions of any individual or group.

In November 2009, the House approved its version of health care reform by a narrow margin, with several compromises and concessions, including reduced federal funding for family-planning services. The following month, despite an attempted GOP filibuster, the Democratic majority pushed its version of the health care reform law through the Senate.

Next, it was on to the Democrat-controlled joint conference committee, where bills of massive scope and complexity are sorted out while disagreements about specific provisions are resolved. This process has been termed by political experts as "making sausage." It's where disparate legislative parts, some written in the House and some in the Senate, are brought together and ground into something that hardly resembles either original bill. The final product is then stuffed into a single casing.

Inside the conference committee, knowledgeable staff and subject-matter experts iron out the exact details in order to create actionable legislation. The president, having taught constitutional law, knew that this was where the real work and hard decisions took place. And it was there that the president hoped to exert major influence on the final bill's design. Once the committee's work was done, the finished bill would come back for one more vote in each chamber before being placed on the president's desk for signature. At least, that was the strategy.

Along the way, the process hit a snag and the president's plan suffered a major setback. Three months before the House passed its version of the law, Senator Ted Kennedy, an avid and career-long proponent of health care reform, died of complications from a malignant brain tumor. Upon his death, the little-known but hard-charging Scott Brown overcame tremendous odds to best Martha Coakley, the Democratic nominee, for Kennedy's vacant Senate seat in January 2010, making Brown the first Republican senator in Massachusetts since 1972. Suddenly, there were only fifty-nine Democrat votes in the Senate, not enough to override a Republican filibuster that would topple the whole deal when it returned for final approval.

Obama, borrowing from his knowledge of history and background in the Illinois and US Senates, accepted that a good law enacted was better than a perfect one killed by partisanship. He knew that if the conference committee made any changes to the Senate's bill, it would need to go up again for debate, where a filibuster would most certainly be waiting. For this reason, the president, along with Democratic congressional leadership, took the simpler path. Instead of modifying the bill further, they passed the Senate's version unchanged.

And that's how the ACA, warts and all, became the law of the land. The signed bill emerged less than ideal in the president's eyes, but it was still a dramatic victory. In the end, it was a mountainous legislative achievement, something no previous president had accomplished.

However, the debate and partisanship were far from over, and the residual tension could be felt in the president's words. After signing the ACA, Obama announced, "I will always work with anyone who is willing to make this law work even better." But he added, "The debate over repealing this law is over. The Affordable Care Act is here to stay."

Of course, strategy and reality don't always align. In October 2016, Donald Trump told supporters at a rally in Florida, "It's over for Obamacare." One month later, he held the future of health care reform in his hands.

A Catalyst for Change

The passage of the Patient Protection and Affordable Care Act in 2010 was, at the time, a strategic inflection point in US health care, a defining moment when the rules of health care delivery and financing changed.

Whether or not you follow health care policy, you likely recall the political angst and the doomsday predictions leading up to and following the signing of the ACA. You might remember the constitutional turmoil surrounding the Supreme Court's ruling—the one mandating that all Americans acquire health insurance or face penalties. And perhaps you remember the technologically rocky launch of the online "health insurance exchanges" in 2013. It all seems like eons ago now. And it will take decades more to put this legislation in full historical context.

To this day, the Affordable Care Act remains a political flashpoint as officials on each side of the aisle have labeled the bill either one of the greatest political decrees in American history or the demise of a once-great nation.

Regardless of political persuasion, nearly all elected officials and pundits came to refer to the Affordable Care Act as "Obamacare." It's a rarity in politics when those who scorn a bill use the same coinage as those who praise it. But no matter what tone they've used, the term itself speaks to the powerful role the president played in shaping and passing this landmark policy.

In 2014, the president joked in a televised interview with retired pro-basketball player Charles Barkley, "I like it (when they call it Obamacare). I don't mind. And I tell ya, five years from now, when everybody's saying, 'Man, I'm sure glad we got health care,' there's going to be a whole bunch of people who don't call it Obamacare anymore because they don't want me to get the credit."

Obama's prediction now seems premature, if not unlikely. But politics in general, and health care in particular, have a unique way of defying expectations. Trump's election as president certainly seemed impossible throughout much of his campaign. In fact, the history of health care is filled with similar surprises. The passage of the Medicare legislation under the Democrat Lyndon Johnson, a process as contentious as the en-actment of the Affordable Care Act, was followed by a rather unexpected twist. Rather than calling for a repeal of Medicare, Richard Nixon, the Republican who succeeded Johnson, called on Congress to expand Medi-care to cover people under the age of sixty-five with long-term disabilities. He even added a new health care law of his own: the HMO Act of 1973, which provided millions of dollars in start-up funding for health mainte-nance organizations (HMOs).

Relevant to the realities of today, Nixon wrote a special message to Congress in 1974, cautioning, "Any program to finance health care for the Nation must take close account of two critical and related problems: cost and quality."

He went on to point out, "When Medicare and Medicaid went into effect, medical prices jumped almost twice as fast as living costs in gen-eral in the next five years." Those cost dilemmas of the past are strikingly similar to the kinds of health care issues President Trump will need to address over the next four years.

At the start of Trump's presidency, there were over 10 million Ameri-cans newly insured through the online health insurance exchanges, with about 7 million more covered through the ACA's expansion of Medic-aid. As a result, seven years after the signing of America's most sweeping health care reform, the rate of uninsured had fallen below 9 percent for the first time ever, about half of what it was prior to the ACA's passage. For those newly insured through the Affordable Care Act, the economic security of coverage has been psychologically liberating. It has also been valuable in improving their overall health and well-being.

Trump campaigned on a platform to "repeal and replace" Obamacare. Doing so, however, poses serious risks for the new president, along with likely congressional challenges. Trying to eliminate coverage for all the newly insured Americans could cost Trump and the Republican-controlled Congress sizable voting blocs in future elections. Without question, it will be difficult for the new administration to strike a balance between its former campaign promises and the political realities in front of them.

Before Obamacare

Several years before the signing of the ACA, I drove to a small community clinic in Delano, California, to volunteer my services as a plastic and reconstructive surgeon. Many of the patients I saw worked the fields, picking a variety of seasonal fruits and vegetables. Unable to afford day care, mothers and fathers brought their children with them to the job site. There, the kids played with their friends until they were old enough to join their parents and work the fields.

The adults I treated during my time in Delano suffered from a variety of conditions. Many had painful hand problems, including damage from injury and advancing age. Others I saw, both old and young, experienced disability and disfigurement from burns or facial trauma. And then there were the children, whose problems were mainly congenital, including cleft lip and cleft palate. In Delano, there was no shortage of people wanting to see the new surgeon at the clinic.

At the end of one especially long day, a little boy no older than six peered into the office where I was working. I was surprised to see him unaccompanied by an adult. Kids knew the clinic as the place where they got vaccination shots. Most tried to avoid it.

When the waiting area emptied out, I called to the boy, his eyes fixed on the floor as he entered the room. I squatted down so that my head and his would be at the same height. As I met his gaze, I could see the boy was in tears.

I knew his problem immediately. Half of his face was covered with a black birthmark (medically, a "congenital nevus"). Still, I asked him why he came. He said the kids at school called him all sorts of names and teased him because of his appearance. The treatment for such a condition requires a series of surgeries to remove the black stain, replacing it either with a skin graft or by rotating skin from the neck. I told the boy that this was a common problem, one that many other kids have. Of course, that didn't help. Nor did it address the reality of his parents' financial situation.

Mothers and fathers in Delano will figure out how to pay for surgery when their child develops appendicitis. But parents who must work sixty hours a week in the fields to survive can't afford to correct a problem that isn't life-threatening. Given their economic reality, the boy's parents—and many other parents like them—had no choice but to hope their son would find a way to cope with the teasing.

For mothers and fathers, this kind of decision is especially heart-wrenching. You know surgery would improve your child's life and diminish the psychological pain. You just can't afford to pay for it. With the passage of the ACA, many hoped that this type of procedure would become affordable and that this type of heartache would be eliminated forever.

After Obamacare

About an hour's drive north from Delano, up Highway 99, you'll pass through the large fruit orchards and vineyards of Fresno, California. The farms there employ thousands of seasonal workers who, like the men and women of Delano, find plentiful jobs when crops need planting or picking. But when the fields are fallow, unemployment runs high.

Prior to the ACA, the seasonality of labor in Fresno left many without employer-sponsored health benefits. Too poor to buy individual insurance but with a combined family income exceeding Medicaid's cutoff, many in this town were caught in the middle of health care's troublesome economics.

In late 2014, six months after the implementation of the ACA, I took my annual site visit to the Kaiser Permanente Fresno Medical Center. As I always do during these trips, I met with physicians in groups and individually to find out what was happening in their practices. I remember this particular set of meetings well. This was the moment when I began to grasp the true impact of health care reform on the lives of Fresno's hardworking inhabitants and on the lives of millions of others like them.

I spoke with an OB-GYN physician who told me about a newly insured woman she had just seen. The patient had an abnormal Pap test, indicative of an early cervical or uterine cancer. Another doctor, a primary-care physician, described a twenty-five-year-old male who complained of a testicular mass that proved cancerous upon removal. Both patients had gone without medical care because they couldn't pay for it. Thanks to the Affordable Care Act, they were both covered and were most likely cured.

In the future, thousands of lives could be saved as more people get the medical care they need and the preventive screenings their doctors recommend. Data from states that have maximized ACA coverage and care show large improvements in population health, especially when compared with states that refused to subsidize increased enrollment. For now, families in Delano and Fresno, and individuals all across the country, wait with trepidation to see what will happen next.

A Lesson in Shifting Perception

Regardless of future changes to the ACA, it's vital to understand its origins, the strategy underlying its design, and the legislation's key provisions. In its final form, the Affordable Care Act and its associated reconciliations exceeded 1,000 pages, an arduous read for even the savviest health care wonk.

The bill's layout—front-loaded with expedited, bipartisan enactments and back-ended by the most controversial provisions—was a politically sensible move for the president and one of the most important reasons the legislation passed Congress. The expedited provisions were ones that just about everyone favored, such as extending coverage to young adults up to age twenty-six, allowing them to stay on their parents' insurance through college. The most problematic parts included a new tax on medical devices, along with major penalties for the most expensive insurance plans (dubbed the "Cadillac tax"). The president knew these controversial pieces would upset both the labor and business sectors, which is why they were pushed to the back of the ACA's implementation timetable, delayed for up to five years.

But there is much more to the ACA than meets the eye. Beyond its layout and between the lines, you'll find the unwritten implications of the law and the strategy President Obama thought stood the best chance of addressing the fundamental challenges of American health care today.

The president knew that unless his bill could help slow the rate of health care inflation, the expansion in coverage wouldn't work for long. To solve that problem, the president had his work cut out for him.

As a nation, Americans spend more on health care than India's 1.3 billion people spend on everything they purchase, from housing to food to transportation, education, infrastructure, and health care. Similarly, we spend more on health care in this country than the entire nation of France spends on everything its people consume, including champagne and truffles. Left unchecked, at the current rate of inflation, health care costs will ultimately bankrupt the United States.

Obama could see that as the total expense of American medical care continued to rise twice as fast as the gross domestic product (GDP), future administrations might look to limit spending on citizens in the lower economic half of the US population. At the same time, he knew that trying to reduce health care spending would not be easy or politically popular. This is where the psychology of perception came into play.

Recognizing that context wields massive influence over perceptions and behavior, the president sought to address health care's financial challenges, not by fiat but by altering its rules and norms. By shifting how care is provided and reimbursed—that is, by changing the context of health care—he believed he could transform the mindset and actions of patients and doctors alike, for good.

The president also recognized that any overt disruption or attempt to force quick change would face heated resistance from the legacy players. It was simple mathematics. Every health care dollar reduced had to come from somewhere, be it a hospital, a drug company, or a physician's pocket. And clearly, none of them would be happy with an approach that led to lost revenue, profit, or income. So rather than trying to reduce their payments on day one, Obama put in place a set of provisions that would influence medical practice over the long haul.

His hope was to convince the legacy players that the government's expansion of coverage would generate enough revenue for them to offset higher taxes or reductions in payment for their services.

In many ways, the role of government represents a fundamental branch point between Presidents Obama and Trump. For Trump, less regulation, increased competition, and the free market serve as the best solutions. For Obama, expansion of coverage through the government was central to his strategy and worldview.

As Obama analyzed the 50 million previously uninsured, he divided them into three groups—those who were economically disadvantaged but didn't qualify for Medicaid, those who had more but still not enough to buy private insurance, and those who had difficulty affording coverage due to preexisting conditions—he embraced different plans and pathways for each.

To address the needs of those in the lower half of the uninsured population, there was Medicaid expansion. For those earning a bit more, there were the insurance exchanges, with major subsidies based on income. And for those previously excluded from coverage based on preexisting conditions, the president encouraged Congress to pass legislation outlawing this discriminatory practice entirely.

In all, the president placed seven "big bets" on the future of health care: two bets on covering America's 50 million uninsured and five bets targeting a combination of cost reduction and improved clinical outcomes.

He hoped that, as a package, the bets would succeed in changing the environment of American health care and the perceptions of everyone in it. Although President Trump and the Republican-controlled Congress may undo some of these bets, it is essential to recognize that the underlying problems won't disappear through repeal alone.

Big Bet 1: Covering the Forgotten

As Obama began structuring the provisions of health care reform, he set his sights first on the 18 million uninsured Americans who couldn't afford health insurance and yet didn't qualify for Medicaid. Although much of the funding for Medicaid is generated at the federal level, the program itself is delivered through the states. Therefore, the president's approach was to offer funding to every state in the union that agreed to expand Medicaid for individuals and families earning up to 138 percent of the federal poverty level. That's up to $15,000 for an individual and $32,000 for a family of four.

The federal poverty level is "a measure of income issued every year by the Department of Health and Human Services." It is *not* a measure for understanding how much money it takes to survive in America. If you're thinking that $32,000 isn't a lot for a family of four, you'd be right. But that's more than what half of all American wage earners take home each year.

The president knew that these are not America's unemployed or unmotivated. Many of them work long hours at tough jobs. They are food preparers and farmers, cashiers and bartenders, personal care aides and nursery workers, desk clerks and auto mechanics, taxi drivers and telemarketers, guidance counselors and security guards, barbers and building cleaners.

These individuals understand health insurance is important. But it's not their only bill in the mailbox. With a gross income of $32,000, these hardworking families also need to pay their taxes, rent, utilities, and transportation costs. They need to purchase food, clothing, and school supplies, along with other basic essentials. That doesn't leave them with much at the end of the month.

For that reason, expanding Medicaid for those least able to afford traditional insurance made the most sense. To accomplish that, the president offered each of the states enough money to fund nearly all of their incremental costs. And, naturally, he assumed all fifty states would jump on board, even knowing the payments would drop to 95 percent of the total cost in 2017 and ultimately 90 percent starting in 2020. But that's when he learned a tough lesson in politics.

Partisanship has a way of undermining even the best ideas and intentions. About twenty states, most of them Republican-controlled, declined the federal subsidy, refusing to expand their Medicaid programs. As a result, less than half of the targeted 18 million uninsured were enrolled in the program. So it is that politics (more than economics) will determine whether big bet number one ever pays out.

Big Bet 2: Covering the Excluded

The infamous paradox of the old health-insurance system was that the people who needed coverage the most—those with preexisting conditions—had the hardest time getting it. For decades, these were the people the health insurance industry tried hardest to avoid.

Barack Obama saw this exclusionary practice as health care's greatest absurdity, an injustice that he took very personally.

He often told the public about his mother in her final days, constantly worrying whether her health plan would cover the bills from her cancer treatments. He spoke of the fear she had waiting for the phone call that would eventually deny her claims, deeming her cancer a "preexisting condition."

In 2009, the president declared, "We need to end the practice of denying coverage on the basis of preexisting conditions . . . cherry-picking who to cover and who to deny, those days are over."

So he placed his second bet on the idea that covering all Americans, particularly those with chronic illnesses, would yield major economic and health benefits in the future.

Obama thought that if more people (even those with preexisting conditions) received preventive screenings, got appropriate treatment for their chronic diseases, had easier access to physicians, and avoided costly Emergency Room visits, the long-term savings would offset the initial expense of covering the millions of Americans that insurers previously denied.

Big bet number two had a name. It was called "guaranteed issue," and it required all insurance companies to accept and cover any individual who applied. What's more, insurers had to charge them a price that is comparable to what others pay.

At the same time, the president realized that if people could obtain coverage at will, then they might delay buying insurance until they became sick. It would mean missing out on the kinds of preventive services that would benefit patients the most. Further, it would unbalance the "risk pool" for insurers, making it impossible to cover all the newly insured sick people at a reasonable price. For this provision to work, there had to be a catch.

So Obama introduced the "individual mandate," requiring nearly everyone to buy health insurance or pay a penalty. After all, imagine being able to buy fire insurance while your home is ablaze, or getting auto insurance right after a collision. No insurer would go for that. Guaranteeing individual coverage would only work if everyone participated. This would prove to be one of the more hotly contested provisions in the ACA, going all the way to the Supreme Court before being upheld in 2012.

Current congressional leaders like guaranteed issue, and so do their voters. A 2012 Reuters-IPSOS poll indicated that 82 percent of Americans favored banning insurance companies from denying coverage to people with preexisting conditions. Upholding this provision was one of the first health care commitments President Trump made after the election. But here's where it gets tricky. The new Congress strongly *dislikes* the idea of forcing people to buy coverage. The question is: Can the two parts be separated without driving the price of insurance sky high?

Big Bet 3: Creating the Insurance Exchanges

The goal of the president's first two bets was relatively straightforward: provide coverage to those who need it the most (the relative poor and those with preexisting conditions) and hope that, over time, the economics of better health would deliver a return on investment for the country.

The next five bets were more like a parlay, linking several bets together in hopes of an even higher future payout—each designed to exert pressure on the health care system to improve clinical outcomes and make care more affordable.

Big bet number three addressed the segment of the population earning between $33,000 and $88,000, along with people working for businesses with fewer than fifty employees that, at the time, did not provide company-sponsored health insurance. Financial incentives included premium subsidies for individuals based on their annual incomes and tax credits for the smallest businesses.

However, the third big bet wasn't just about throwing credits and subsidies at the problem. It was about creating a whole new way to compare, understand, and buy health insurance.

Seeing how Amazon and Expedia had disrupted the retail and travel sectors, the president envisioned an online marketplace that could do the same for health insurance. These "insurance exchanges," elegant in their design, offer a broad array of plans with standardized benefits, creating the kind of information and cost transparency that encouraged enrollees to pick programs with the highest value to them.

If you've never been on an insurance exchange website, imagine a checkerboard. Along the top of the benefits page, you'll find a list of participating health plans. Vertically down the page, you can comparison shop across four "metal tiers," from platinum on down to bronze.

Horizontally, you can compare prices for the same type of product by insurance company and, in the small print, the providers (doctors and hospitals) available in each network. Vertically, the only difference from one metal tier to the next is how much of your health care cost is paid through your monthly premiums versus out-of-pocket payment. Details about the available plans make up the middle squares.

Like auto insurance, if you choose to pay a higher premium up front (the gold and platinum plans), you pay less out of pocket if something bad happens. However, if you want the basic package, you choose silver or bronze. With it, you have a more affordable premium, but you pay a lot more should you become sick and need to use your insurance. And by tying the subsidies to the two lower tiers, Obama hoped to provide incentives for people to take better care of themselves and be more demanding in their choice of providers.

In each square on the website, you'll find a price that can be easily compared to all the others and, in the margins, information on quality and user satisfaction, similar to the ratings you'd find on TripAdvisor or Hotels.com. And just as in the travel world, the exchanges let you pay more for a particular brand, if you wish, or select an alternative with more value. The choice is yours.

Looking back, the president could have taken a different tack. He could have established a review board, a selection process, and a predetermined price point, ultimately giving people a limited set of "government approved options." Instead, he bet on broad competition with a common set of benefits, transparent prices, and the freedom of choice. In other words, Obama chose consumerism.

He was optimistic that over time, the programs with the highest quality and lowest cost would dominate and the others would therefore disappear. And in the first few years, people did choose the lower-priced options while putting pressure on the companies that couldn't compete on overall performance.

But that's not all he hoped big bet number three would accomplish. The president was also banking on something even bigger happening down the road. That is, once employers saw people enjoying more choices and competitive prices on the individual exchanges, perhaps they would begin migrating all of their employees to this new model as well. And if that happened, competition on the exchanges would intensify, lowering prices even further while boosting quality and accelerating the impact of health care reform.

From a political perspective, this turned out to be a bad bet. The rapid rise in insurance-exchange prices just before the 2016 elections gave political ammunition to candidates who campaigned on the promise to repeal the ACA.

But with Obama's first three bets in place, President Trump inherited upon his election: (1) about 17 million newly insured Americans, (2) a guaranteed issue law prohibiting insurers from denying those with preexisting conditions, and (3) an established health insurance exchange tool in place.

Trump knew these provisions would be hard to repeal and even harder to replace, given the threat of a Democratic filibuster in the Senate. However, as I'll explain later, the exchange subsidies, the individual mandate, and funding for Medicaid expansion could be reduced through a simple majority vote (even without a replacement plan), moves that would greatly diminish the impact of these bets.

Big Bet 4: Caring for Seniors and Rewarding Excellence

Americans fifty to sixty-four years old spend an average of $3,869 out of pocket each year on insurance premiums and health care services. Over this fourteen-year stretch of their lives, out-of-pocket medical expenses amount to about $54,000. And unless you're on a publicly funded health plan, the federal government pays nothing toward it. However, on the day you turn sixty-five, the fed covers almost all of it.

One thing demographers know for sure is that twelve months from now, everyone who is alive will be a year older. Therefore, we know that roughly 3.65 million baby boomers will cross the Medicare threshold each year for the next fifteen years. Today, baby boomers are marching toward mandatory federal coverage at the astounding rate of 10,000 new enrollees each day. From the perspective of Medicare's budget, this is not the foretelling of a smooth transition. This has all the makings of a fiscal cliff.

The government has been insuring seniors ever since Congress enacted Medicare in 1965. The original form of this federal health insurance program, what is now called "traditional Medicare," was and remains a "fee-for-service" package. Seniors who enroll can go to any participating provider and the Centers for Medicare and Medicaid Services (the agency that administers the program) pays the physician directly, based on the number and complexity of services provided.

But beginning in 1978, Medicare beneficiaries were given a second option. Unlike traditional Medicare, patients enrolling in what would eventually be renamed "Medicare Advantage" pay an average monthly premium of $49 and receive their care through a health plan. In turn, CMS pays the insurance company an annual fee, based on the person's age and severity of underlying medical conditions.

Under Medicare Advantage, it's the health plan's responsibility to select the physician network or the specific medical group that will provide the care. And therefore, it's the insurance company that takes the risk, should the total cost of care exceed the $49 fee, plus the monthly payment from Medicare.

Obama appreciated the prepaid nature of this approach and perceived Medicare Advantage as a potential reform model for all of health care delivery. That's why he placed his fourth big bet on making an unprecedented modification to the program.

Shifting Perceptions Through Medicare Advantage

Through the Affordable Care Act, the president introduced "differential payments" into Medicare Advantage based on quality outcomes and patient satisfaction. And to measure the difference in quality and satisfaction, the administration introduced the "Five-Star Quality Rating System."

Organizations participating in the Medicare Advantage program are required to report quality and patient-satisfaction data to CMS annually. Based on this information, each Medicare Advantage plan is awarded one to five stars, information that is made readily available to seniors enrolling in the program.

Through the Medicare stars program, health plans with the highest quality and best customer service receive large, additional payments at the expense of the lower-rated programs. Most important, instead of doling out the added dollars incrementally (a little for one star, a bit more for two, and so on), all of the payments were targeted to those programs at or near the top. The president's big bet was that each year, more enrollees would select the four- and five-star programs. Consequently, the low performers would either have to improve dramatically or exit the market.

Big Bet 5: Integrating a Fragmented System

It took fifteen years after Medicare was passed by Congress for the major kinks to be ironed out. Policy experts predicted that would be a reasonable timeline for the Affordable Care Act, too. And there was a good reason for that. We can't, as a nation, structure the current delivery system from scratch. It needs to evolve from the existing design. But fifteen years is a very long time, politically speaking.

Just as Nixon had recognized decades earlier, President Obama understood that expanding coverage to millions of Americans would increase total health care costs, at least in the short run. By opening the exchanges to patients with preexisting conditions, Obama had flipped the old insurance practice of cherry-picking and lemon-dropping on its head. In doing so, he knew the exchanges would become a magnet for the nation's sickest (and most expensive) patients. As a result, he had to drive delivery-system improvement over the long haul, hoping that health care prices didn't become so unaffordable in the meantime as to threaten the solvency of the entire program. The president knew he was taking a chance and working with a delicate timeline. But he failed to understand how truly great the risk was, politically.

We can liken President Obama's strategy to surgery. Sometimes, doctors perform operations that make the patient sicker at first. They do this with the expectation that the patient will recover and be healthier in the future. The same approach was embedded in big bet number five: suffer through high costs in the short term with the expectation that, over time, clinical outcomes will improve and greater efficiency will bring costs back down. But in politics, as in surgery, things don't always happen according to plan. And unfortunately for Obama, this bet suffered two significant blows.

First, he miscalculated the financial impact of the exchanges on large insurers. Over the first two years of ACA implementation, most of the major health insurers struggled with the high costs associated with new enrollees. In 2017, insurers on the exchanges raised premiums for state-based plans by an average of 25 percent, according to the US Health and Human Services Department.

Second, Obama was forced to realize that even those rate increases wouldn't be enough to keep all insurers satisfied. The nation's largest insurer, UnitedHealthcare, dropped out of most of the exchanges, pointing to the higher risks and increased cost of insuring a sicker population of newly covered Americans. Indeed, the company had been taking a hit, reportedly losing $475 million from the exchanges in 2015, with an estimated loss of $500 million more the following year.

But United's exit from the exchanges wasn't even the most shocking development for the insurance marketplace. In a 2016 letter to the Department of Justice, Aetna's CEO wrote, "We believe it is very likely that we would need to leave the public exchange business entirely . . . should our deal ultimately be blocked."

The deal he referred to was the proposed merger of insurance giants Aetna and Humana, a consolidation effort that would likely ratchet up premiums and hurt competition, according to a lawsuit filed by the DOJ.

With the department's decision to block the merger, Aetna made good on its threat, announcing it would reduce its participation in the exchanges from eleven states to four, which is sixteen fewer than it had been planning for 2017. Similar to United, Aetna pointed to $430 million in losses since joining the exchanges in 2014. It's still unclear how much of this was hardball negotiations and how much was real economics. What's certain is that insurance choices are, as a result, considerably fewer. Observers estimated the number of insurance options offered through the online exchanges would drop from 232 to 167 in 2017.

Compounding this failure, the president's plan to spur competition at the delivery-system level experienced a major setback. As part of big bet number five, Obama's goal was to integrate care delivery through the introduction of an innovative new approach called Accountable Care Organizations, or ACOs.

Here's the concept in a nutshell: the ACO model pairs up independent primary- and specialty-care physicians with a hospital and aligns their financial incentives for greater efficiency through a single "capitated payment," that is, a payment in advance—made out to the combined hospital-and-physician organization—to cover all of the care required for a defined patient population.

Ideally, this new payment model would motivate providers to improve preventive- and acute-care services, eliminate waste, and prevent unnecessary hospitalizations. Then with the savings generated from this more efficient care, doctors, hospitals, and the government could reinvest those dollars toward even better care down the road.

It's a wonderful model, in theory. But as Mark Smith, president and CEO of the California Healthcare Foundation, says, "ACOs are like unicorns, beautiful in concept but yet to be seen in reality."

The ACOs that formed were different than the ones policy makers recommended to President Obama. Part of the mix-up was not the president's fault. For something so new and different, the best place to get the legislative details right would have been in the joint-conference committee. But because that option was null and void after the death of Senator Kennedy, the Senate's incomplete version of the ACO legislation passed, essentially unchanged.

That's been problematic for two reasons. The version that was enacted failed to clearly define which patients were assigned to a particular ACO, making population management difficult. It also failed to include restrictions on where and with whom patients could obtain care, forcing ACO providers to take on responsibility for the cost of care provided by those outside their organization.

The ACO Experiment

Based on the early returns, the ACO model has achieved mixed results. On the one hand, it has led to better quality outcomes at lower operational costs. That's the good news.

On the other hand, building an ACO requires major investments in new systems, technology, and leadership, which so far have offset the reductions in operating costs. So, although ACOs reported more than $460 million in savings in 2015 (the latest data available), the bottom-line impact is unclear.

Take a look at the Medicare Pioneer ACOs, the product of the Center for Medicare and Medicaid Innovation skunkworks. They exemplify how difficult the transition proves to be in practice. This particular ACO program was designed to attract the more sophisticated medical groups with existing prepayment experience and with much of the necessary infrastructure already in place. But of the thirty-two original Pioneer ACO participants, almost one-third left the program after one year, citing that the investment costs dwarfed the added incentive payments they received.

Following that effort, many groups participating in the Pioneer ACO program joined the Next Generation cohort, Medicare's newest ACO testing ground. Less than a year into the program, three of the twenty-one participants bailed.

The biggest problem for doctors and hospitals wanting to form an ACO is the transition period. When you try to create an ACO in a previously fragmented and bloated fee-for-service community, you start with far too many physicians. There may be eight orthopedic surgeons and six cardiologists on a staff to begin with, but as care gets more efficient, the ACO may only need four or five of each going forward. Imagine the ire of those left out.

The day after announcing the reduced staffing, any doctors excluded from the ACO would likely take their patients elsewhere. The hospital would see its revenues plummet and be forced to lay off staff. To avoid these problems, hospitals tend to keep everyone on the roster, thus limiting the probability of true delivery-system transformation. When the cost accounting is complete, the dollars saved through improvements in performance are more than offset by the added inefficiency and costs of retaining the extra physicians. In short, these programs have been a lot of work without much to show for it.

The future of ACOs is unclear, particularly during this political transition period. ACOs could compete on exchanges and in Medicare Advantage, offering more opportunities to improve the efficiency of health care delivery. Then again, doctors and hospitals may find the rigors of lowering costs too daunting. If that happens, they could just pivot and use their newfound size and market power to demand even higher rates of reimbursement, ultimately raising, not lowering, the total cost of health care.

Big Bet 6: Finding a Meaningful Use for Technology

Fortunately for the president, the need to digitize health care, his sixth big bet, brought out a rare form of bipartisanship on Capitol Hill. Most politicians agreed that to improve patient care, doctors need to have comprehensive, electronic access to patient information.

Obama believed that patients shouldn't have to restate their entire medical history or reiterate their prescriptions to every new doctor simply because the answers they had already given were stored in a different doctor's paper folders. Likewise, patients shouldn't have to repeat costly tests just because their new doctor can't easily access the previous ones. Paper records, he realized, lead to mistakes and inefficiencies.

The president insisted this information should be stored securely in a private medical record, available to all doctors for meaningful purposes. These systems would allow care providers to communicate with their colleagues and transmit prescription requests. And they would allow patients to schedule office visits easily and review their clinical information online.

A law designed to do all of that had already passed earlier in 2009. The Health Information Technology for Economic and Clinical Health (or "HITECH") Act offered doctors $44,000 in subsidies to install a computer system in their office, under one condition. They had to agree to use the computer system for "meaningful uses" that improve patient care rather than just helping doctors manage their back-office billing and accounting.

Had the HITECH Act not passed in parallel with the ACA, it would no doubt have been among President Obama's most pressing reform matters. In his speeches, Obama often cited a quip from his political rival Newt Gingrich: "We do a better job tracking a FedEx package in this country than we do tracking a patient's health records." They both understood that something had to change.

The Impact of Meaningful Use

Although technology drives nearly every aspect of American industry, look behind the reception desk in nearly half of all American doctors' offices and you'll find a maze of file folders stuffed with patient information, just as it was twenty, thirty, and forty years ago. The president recognized both the potential for better care with modern computer systems and health care's inability to progress without them.

Back in 2007, then presidential candidate Barack Obama pointed out, "At the Veterans Administration, where it used to cost $9 to pull up your medical record, new technology means you can call up the same record on the Internet for next to nothing. But because we haven't updated technology in the rest of the health care industry, a single transaction still costs up to $25, not one dime of which goes toward improving the quality of our health care."

If we brought our entire health care system online and did so securely, the president added that America "would be saving over $600 million a year on health care costs." It's not entirely clear where he got that number. But if he had included the computerized benefits that come with improved prevention, the impact of seamlessly coordinating care, and the advantages of rapid intervention, the actual savings would be an order of magnitude greater—more like $600 billion.

Almost a decade later, in spite of the vast amounts of money invested in information technology, net-dollar savings haven't materialized. The reality is that without transforming care delivery, computer upgrades themselves don't add much value. Today, rather than improving physician performance, electronic health records mostly just slow doctors down.

Enter "Meaningful Use Stage 2," with incentives for enhancing the interoperability of computer systems in the future.

It's a promising next step, but, as you'll see in the next chapter, unless the large electronic health-record companies are willing to open up their systems to third-party developers, the effects will be limited. And until the medical records from all doctors are linked together and made easily viewable, digital systems will remain relatively ineffective. Physicians are too busy to manually input another doctor's records. It just takes too much time.

What the Republican Congress and President Trump will do in this area is not yet clear. Forcing change through regulation is antithetical to their proposed economic plans, and yet without moving health care into the modern world, the dollars generated through their economic programs will be consumed by the rising costs of medical coverage, something businesses across the country won't be able to overcome.

Until a truly comprehensive set of medical information is made available to all doctors and hospitals rendering care, these computer systems will continue to increase health care expenses, not diminish them. The nation had no choice but to make this bet. So far, we have yet to collect on it.

Big Bet 7: Measuring Quality and Effectiveness

"We have the best medical schools, the most sophisticated labs, the most advanced training of any nation on the globe," the president said in one of his final ACA sales pitches. "Yet we're not doing a very good job harnessing our collective knowledge and experience on behalf of better medicine."

Indeed we are not. Less than 1 percent of US health care spending goes toward examining the most effective treatments, leaving too many doctors and patients to make life-altering decisions without the information they require.

We can't expect drug and device companies to provide objective information on drug and device effectiveness or value. And there's little chance the medical-specialty societies will voluntarily commit to evidence-based approaches to care delivery, not when more efficient and effective approaches reduce the incomes of their members.

To address this vacuum, the president placed one final big bet: the Patient Centered Outcomes Research Institute (PCORI). Using public and private funding, this program selects, designs, and conducts clinical effectiveness research that compares drugs, devices, medical interventions, and different delivery-system approaches.

This was a massive wager. It was also a hedge against his other bets. Even if the United States fell short in its efforts to change the structure of health care through the insurance exchanges, Medicare Advantage, or the ACOs, this bet could still have an enormous impact on American health.

The president expected PCORI to clarify which approaches achieve better health outcomes for patients at a lower cost. He hoped that all doctors would follow its recommendations and embrace the approaches shown to be most effective. But in retrospect, President Obama and his staff underestimated the power of the legacy players to resist change.

Today, when drug or device companies want to introduce a new (and often expensive) medication or technology, they must demonstrate that it's safe and effective. That's it. They're not required to prove it's any better than products that already exist.

PCORI is tasked with stepping in and making that type of comparison, disseminating the results, and recommending the best options.

Doctors recognize that a brand-name drug is identical to and no better than its generic counterpart. Nonetheless, physicians often end up prescribing the name-brand version, thanks to a combination of drug-company advertising (which drives consumer preference and demand for the more expensive medications) and something called "drug detailing" (when pharmaceutical representatives come to doctors' offices to promote their products and leave samples). Drug reps will tell you these detailing visits are about offering clinical expertise. Watch them in action, and you'll conclude their true desire is to market their company's most expensive options.

Today, the pharmaceutical industry enjoys massive profits and minimal interference, thanks to long periods of patent protection for name-brand drugs, the freedom to introduce them without any proof of added efficacy. And for the drugs that already exist, monopolistic pricing has become the norm.

For example, take Avastin, a medication approved for cancer treatment by the Food and Drug Administration. It slows the growth of new blood vessels that feed tumors. A while back, a thoughtful group of ophthalmologists recognized that if this drug could limit blood-vessel proliferation to stop tumor growth, it might also be useful in slowing a medical problem called wet macular degeneration, a chronic eye disease that blurs vision and leads to blindness, particularly in older patients. It happens because of an overgrowth of abnormal blood vessels in the back of the eye.

The ophthalmologists were injecting a very small dose of Avastin in their macular-degeneration patients with excellent clinical results and an average cost per treatment of about $60.

Here's where it gets interesting. Genentech, the manufacturer of Avastin, recognized the same opportunity at about the same time as the ophthalmologists. But instead of seeking FDA approval of Avastin for wet macular degeneration, Genentech created Lucentis, a drug with a biologically active component identical to Avastin. Once Genentech received FDA approval for Lucentis, it priced the drug at $2,300 a dose and tried to prohibit ophthalmologists (or anyone else with a low-cost solution) from obtaining or administering the much cheaper option, Avastin.

Ophthalmologists were outraged. Not surprisingly, when the National Eye Institute tested Lucentis against Avastin, it found essentially no difference for a drug priced nearly forty times higher.

"It's perfectly understandable for a corporation to try and make a profit," President Obama said, "but when those profits are soaring higher and higher each year while millions lose their coverage and premiums skyrocket, we have a responsibility to ask why."

Will PCORI Succeed? Will It Survive?

There are legitimate reasons that some drugs and devices cost more. But it's now more and more common for manufacturers to dramatically hike up prices even when the magnitude of clinical improvement is minimal or, in the case of Lucentis, nonexistent. Increasingly, drug companies are buying the rights to medications that have been in use for decades for the sole purpose of raising their prices, often between 200 and 500 percent, and effectively shutting out the competition.

We can begin to rein in these practices, the president said, by demanding that pharmaceutical companies disclose the true cost of drug development as part of the FDA-approval process. If they did, regulatory agencies and PCORI could then use that information to evaluate the appropriateness of the price in the context of the medication's value and the R&D dollars spent. Further, the FDA could require that all new agents and devices be tested against existing approaches so that pricing and incremental value can be measured, and thus make that information available to consumers.

It all seems very logical. However, it's unlikely we're going to see any of this come to fruition, because the legacy players, particularly big drug companies, will fight it tooth and nail, flexing their political and economic muscle to impede the legislative process.

President Obama thought that by creating a comparative evaluation tool, he could persuade America's most profitable companies—those with ample R&D budgets—to dedicate more of their research dollars toward finding the best treatments for patients, including those with rare and neglected diseases. That hasn't happened.

To put the consequences of this problem in perspective, here's an excerpt from an e-mail I received a couple of years back. It came from Susan Fiorella, a colleague of mine and mother of three:

> Nineteen months ago, I thought I was the mother of three healthy children. Suddenly our lives changed forever. One day, my beautiful, playful 2½-year-old son Jacob seemed to be suffering from a stomach bug. As the hours passed, he grew increasingly lethargic. We took him to his doctor's office where we were told that Jacob's vital signs were abnormal. Moments later an ambulance was called.

We raced to our local Children's hospital, where we were met by a team of exceptional physicians and nurses. We learned that Jacob was suffering from hydrocephalus—a word we had never heard before.

As Susan goes on to explain, hydrocephalus literally means "water on the brain." As fluid accumulates in the brain's ventricles, the pressure intensifies.

"Jacob's brain was being crushed against the inside of his skull," she wrote.

Her son was dying and required emergency surgery, which helped to bring his intracranial pressure down to a safe level. But the experience damaged the areas of Jacob's brain that control his lower extremities and sense of balance. Susan hoped that after months in the hospital, and hundreds of physical- and occupational-therapy appointments, her son would recover and that their lives could return to normal. Then she shared some unfortunate news.

"Four months ago he started vomiting and required another emergency brain surgery to reduce the rising pressure. We now realize that there is no permanent cure for hydrocephalus. At any moment, without warning, excessive fluid can accumulate again, threatening his life."

Susan was shocked to learn that there's very little government funding to treat or even research new approaches for Jacob's condition.

As a physician and surgeon who has cared for hundreds of children with major congenital problems, I know that many mothers share Susan's concern and empathize with how helpless she feels. They, too, worry their child's problem will be ignored by the large drug and device manufacturers.

In the United States, 6,000 babies are born with or develop hydrocephalus each year. It affects more than 1 million Americans, from children to adults.

There are currently two treatment options for hydrocephalus but no cure. One is a surgery that was developed half a century ago. It requires a neurosurgeon to insert a silicone tube into the fluid-filled space inside the brain (or "ventricle") before tunneling under the skin to the abdomen. Using a valve, this shunt system diverts excess fluid to the abdominal area, where it can be resorbed back into circulation. However, approximately 40 percent of these shunts fail within two years, and 98 percent fail within ten years. When that happens, doctors are forced to replace the entire system.

The second approach is newer, but applicable only to a small subset of children. And although the alternative procedure eliminates the need for a permanent tube, the risk of obstruction can be life-threatening, as in Jacob's case.

Given the reach of this medical problem and its subpar treatment options, one might expect that finding a better solution would be a high research priority. It's not. What frustrates Susan and her family is that hydrocephalus is as common as Down's syndrome but gets one-thirtieth the public research funding. Parkinson's disease, which affects a population comparable to that of hydrocephalus, receives $200 million in National Institutes of Health funding, more than triple the amount for hydrocephalus research.

It is not clear why the government isn't funding more research for this devastating medical problem, but it is clear why medical-device manufacturers aren't. The reason is purely economic.

In the United States, publicly traded drug and device companies fund almost two-thirds of all medical research. When deciding which investments to make, they consider three strategic priorities: money, volume, and risk.

First, they ask which drugs are likely to command the highest prices, which can be protected through a combination of patents and aggressive marketing tactics. This criterion eliminates any clinical problem with relatively inexpensive solutions, particularly ones that are easy to copy. Second, they ask which diseases affect a large population of patients. This allows companies to maximize their total drug or device revenue, even when their unit price is not exorbitant. And third, they ask which solutions can be created with the least amount of investment and with the highest probability of finding a receptive market. That means instead of trying to solve difficult clinical issues through major R&D investments, drug and device companies prefer to make a minor modification to an existing drug, patent its successor, and invest most of the dollars in marketing and sales.

These three priorities are why developing a newer "smart valve" to treat Jacob's problem won't be attractive to most medical-device companies.

The president knew that to improve quality of life and control the expense of medical treatment for all Americans, we would need a better system for identifying, prioritizing, and funding medical research. But he also knew that taxing these drug and device companies to generate the dollars needed for an independent research group would be heavily resisted.

The new Congress and president are likely to move away from greater governmental regulations and restrictions for the drug industry, viewing the development of new medications and devices as essential for the country. At the same time, if Trump and congressional leaders want to improve the health of more Americans, they will need to make sure drug and device companies actually invest in research and development, and lower their prices when they don't.

Perception and Health Care Reform

Major legislation tends to undergo modification and improvement over several years. That was President Obama's long-term plan for the Affordable Care Act. Rather than "repeal and replace," as his successor promised, Obama envisioned something more along the lines of "modify and improve."

In a 2016 article written for the *Journal of the American Medical Association*, Obama assessed the headway of his signature legislation. "I am proud of the policy changes in the ACA and the progress that has been made toward a more affordable, high quality, and accessible health care system," he wrote. "Despite this progress, too many Americans still strain to pay for their physician visits and prescriptions, cover their deductibles, or pay their monthly insurance bills; struggle to navigate a complex, sometimes bewildering system; and remain uninsured."

It was a candid critique for a sitting president, and a very accurate reflection of the challenges that remain.

Looking back on his landmark legislation, perhaps Obama wishes he had taken a less diplomatic and collaborative approach. Had he tried to drive health care reform by fiat, rather than with compromise and incentives, he would have had the congressional mathematics to pull it off. Such an approach would likely have made it more difficult for the new president to reverse key provisions. Most likely, Obama is now second-guessing his decision.

In all, the former president made seven big bets on the future of health care. Some of them promised quick payoffs. Others were designed to pay out over a decade or more.

Looking at the "win" column, we see coverage expansions for three groups: the poor through Medicaid, young adults up to age twenty-six under their parents' plan, and patients with preexisting medical problems. In addition, Medicare's five-star system has achieved the goal of moving enrollees into the higher-performing programs, while the online exchanges have given health insurance coverage to 10 million individuals.

The president's bet on technology has been more of a "push." Computers are more prevalent in doctors' offices today, but improvements in patient care have been relatively minimal. For other bets, including ACOs and comparative research efforts, little has been achieved, and the future of these programs is in serious doubt under the new administration.

The Affordable Care Act and Beyond

The 2016 general election campaign will go down in history as one of the most contentious and polarizing ever. The ACA legislation has been a lightning rod since its implementation, attracting powerful surges of emotion from all sides of the American political spectrum.

Historians will debate for years how the 2016 election could have ended as it did, given that polls overwhelmingly predicted a different outcome. In many ways, the outcome was analogous to what happened in England during the so-called Brexit debate, which led to Britain's withdrawal from the European Union, despite the strong urging of most governmental leaders to stay.

The best explanation for the unexpected results in the United States boils down to a combination of general discontent among many citizens and their deep-seated distrust of the traditional political process.

I realized the full depth of these emotions when I participated in a panel discussion at the University of Chicago. Held on Halloween of 2016, just days before the election, the session was titled, "The Affordable Care Act: Trick or Treat?" As I listened to others on the panel and fielded questions from the audience, I was shocked by how inaccurately some in the medical community were describing the legislation some six and a half years after it had been signed. The gap between perception and the reality of the Affordable Care Act was far wider than I previously imagined.

The first misperception concerned the impact of the ACA on patient health. Even though the legislation had effectively lowered the rate of uninsured to the lowest in our nation's history, the tally of all of the beneficiaries amounted to only 5 percent of the US population.

So when the audience in Chicago questioned why the legislation has not yet had a greater impact on the country's overall health, the answer lay in simple mathematics. Even a 30 percent improvement in the health of the 17 million newly insured would result in almost no statistical change in the health of the country as a whole.

Equally straightforward was the answer to why policyholders were projected to experience large premium increases in 2017. When you insure millions of people with preexisting medical conditions and price their care as if they were of average or even reduced risk, the initial rates would surely be unsustainable. Ultimately, prices had to reflect the cost of providing care to the newly insured.

These realities were relatively easy to understand, and yet few of the critics acknowledged either the calculus or the consequences of guaranteed issue. It was then I realized opposition to President Obama's health care reform law was as much about people's dissatisfaction with their own health care experience—the high costs, inconveniences, and lack of transparency—as it was about the legislation itself.

When out-of-pocket costs continued to rise for people, many faulted the ACA, rather than the underlying cost inflation. When doctors were forced to see more patients than before to maintain their incomes, they too pointed at the ACA, rather than the underlying inefficiencies of the health care system. And when insurers narrowed their networks, everyone concluded the ACA was the culprit, if only because both changes happened at around the same time.

As such, the ACA proved to be a bellwether for much of the country's mood and mindset leading up to the general election. For doctors and patients alike, it had become a convenient target for their political and economic frustrations. Indeed, the ongoing and vitriolic dialogue that suffused the first few years of Obamacare implementation served as a metaphor for many of the problems in America, a symbol of the nation's broad unhappiness with the status quo.

This is the struggle our new president now inherits: Address the cost issues, and unhappiness will grow. Ignore them, and many of the economic plans he seeks to accomplish will be impossible as dollars continue to get shifted from American workers back to health care's legacy players.

In general, candidates support legislative changes that are favorable to the constituency that elected them. Many of President Trump's supporters—particularly in states such as Pennsylvania, Michigan, Ohio, and Wisconsin—will face serious economic challenges if insurance coverage is reduced in breadth, if deductibles continue to rise, or if subsidies are lowered or eliminated.

That's why repealing the ACA without a carefully crafted replacement plan will be politically dangerous for President Trump. But in the context of a president elected to create jobs, lower taxes, and weed out government interference, the prospect of a financially viable replacement remains, at best, an uncertainty.

The New President's Plan

As the 2016 presidential election taught us, prognostication is a dangerous endeavor. However, we can make a few reasonable guesses about the factors influencing Trump's key health care decisions. First, any plan that threatens to take away coverage from newly insured Americans will face stiff resistance. Second, the oft-recited mantra "repeal and replace" will prove easier said than done. Third, in light of that fact, Congress will stop short of attempting a complete ACA overhaul. Instead, it will likely take steps to reshape key ACA provisions. Many policy experts predict that "repeal but delay" (or, perhaps, "repair without repeal") will be the safest middle ground. It would give Congress and the president two to three years to reach a compromise with Democrats while delaying the impact of major changes until after the 2018 midterm elections.

I write this chapter amid the transition of power to President Trump. Readers will have the advantage of knowing what the new president actually does in the months and years ahead. At the same time, we should remember that today's health care difficulties evolved over a half century. Therefore, we need to be cautious when assuming that short-term happenings portend future events. If you have any doubt, just ask the previous commander in chief.

Whichever path President Trump and the new Congress choose, we can expect that solving the political calculus will prove more difficult than delivering campaign rhetoric. There is a well-known political aphorism that candidates campaign differently than they govern once elected. And so it will be as the next chapter in American health care policy is written.

The election of Donald Trump affects all of Barack Obama's big bets. As with the former president, Trump's background and life experiences have shaped his perceptions. This will no doubt influence his health care approaches and policies.

In many ways, the current president is unlike any other in our nation's history. At age seventy, he is the oldest first-time president and the only person to assume the role having never served an elected public position. He is a businessman and a reality TV host with both huge successes and multibillion-dollar failures. Although he ran as a Republican, he has at different times in his life been a registered Democrat and even considered running for president under the Reform Party ticket in 2000, eventually withdrawing his candidacy well before Election Day.

Trump has been described by *Politico* as "eclectic, improvisational and often contradictory." He has taken up differing positions on progressive taxation, abortion, and the role of government in health care. Unlike Barack Obama, whose positions on most issues had been consistent and predictable from the outset, Trump's plans for the next four years remain largely speculative.

The one certainty is that change will happen. And even if we can't be sure at this moment exactly what change will look like, we can predict the most likely overall direction.

Trump's Take on the Big Bets

Starting with FDR, decades of former presidents have talked about health care as a fundamental human need. When I awoke the morning after the 2016 presidential election, I had dozens of messages from concerned patients, all of them asking me whether they would be able to maintain or afford health coverage for themselves and their families in the future.

Given his approach to business, President Trump will likely look for ways to reduce the federal government's role in the health care process.

For example, Trump has indicated that he may try to reverse the Medicaid expansion implemented through the ACA and replace it with "block grants," money from the national government handed over to state authorities with fewer stipulations for its use.

On the other hand, as a pragmatist, Trump is likely to retain two of the most popular parts of the ACA: coverage provided for children and young adults up to age twenty-six under their parents' insurance plan, and the prohibitions that prevent insurers from excluding individuals with preexisting disease.

Still up in the air are policies Trump championed during the election campaign that would face heated resistance from the legacy players and potential filibuster on Capitol Hill. Examples include (1) legalizing the interstate sale of insurance products, (2) reversing the ban on patients buying medications from other countries, and (3) allowing the federal government to negotiate lower drug prices on behalf of Medicare beneficiaries.

Reconciliation Versus New Legislation

If you recall what happened when the Affordable Care Act first passed the House in 2009, President Obama had sixty votes in the Senate, a "supermajority," which effectively shut down Republican opposition. But when the late Senator Kennedy's seat was replaced by Scott Brown, the number of Democratic votes remaining dropped to a level that would subject the ACA to certain Republican filibuster and likely failure. Without the sixtieth vote needed, Senate and House Democrats opted for the alternative path of budget reconciliation, needing only fifty-one votes in the Senate to enact the legislation but requiring the House to pass the Senate's version unchanged.

Now the tables have turned, and President Trump will need to think through the same political calculations. Under the new administration, Republicans can't repeal the Affordable Care Act outright without a supermajority in the Senate, which currently seats fifty-two Republican senators. If they try to pass entirely new legislation and replace what exists without recruiting Democratic votes, the attempt will surely be blocked. However, through reconciliation, the US Congress can undo several of Obama's big bets.

Reconciliation only applies to legislation that is solely dependent on tax revenue or other forms of governmental expense. As such, the ACA policies most at risk are the expansion of Medicaid, subsidies provided through the exchanges, the individual mandate, the medical-device tax, and the Cadillac tax, that 40 percent excise tax on high-end health-insurance plans.

In the end, both Presidents Obama and Trump understand that health-insurance coverage, although essential, is not the fundamental problem facing American medicine. The most important challenge for the nation is health care's rising cost. Trump knows these costs have hurt American jobs and wages. For the rest of his agenda to be successful, he will need to figure out a path to flatten the rate of health care inflation. As business professors like to say, "Unsustainable trends can't continue forever." It is simply a mathematical and economic reality.

Beyond Politics: What Tomorrow Will Bring

It would be understandable, given the emotional roller-coaster ride of the 2016 elections, to assume that the fate of American health care—if not all of America—hinges almost entirely on the policies shaped inside the White House and on Capitol Hill. No doubt, the decisions President Trump and the 114th US Congress make will have a tremendous influence on the future. But we would be remiss to discount the decisions facing doctors and patients, many of which are free from the happenings in Washington, DC. Ultimately, four questions will determine the health and well-being of our nation.

1. Will the Expectations of Patients Change in the Future?

Across the United States, fragmented, inconvenient, and episodic health care has been the norm. Advances in health information technology have lagged, forcing patients to accept inconveniences they wouldn't from almost all other major industries. Doctors continue to practice in small offices and without the economies of scale necessary to simultaneously raise quality and lower costs.

As such, the price for America's outdated care-delivery system continues to escalate, putting the squeeze on more patients each year. Although the new administration has the power to affect the models of care delivery and insurance coverage, patients will need to decide whether to select the highest-rated programs through Medicare Advantage and the exchanges, or cling instead to the failed models of the past.

2. Will Care Providers and Insurance Companies Embrace New Reimbursement Models?

For transformation to occur, health care will have to move from a fee-for-service reimbursement model to one with prospective payment. There are two options to do so, both of which have been proven to emphasize the quality, rather than the quantity, of patient care.

The first option is a bundled payment. That's a single payment made on the basis of expected costs for clinically defined episodes of care. The financial equivalent would be purchasing an all-expense-paid vacation, including airfare, hotels, meals, and tips. Under this approach, when a patient is admitted to a hospital for a total-hip replacement or heart surgery, all the services provided during that admission are lumped into one payment instead of being billed separately. Advocates of bundled payment say the reimbursement method discourages delays in care for hospitalized patients, encourages coordination across providers, and improves quality.

The second option is capitation. This is a payment that funds all of the medical care needed by a population of patients for a specific time period, usually a year. It's like a maintenance program for your car that covers everything from routine services to "end-to-end" repairs if something goes wrong.

Both options make more sense and align incentives better than the traditional fee-for-service model. But each is likely to prove far more contentious than today's system. Physicians and hospitals will need to agree on how to divvy up the dollars. And they will inevitably need to move dollars from specialists who treat medical problems when they arise to primary-care physicians who help patients avoid medical problems in the first place. And when it comes to money, what seems fair to one person is perceived as problematic to another, particularly to those who will personally lose income.

3. Will Doctors Make the Changes Necessary to Realize the Benefits of Technology?

The advantages of technology are obvious. Health-IT allows patients to actively participate in their own care and the decisions that affect them the most. Comprehensive electronic health records provide physicians

with the information they need to treat patients without delay and with
maximal regard for patient safety. Secure e-mail allows patients and physicians to communicate more easily. Video care enables patients to receive
medical treatment conveniently and at a lower cost.

Few patients today have these benefits and conveniences available to
them. Only half of all physicians have installed an electronic health-record
system, and few use it to enable secure e-mail, video, or direct scheduling
of office visits. Often, office computers serve mainly as a billing tool or an
expensive paper record, and they will do so until physicians are willing to
modify how they practice.

4. Will Our Definition of the "Best" Medical Care Reflect Our Modern Realities?

A decade ago, solo practitioners and small community hospitals were
thought to be the acme of medical-care delivery. We now understand
that teams of doctors working together achieve superior outcomes, provide expanded specialization and expertise, and offer greater convenience
and more rapid access.

In the past, we thought care "close to home" produced the best results.
We now know that higher-volume facilities drive better outcomes and
that consolidation of smaller hospitals into larger centers-of-excellence
improves results. So far, hospitals that have closed their doors did so for
financial reasons, not as an approach to raise volume and improve quality
outcomes.

The history of health care is that of a rigid culture and slow-changing
perceptions. But perceptions can shift, particularly when context and circumstances allow. President Obama understood this and took the long
view on improving clinical outcomes. His big bets were designed to (1)
move the nation toward greater integration through programs like ACOs,
(2) reward care providers more for value than volume through Medicare
Advantage, and (3) increase consumerism through the exchanges.

So far, doctors and hospitals have struggled with making these transi-
tions, and with investing the time and resources necessary to see returns.

As we look toward the future, the economics of health care are shaping
up to be a classic example of the unstoppable force meeting the immovable object. The rising percentage of total dollars spent on health care
(unstoppable force) and the limited ability of government, businesses,

and individuals to pay for it (immovable object) are on a collision course. Something will need to give.

Compared to our GDP, health care costs are rising at a much faster clip. Twenty years from now, if nothing changes, health care will consume over 30 percent of our total expenditures. As Americans, we simply can't spend one-third of our gross income on our medical care. And with baby boomers qualifying for Medicare significantly faster than tax revenues can support, the federal government will have no choice but to use more of its budget on health care and Social Security, leaving less money for investments in other areas of our society.

Legacy players recognize the immense pressures they will experience as this happens. That's why large insurers are trying to consolidate. That's why drug companies are aggressively raising prices to maximize profits in the short run. And among doctors, that's why a growing percentage of them are opting for the protection and added clout of working in a hospital system or medical group.

The collision of these economic forces is inevitable. The next chapter offers a four-point plan for the future, one that has the potential to increase clinical quality, make care more convenient, and flatten the health care inflation curve. Each part of this plan will be difficult to achieve. But in total, it has the potential to effectively address our nation's (and our new president's) biggest health care challenges.

Chapter Seven

THE FOUR PILLARS
OF TRANSFORMATION

Two mothers need surgery. Both have problems with their hands. Both of their surgeons will fail to ask a crucial question. These omissions will cost each woman her life. Because of the error, one physician will face intense scrutiny, lose his license, and be sued for malpractice. The other will face no ramifications. When it's all said and done, two similar mistakes with the same tragic result will hurl the fates of two doctors in opposite directions.

American medical culture has a commanding and contradictory influence over how physicians perceive medical care and its consequences. When patients die, some omissions are seen as terrible, while others aren't. Some doctors are punished and others walk free.

I learned of one mother's death during my residency at Stanford. I was attending a surgical mortality and morbidity conference. There, we watched as a hand surgeon presented a series of clinical events in great detail, reliving the experience that killed his patient.

These conferences are meant to be objective, led by chiefs of quality for the betterment of medical practice. But to a physician whose patient suffered a complication, the experience feels deeply personal. At these proceedings, reputations and careers can be destroyed. As a junior resident, I could feel the intensity of the atmosphere, sensing the doctor's anxiety as he stood in front of his colleagues and began the narrative.

The woman had been washing dishes after dinner one evening while her kids were doing their homework, the doctor recalled from his notes. A glass broke in the sink, and as she reached for it, a shard lacerated her left hand, severing the flexor tendons to her ring finger. Inside the Emergency Department, a physician stopped the bleeding, and with the wound sewn up, the woman was told that because she had eaten dinner that night, she could not undergo surgery until the following day. She had already eaten dinner that night. She was referred to the hand surgeon for evaluation.

Well-trained, reputable, and respected, the physician who stood before us at the conference had performed this procedure hundreds of times. He scheduled her for outpatient surgery that afternoon. His plan was to do an axillary block for anesthesia, a technique used to numb the limb. (In today's age, an anesthesiologist would have been assigned to do the axillary block. In the 1970s, it was acceptable for a surgeon to do the entire procedure without additional anesthesia assistance.)

As the surgeon described the scene, everything in the Operating Room seemed in order. As he began the axillary block, ideal for operations of the hand, the physician identified an artery high up in the armpit area and placed a needle inside the sheath that surrounds both the artery and nerve. The doctor injected an anesthetic, which included adrenaline to prolong the agent's numbing effect. The doctor then placed a tourniquet about the upper arm, inflating it to stop blood flow to the hand.

In the Operating Room, a heart monitor positioned near his patient showed a regular, normal rhythm, or so the doctor thought.

Suddenly, the patient's heart overreacted. The ventricles started to contract faster and faster, and the beeping of the monitor accelerated until the woman's heart stopped beating altogether. An emergency team rushed in to resuscitate her, but it was too late.

At this point in the mortality and morbidity conference, the surgeon was being grilled with questions. I could feel the room getting warmer.

For physicians, it's not always clear what went wrong, even in hindsight. One of the surgeon's colleagues suggested that maybe, when placing the needle, he had injected the anesthetic with the adrenaline directly into a blood vessel, flooding the body and the heart with the stimulant. The surgeon assured the room that it could not have happened, as he had drawn back on the syringe to prevent this well-known complication.

No, this wasn't an intraoperative error. Rather, the error happened earlier that day in the surgeon's office, before the patient signed the form giving him consent to operate.

As the surgeon sat down with the woman for the preoperative visit, he asked almost all the right questions. He asked her which hand was her dominant. He asked her whether she had allergies and what she did for a living, all standard. But he forgot one.

The surgeon didn't ask whether she'd ever experienced heart palpitations. If he had, the woman would have said yes. And when she said yes, the surgeon would have contacted her primary-care physician and learned that the patient had an abnormality in the electrical system of her heart. It was mild, but present.

But he didn't ask. And not knowing she had an underlying heart problem, he didn't request that an anesthesiologist be present with him in the Operating Room. Most of the time, not asking a patient about heart palpitations wouldn't be a problem. This time, forgetting to ask proved fatal. To this day, the doctor no doubt regrets not asking that question.

The second mother was a neighbor of mine, a woman in her mid-fifties. She knocked on my door one afternoon. "I hate to bother you on your day off," she began.

A lot of conversations begin this way when you're a physician. It was no bother at all. I admit I enjoy informal consultations—an opportunity to share my expertise. Besides, people in my neighborhood often reciprocate whenever I'm stumped by handyman work or house repairs.

That day, however, I was worried by the visit. My neighbor and her husband weren't the kind to go to a doctor unless something really bothered them. Fortunately, my neighbor's medical problem was an easy one to diagnose and solve. While driving long distances, she said she experienced numbness in her thumb, index, middle, and half of her ring finger. Occasionally, these same symptoms would wake her up in the middle of the night.

Carpal tunnel syndrome, I told her. I gave her the names of a few hand surgeons I knew in the area. A couple of months later, she returned to my door with a pie she had baked and filled with blackberries from her garden. She smiled and thanked me, her symptoms now completely relieved.

Two years later, she knocked again with a different medical problem. "I hate to bother you."

This time, she looked different, not well. Her face had narrowed and her blouse hung loose. She told me a chest X-ray had shown an abnormality, which had been diagnosed as metastatic colon cancer. My neighbor stopped by, hoping I could give her a more optimistic opinion than the one her oncologist did. Unfortunately, I couldn't. Six months later, she died, leaving behind her husband and two sons.

Prevention experts recommend screening for colorectal cancer beginning at age fifty. Because my neighbor rarely went to the doctor, no physician had ordered one. But the hand surgeon who fixed her carpal tunnel could have. He just didn't ask. If he had, he would have learned she had not been screened. He would have referred her to a gastroenterologist, who would have found the tumor two years ago, back when it might have been curable. From afar, this death and the previous one should have been judged equally negligent, as both were preventable.

But in the second case involving my neighbor, there was no morbidity and mortality conference for the surgeon, no review of her death, and no malpractice suit. Perhaps the surgeon saw my neighbor's obituary in the newspaper. If he remembered her, he would likely have been saddened. But I doubt he would have considered himself responsible.

We could criticize both surgeons for their omissions and blame these unfortunate deaths on their individual failures. Had they asked the right questions, both patients would have lived and two tragedies would have been avoided. But each doctor acted no differently than his colleagues would have under the same circumstances. These two just were unlucky.

Rather than blaming these individual physicians, we need to address the real culprit: the health care system in which they operated. The care structure and information systems that could have saved these women's lives should be readily available in every physician's office today. Unfortunately, they're not. In most parts of the country, the health care system remains relatively unchanged from the past.

Christy Saved a Life

In 2006, we began installing a comprehensive electronic health record system in every Kaiser Permanente medical center and hospital in the United States. The goal was to provide all 17,000 of our physicians with immediate access to the medical records of our 10 million patients coast to coast. It was a bold and challenging task at the time.

Although the physicians could recognize how this information would improve care delivery, motivating the support staff to embrace the new system proved a much harder task.

Medical assistants in every office are expected to greet patients, escort them to the exam rooms, check their vital signs, and complete any necessary paperwork. With the introduction of the computer, they now had to update each patient's medical record, check the status of the person's preventive services, and schedule any outstanding screening tests.

Prior to the introduction of the computer system, medical assistants had far fewer steps to follow. They wrote down the patient's pulse, blood pressure, and weight on the front of the paper record, and then told the doctor the reason for the patient's visit. Now they had to spend several more minutes each time they brought a patient into an exam room to make sure everything was complete. Reviewing and updating the electronic health record seemed like a lot of extra work.

I knew these improvements in patient care were essential, but I wasn't sure how to win the hearts of the staff. About a year after the switch, I got my answer.

I was walking through the ophthalmology department at our Stockton Medical Center around lunchtime. I could see a meeting had begun. Several doctors had gathered in a large conference room, joined by dozens of medical assistants, receptionists, and nurses.

Discreetly, I took a seat in the back. Up in the front row, a woman caught my eye. She was dressed up and wearing a corsage. The chief of ophthalmology asked her to join him at the front of the room. He began telling a story about a patient named Sarah with glaucoma.

He explained that Sarah came to the medical center every few months to have her eye pressure measured and her medications renewed. Each time Sarah visited the department, a medical assistant named Christy was there to check her in and obtain the important ocular-pressure measurements. I quickly realized that Christy, the medical assistant he was talking about, was the woman with the flowers on her wrist. I then noticed Christy's husband and kids sitting in the front row.

The chief of ophthalmology went on to describe a recent afternoon when Sarah arrived for her regular appointment. Christy asked Sarah to put her face into a machine and look at an image in the distance. Suddenly, a puff of air shot at her eyeball, allowing the device to calculate the pressure in the eye's anterior chamber. And as she had recently been taught, Christy entered the information—not on a piece of paper but into the new electronic health record. And when she did, she also reviewed Sarah's preventive screening information.

Christy could see that Sarah was due for a mammogram, a test recommended every one to two years for women in her age group. With a friendly smile, Christy informed Sarah she did not need an appointment. Rather, she could just walk one floor down to the radiology department and have it done as soon as her ophthalmology visit was over.

"But the next time Sarah came back," the ophthalmologist continued, "Christy saw that the preventive screening test had remained undone. So, she asked Sarah's doctor to let her know when the eye exam was complete. Afterward, Christy walked Sarah down to the radiology department and waited with her until she had gone into the mammography suite."

To some people, what Christy did might seem a bit pushy. And to her fellow medical assistants, this probably would have felt overly time-consuming and beyond the normal scope of their work.

But Christy realized that Sarah's problem wasn't that she was lazy or forgetful. Clearly, the two-minute walk down to the radiology department wasn't the barrier. And neither was the cost, as the preventive test was covered by her insurance.

Christy understood that Sarah was afraid. So she did what was needed to quell Sarah's fear. And it proved to be an incredibly important choice.

Although most screening mammograms don't show cancer, Sarah's did. Within forty-eight hours, she had a biopsy done and her cancer was diagnosed. The surgery went well. And with no evidence of spread to the lymph nodes, the chances of Sarah being cured were excellent.

As the ophthalmologist handed the microphone over to Christy, he asked her to describe the experience in her own words. She looked embarrassed, uncomfortable in the spotlight. Christy said, "I was only doing my job. I just checked the preventive screening list and made sure that Sarah got what she needed."

The ophthalmologist quickly pointed out, however, that nowhere in Christy's job description was she expected to personally escort a patient down to radiology for a mammogram.

He then handed her a medallion. On it was an engraving that read "I Saved A Life." Christy's eyes welled up with tears. She took a moment to collect herself and thanked her colleagues, explaining how much this recognition meant to her. Christy confessed that she hadn't had an easy life. In her late teens, she became a young mom and never had the opportunity to attend a four-year college. She later enrolled in a medical-assistant training program, convinced that it was the only way to get a job with a steady income and benefits for her family.

"I really never imagined I would have the chance to save a life one day."

Most doctors aren't comfortable showing their emotions in the workplace. But that day, even some of the crustiest and most curmudgeonly physicians were wiping tears from their eyes. I could tell this was no small event. And it's one I'll never forget.

As physicians, we sometimes take for granted experiences like these. For Christy, after the birth of her children, this recognition was the highlight of her life. And for Sarah, Christy is someone she will remember, gratefully, for decades to come.

Christy's story teaches us that health care must be both "high tech" and "high touch," virtues that in the right setting are complementary, not contradictory. Without the technology, Christy would not have known that Sarah needed the screening. Without the personal touch, Sarah might not have overcome her fears.

But there's more to this story. If Christy's celebration had been the only one that ever happened, we might conclude that her personal commitment was head and shoulders above that of her colleagues. But on my most recent visit to the Stockton Medical Center, I asked the physician in chief how many of these celebrations there have been. Almost two hundred last year alone, he said. Translate that across the nation, and we're talking about tens of thousands of lives saved every year.

Dedicated, caring people like Christy are attracted to health care. But how they act in a health care environment reflects as much on the system and culture in which they work as it does their personality, work ethic, or values.

Taking nothing away from individuals like Christy who go the extra mile, there's something bigger happening here—something that offers us a glimpse into what the future of health care might look like if we were to alter the context of medical-care provision across the United States.

Let's imagine that Christy and Sarah had met somewhere else, in a small doctor's office perhaps. Christy, with the same friendly disposition, same passion for her patients, and same medical-assistant skills she learned in school, would most likely not have saved Sarah's life.

Even if Christy had asked about the screening and described the location of the mammography center, she wouldn't know whether Sarah went or not. And if the ophthalmologist in Christy's office was paid on a fee-for-service basis—reimbursing him only to perform ophthalmology-related services—then Christy would not have been permitted to escort her to radiology.

After Christy's ceremony, saving a life became contagious for the medical assistants in Stockton. They couldn't wait for their opportunity.

Context makes a world of difference in what we see and what we do. It influences what we deem is important and what is not. This is as true for medical assistants and physicians as it is for patients and Uber drivers. Context can alter our perceptions and behaviors. It can inspire meaningful change in the right settings and hold people back in others.

A System from Scratch

Type "design your own running shoe" into a search browser and up pops a long list of websites offering that service. Designing your own shoe gives you the freedom to determine the stiffness, fabric, and color that's right for you. Of course, consumer customization isn't limited to sneakers. Type "design your own clothes" or "custom wedding rings" or "bespoke suits" and scores of personalized choices will cascade in front of you.

Unfortunately, we know by now that when it comes to something as complex and expensive as the American health care system, designing it from scratch simply isn't an option. That's the reality President Obama faced and the one President Trump now must confront as well. Still, let's imagine for a moment that it is possible. How would we proceed?

Would we want all of the doctors working in their own offices independently, or would we bring physicians from multiple specialties together in one place and encourage them to collaborate? Would we instruct them to write our medical information down on a piece of paper and file it away on a shelf, or would we prefer they compile all that information safely and securely into a comprehensive electronic system that's available to all physicians? Would we decide to pay doctors and hospitals based solely on how many procedures they perform, or would we pay them more for achieving superior outcomes? And would we prefer for our health care system to be led by the clinicians who provide our care, or by the legacy players?

Let's examine how differently things might have gone for the two mothers who died had they received their care in a health system designed from scratch.

The first patient's EKG (and the cardiologist's interpretation of it) would have been available digitally for all doctors throughout the system to see, probably with a treatment warning. And so, when she came in for her hand surgery, the system would have alerted the surgeon to her heart abnormality. In the case of the second patient, the physicians and staff caring for her would have been alerted that she required colon-cancer screening. And if they failed to order it, or if the patient didn't follow up on the referral, there would have been a follow-up message. As a result, both medical errors would have been avoided and, most likely, both of these women would have lived.

Putting the pieces together, if we were able to start all over and build a health care system from scratch for ourselves and our family, we'd begin by constructing moderately large medical office buildings, co-locating physicians from a variety of specialties, and bringing in services like laboratories and X-rays. We would install a computer system that's connected to all of the clinicians and diagnostic departments. We would pay physicians based on the excellence of their clinical outcomes—not just for treating acute and chronic illnesses, but also for avoiding medical problems and disease complications in the first place. And we would engage physician leaders like Drs. Diane Craig, Manny Rivers, Edward Greene, and Mona Hanna-Attisha to organize and coordinate the best possible care on behalf of ourselves and our families.

This last point is important. Leadership in health care demands that doctors figure out ways to make innovative and positive things happen that otherwise wouldn't.

Overcoming resistance and making change happen is what distinguishes leadership from management. Invariably, people will resist the transformation of health care. For doctors, resistance arises from the fear that too much will be asked of them. Skilled leaders understand that most people overestimate the difficulty and problems resulting from change. In turn, they underestimate the benefits. That's why the true test of successful leadership is best measured months or even years later. It is defined by whether those who dragged their feet at first would ever choose to go back to how things were done before. When leaders make the right things happen, the answer is always the same: let's leave the past in the past.

The Four Pillars of Health Care Transformation

As noted throughout *Mistreated*, the current health care system is broken. It most closely resembles a nineteenth-century cottage industry, with doctors working alone in small offices, disconnected from others, unaided by modern technology, and paid piecemeal for each service they render.

President Obama, consistent with his personal style, addressed this challenge by "tilting the board" in a new and particular direction. President Trump has a very different personality. He would like to overturn the board and start over. But if he approaches health care's economic problems through repeal without a sound replacement, some of the constituents who helped put him in office will redirect their anger toward him.

Patients are mistreated not because doctors or politicians want to do them harm. They're mistreated because the systems and cultures of medicine influence doctors to make decisions that don't produce the best clinical results. Phrased differently, if we put the same doctor in two different systems—the current one and the one we would create from scratch—a doctor in the current setting will harm many more patients than need be. And at the end of the day, the physician will go home feeling frustrated and unfulfilled.

The transformation of American health care into a more ideal system will be dependent on four major shifts. Each pillar of transformation can stand on its own. But most important is understanding how they work together, synergistically, to create a more efficient and effective model of care delivery in the future.

1. Health care will need to be integrated, both horizontally within specialties and vertically across primary, specialty, and diagnostic care.
2. Health care will need to be prepaid, moving away from pay-for-volume toward paying for value and superior outcomes.
3. Health care will need to be technologically enabled, with comprehensive electronic health record systems, patient access to medical information, and the ability to obtain care using mobile and video technologies.

4. Health care will need to be physician led, which will require greater leadership training and development.

These four pillars, simple in concept and design, can deliver the best outcomes for patients, enabling our nation to lead the world in quality outcomes, convenience, and service. And they can make health care more affordable for both individuals and the country as a whole.

Pillar 1: Physicians Working Together on Your Behalf

Health care will need to be integrated, both horizontally within specialties and vertically across primary, specialty, and diagnostic care.

The perfect model for health care delivery doesn't exist today. The leading systems and alternatives were all designed decades ago, each with its share of benefits and challenges.

In their 1995 book, *The Discipline of Market Leaders*, authors Michael Treacy and Fred Wiersema concluded that organizations must make one of three choices to be successful. They can focus on (1) customer intimacy, (2) product differentiation, or (3) operational excellence. Most health care organizations today have made their choice. In the future, the best organizations, those that will dominate American health care, will figure out how to lead in all three market disciplines.

Today's health care delivery happens in one of three venues, each with a history and culture that emphasizes a particular discipline.

There are community-based providers, mostly working in individual doctors' offices and smaller hospitals. Then there are the traditional academic medical centers (university clinics and hospitals) with their associated basic-science research laboratories. Finally, there are relatively large, integrated delivery systems with multispecialty medical groups and associated hospitals. These include such systems as the Mayo Clinic, Ochsner Health and Virginia Mason.

Let's take a closer look at each of these three models to better understand the context in which they operate.

Model 1: Community-Based Providers

The typical community doctor works alone or in a small group. This structure is conducive to Treacy and Wiersema's market discipline of "customer intimacy." In this setting, the doctor-patient relationship is personal and often long-lasting. The physician's office staff knows every patient by name.

The challenge is that the office's humble size limits (1) investments in technology, (2) broad collaboration with colleagues, and (3) "economies of scale," a factor that raises quality and drives down costs in the higher-volume health care settings.

Model 2: Academic Medical Centers

By contrast, university hospitals have relied on the value discipline of "product differentiation" above all else. Their buildings are huge. They attract patients with the promise of miracle cures from their research laboratories (even when little of the work itself is medically applicable). To accentuate their product differentiation, academic medical centers purchase the latest medical technologies and newest machines, which they advertise broadly.

Their challenges include the impersonal nature of a large, academic environment and the relative inefficiency of an academic model. Furthermore, over the past decade, university hospitals have lost a major competitive advantage in that recently trained specialists and many community hospitals can now perform the kinds of complex procedures once exclusive to academic medical centers.

As the authors point out in *The Discipline of Market Leaders*, organizations with greater customer intimacy (community doctors) and product differentiation (academic medical centers) have historically been able to charge a higher premium for their services. But as health care costs continue to rise, insurers are squeezing these two groups to lower prices. Both are having trouble responding to these changes and now face the threat of being excluded from insurers' ever-narrowing networks.

Model 3: Integrated Delivery Systems

The third group takes a different path than the other two, focusing mainly on "operational excellence." The structure of integrated delivery systems helps maximize collaboration and cooperation, thereby making the provision of care more efficient and effective. These delivery systems typically include a variety of physicians from different specialties who practice together in big, centralized medical buildings, often more functional than ornate. Their combination of greater size and fewer locations succeeds in lowering their costs, while higher patient volumes allow specialists to perfect their skills and improve outcomes.

Size has its disadvantages, too. A large integrated system can make the patient's experience seem less personal, more institutional. Meanwhile, the incomes of its doctors aren't dependent on generating patient referrals. This helps doctors focus their time on direct patient care, but it can also cause doctors to be less concerned with the patient's satisfaction than physicians who work for themselves.

There's tension among the three market disciplines. They are, in many ways, competing priorities, which makes it difficult for care providers to excel in all three. Twenty years ago, while visiting a community public health building in Oregon, I saw a sign posted in the lobby. In bold capital letters it read "QUALITY. SERVICE. COST." And below that, in a much smaller font, "Pick any two."

This was the reality of American medicine for most of its history. It's not what patients want or need today.

Fortunately, advances in medical practice and technology now make it possible for people to enjoy the best of all three market disciplines. And in the future, each type of health care organization will be required to provide the best of all three to survive.

"Customer intimacy" requires doctors and medical staff to know you as a patient and respond to your preferences. In the future, doctors will be able to respond to your preferences through the use of information technology and convenient computer applications. Patients will have the ability to communicate with their personal physician through secure e-mail and consult a specialist virtually, regardless of where they are at the time or the specific medical problem they have.

"Product differentiation" doesn't have to be more expensive, provided doctors are willing to embrace technology that does more than glitter. In particular, mobile and video technologies will allow physicians in the future to offer sophisticated treatments and coordinate care while eliminating redundancy and inefficiency.

"Operational excellence" results from improved systems of care. When doctors work together for the benefit of the patient, they more consistently avoid medical error, provide preventive services, and maximize performance in both the outpatient and hospital arenas. When done well, the combination increases quality and reduces cost.

Advances in medical knowledge and modern technology now allow doctors and hospitals to achieve success in all three market disciplines. But none of these changes will happen without the right motivation and direction. That is why physician leadership will be so essential.

The Advantages of Integration

A powerful example of how an integrated approach can improve the health of individuals and communities emerged from the Camden Coalition of Healthcare Providers, a group of clinicians in one of America's most impoverished and crime-laden cities. Recognizing the opportunity to lower cost by increasing quality and access, the New Jersey–based group analyzed health care spending among all of its patients.

As Atul Gawande explained in an eye-opening *New Yorker* article, "between January of 2002 and June of 2008 some nine hundred people in two buildings accounted for more than 4,000 hospital visits and about two hundred million dollars in health care bills." One patient alone accounted for 324 admissions and ER visits in five years. Another patient cost insurers $3.5 million in medical reimbursements.

So, what was the coalition's solution? The group decided to offer medical care *inside* the two buildings that accounted for the most hospital visits. By bringing health care into the homes of the community's "worst of the worst" medical cases, the Camden group cut hospital bills in half.

A single physician could not have done this. And it's likely an academic medical center wouldn't have done this. But a coalition of doctors working in conjunction with a hospital did. This remarkable turnaround in Camden is just one proof point that speaks to what is possible when doctors and hospitals share common systems, incentives, and leadership.

Regardless of the health care setting in which doctors practice, they tend to overvalue the advantages of their own environment while overlooking its shortcomings.

Doctors in community practice, for example, are proud of their offices and talk up the importance of having personal relationships with their patients. Yet they can't see how their small size, fragmentation, and lack of information technology harms quality and raises costs. To improve, they will need to integrate directly or virtually with their colleagues, something that will require them to forgo some of their independence.

Physicians in academia, on the other hand, value their CVs filled with published articles and teaching accolades. But they don't see the redundancy and inefficiency in their care-delivery systems. They resist change when it competes with other priorities like conducting research and teaching. To increase operational excellence and customer satisfaction in this setting, doctors and researchers will need to be less "ivory tower" and more business savvy.

Already, American hospitals are seeing an uptick in doctors pursuing MBAs. Today, more than 50 percent of medical schools offer a joint degree in business and medicine.

Integrated delivery systems have a leg up on the other two models when it comes to cost effectiveness, but until they emphasize customer intimacy as much as they do operational excellence and quality outcomes, they'll have trouble expanding their footprint. Physicians in solo practices understand from day one that their income is dependent on pleasing patients, so they go out of their way to do so. When you're part of a larger group, it's easier to hide. As community providers and academic institutions become more efficient—figuring out how to leverage information technology and lower costs—integrated systems will experience increased competition.

In the past, all three approaches to care delivery could survive on one market discipline. Community doctors and academic institutions were able to offset their inefficiencies by passing costs onto purchasers and patients. But as government and commercial payers increasingly refuse to accede to these increases, and as patients feel the strain of rapidly rising out-of-pocket expenses, both groups will need to ratchet up their operational improvements. And once they do, integrated delivery systems won't be able to succeed through economies of scale and reduced costs alone.

In this new world of health care, excelling in just one discipline won't be enough. Physicians will find the transition difficult, but they will face major repercussions if they don't.

The Death of Community Hospitals

When health systems integrate, they have the ability to increase collaboration, maximize economies of scale, and provide more preventive services. And when that happens, patients will occupy fewer hospital beds. And when *that* happens, we'll need fewer hospitals altogether.

To most people, the thought of losing their local hospital is a scary proposition. For more than a century now, these care facilities have carried deep emotional associations.

When we hear the word "hospital," some of us feel a sense of gratitude for the birth of a child or the treatment of an acute condition. Others feel sorrow, remembering a loved one who passed away in a hospital. Regardless of our experiences, many of us assume the closer we live to a hospital, the safer and better off we are.

That was true long ago. But that's just not the case anymore. Reviewing the history of the American hospital will help us understand why we'd be better off with fewer of them.

In the early 1700s, hospitals in the New World provided very little medical care. They served primarily as isolation facilities for those with contagious illnesses, as shelters for vagrants and people with mental illness, and on occasion as almshouses for the poor.

That's because those who could afford medical care received it in their own homes. But by the end of the nineteenth century, with the introduction of general anesthesia, medical care was becoming too complex to be delivered by house call alone. As a result, care shifted to centralized facilities where patients benefited from the latest medical advancements, and around-the-clock physician and nursing care.

Before long, hospitals were turning up in nearly every community. And though the surge in hospital construction signaled an advance in medical care, it also mirrored the difficulty, high cost, and slowness of travel at the time. Building a hospital in every town made sense in that context. Hospitals became major employers and a source of great civic pride for local leaders who sat on their governing boards.

And thus, the "community hospital" was born. Founded by physicians, religious groups, and public municipalities, US hospital growth boomed from a few hundred in the 1870s to upward of 6,000 by the mid-twentieth century.

Fast-forward to the 1990s, when high-margin procedures such as heart bypass surgery and total joint replacement were being performed in nearly every hospital and advertised by most. Suddenly, with the introduction of more restrictive managed-care programs and the expansion of outpatient alternatives, the demand for inpatient (hospital) services declined sharply. Some hospitals were forced to merge. Others had no choice but to close their doors for good.

Since the year 2000, the number of acute-care hospitals has held steady at around 5,700. The nationwide effort to avoid unnecessary hospital use now has many low-volume hospitals struggling to survive.

Over the past decade, 16 percent of hospitals have consolidated by joining a health system. That trend is accelerating nationwide in the context of health care reform. Ambulatory surgery centers, which use innovative technology and new surgical approaches, have taken over many of the high-margin procedures that were once under the exclusive purview of inpatient facilities.

It's easy to understand why community leaders would mourn the loss of hospitals, the jobs they created, and the status they symbolized. But as patients, we should welcome this change.

Donald Trump, who brings a business mindset to the presidency, should be able to recognize opportunities to convert expenses that add little value into ones that contribute more broadly to the economics of the nation. For example, eliminating inefficient hospitals could, in turn, help him fund the infrastructure programs he favors. At the same time, doing so will cost jobs in the short-term, something he has promised to avoid. No one should underestimate the unhappiness hospital closures would cause, but the benefits of consolidation on quality and cost would be significant.

When hospitals consolidate, patient volumes increase in the ones that remain. As a result, these institutions and their physicians will be able to further specialize, leading to improvements in overall quality. To put it another way, less will be more (or at least better). Fewer hospitals will require fewer surgeons, and when that happens, surgeons who do more of a specific procedure will get better at doing it and make fewer mistakes.

Given the chance to go to your local low-volume community hospital or drive an extra twenty minutes to one with twice the volume, always pick the latter. As more patients do, our country will see not only improved clinical outcomes but lower costs. If you doubt it, just look at every other industry. Most of them embraced this mentality decades ago.

The Resurrection of Primary Care

In the future, greater integration along with a heightened focus on prevention in medical practice will make the role of the primary-care physician more important than it has been in quite some time. That's a good thing for patients.

Until the late 1980s, the primary-care physician's unique diagnostic skills made internal medicine the pinnacle of the medical profession, a specialty preferred by the top graduating students. However, three events altered the pecking order.

First came the introduction of sophisticated diagnostic machines, which made figuring out what was wrong with patients more routine, thus diminishing the importance of individual acumen. Second, surgical procedures—from total joints to heart surgery to cataract removal—became safer and more common. This produced a rapid rise in surgical specialty jobs and incomes, leaving primary-care reimbursements far behind. Finally, job satisfaction of primary-care physicians plummeted as insurers began implementing new and cumbersome authorization processes.

"Prior authorization," as it's known, is an added step the insurance company requires physicians to complete prior to ordering expensive tests or sending a patient to get a specialty consultation. Its purpose is to discourage physicians from recommending expensive medical care. In parallel, in the 1990s, insurance companies put primary-care physicians in the role of "gatekeeper." As gatekeepers, they were the sole referring agents to specialists and also personally responsible for the added costs of specialty care. This new task undermined the mission-driven spirit that led them to choose medicine for their profession. It's understandable then why the previously desirable role of a primary-care physician fell off dramatically.

Today, for every 100,000 US patients, there are sixty-six specialists and forty-six primary-care physicians. In the global health systems with the best outcomes, that ratio is reversed. Primary care, through disease prevention and the management of chronic illnesses, can claim credit for 80 percent of the superior clinical outcomes in health care today. If our country wants to improve health care performance and outcomes in the fastest and simplest way possible, a great place to start would be addressing this workforce imbalance.

The first step will be to shift financial rewards. Physicians who perform complex procedures currently earn two to three times more than those in primary care who focus on preventing and managing chronic illnesses.

The second step will be to increase the connectivity between primary and specialty physicians through technology. This change offers dual positives for patients. By facilitating physician communication, patients will receive better medical care sooner. And when patients have complex medical problems that require the expertise of multiple specialists, the primary-care physician can make certain these patients don't "fall through the cracks," as so often happens today.

When their overall head count increases, primary-care physicians will have the time to become even more adept at helping patients deal with difficult lifestyle issues (smoking, obesity, drug abuse, and so on), and they'll find better ways to help patients avoid the ravages of chronic illness in the first place. Today, seven in ten deaths in America each year are caused by chronic—often preventable—illnesses. It doesn't have to be this way.

Integration Matters

Moving from fragmentation to integration is difficult. It requires investments in technology. It demands a restructuring of how care is reimbursed and a commitment by all physicians to work as a single team. But without question, these changes are worth it.

When independent organizations such as the National Committee for Quality Assurance and J.D. Power and Associates measure quality and service outcomes, time and again the integrated medical groups score the highest. And when the best of these physician-led multispecialty organizations are measured against the fragmented community providers around them, the results are telling. Go to the NCQA website and see for yourself. The organizations that earned a five-star rating for exceptional patient satisfaction, prevention, and treatment are the same health care–delivery organizations you'll find on the J.D. Power site.

Meanwhile, patients in the highest-performing integrated care settings are, on average, 30 percent less likely to die of a heart attack or stroke, 40 percent less likely to die from sepsis, and 50 percent less likely to die from HIV or AIDS.

Integration is a crucial pillar for transforming health care. It's perhaps better thought of as the foundation upon which all the other elements rest. But without the other pillars, change won't happen. Next, we need to fix health care's money problem.

Pillar 2: It's Better and Cheaper Not to Get Sick in the First Place

Health care will need to be prepaid, moving away from pay-for-volume toward paying for value and superior outcomes.

Americans appreciate a doctor who can rescue them from a catastrophic event. But of course all patients would prefer not to have a heart attack, develop colon cancer, or suffer a stroke in the first place. Unfortunately, that's not what the current reimbursement system is designed to achieve. If the physician taking care of you is paid on a fee-for-service basis, it's likely your care isn't optimal. The reason is simple.

Fee-for-service medicine pays health care providers to do more, not better. Doctors are rewarded many times more for treating the catastrophic event than preventing it. If you have any doubt, look at the data from the nationally reported *Healthcare Effectiveness Data and Information Set* published annually by the federal government. Depending on the specific quality measure you examine, you'll see a 20 to 30 percent gap between the organizations performing the best (most of which are prepaid) and the lower-performing organizations (reimbursed primarily through fee-for-service models).

Doctors aren't the only ones falling into this quality gap. When hospitals can charge whatever they want for an operative procedure or a day in the hospital, many do. That is, until someone does something about it.

Pacific Business Group on Health (PBGH) is one of the nation's leading nonprofit business coalitions, and it focuses on improving the quality and affordability of health care. When the group's leaders looked at ways to increase quality and reduce costs, they honed in on the operations that replace worn-out hips and knees using prosthetic joints. They started by calculating the total expense for everything involved, including the surgeon, anesthesia, the Operating Room, and the hospital's costs.

They were shocked to discover that prices for this "bundled service" varied from as low as $20,000 to upward of $120,000, depending on the hospital in which these procedures were performed. Even more astounding was the realization that clinical outcomes at the most expensive facilities were no better than at the hospitals charging one-fifth as much. In measuring outcomes against cost, they found hospitals that charged $50,000 or $70,000 or even $100,000 for a total joint surgery achieved no better results for their patients than those charging $30,000. Although the more expensive locations had sterling reputations, big marketing budgets, and beautiful lobbies, the operations and postoperative outcomes were identical across the price continuum.

So, guess what happened when PBGH announced it would only include in its network the hospitals charging no more than $30,000 per total joint? Even the locations that once charged $100,000 lowered their costs to meet this single bundled-payment cap. And you can rest assured that any hospital agreeing to this price wasn't losing money.

The "fee-for-service" reimbursement model works well in retail. If you choose to pay more for a particular brand, be it Gucci or Tesla, or for a particular service, say a limo over a cab, you're free to do so. Consumers buy these products and services based on the added quality they associate with them.

But in health care's fee-for-service model, higher pricing doesn't equate to higher quality. And when an individual's health is in immediate danger, costs go up in fee-for-service medicine while the patient's choices go down.

This is why the federal government, through the Medicare Advantage program, has moved reimbursements in the direction of pay-for-value. As PBGH describes it, paying for value is about "[e]nsuring providers of health care are rewarded for quality and efficiency."

Changing what hospitals and doctors earn (and how they earn it) is always a contentious issue. Those succeeding under the current rules are hardly eager to move to a different payment method. But to improve American health care, we need to recognize that fee-for-service reimbursement leads to mistreatment. It doesn't adequately reward physicians who prevent problems. It doesn't maximize patient safety. It doesn't deliver higher-quality care. Rather, it enables unnecessary "utilization" and even rewards medical errors. It tolerates and perpetuates sky-high prices. In the future of health care, this form of reimbursement simply won't fly.

Pillar 3: What Your Doctor Doesn't Know Can Hurt You

Health care will need to be technologically enabled, with comprehensive electronic health-record systems, patient access to medical information, and the ability to obtain care using mobile and video technologies.

No business today can afford to ignore the importance of information technology. And most have embraced IT. From large-scale food makers to cutting-edge communications firms, organizations rely on the latest technology to climb to the top of their industries. The lone industry exception: health care.

I am shocked when doctors claim they can deliver the best quality or service without twenty-first-century information-technology systems. The reality: they can't.

Unleashing Digital Data

The data revolution of the past decade has led to an almost universal appreciation for the power of information. Professionals today marvel at all the ways data analytics can boost decision making and results.

My colleagues and I are fortunate to have access to information from more than 10 million medical records. Through algorithms devised by our division of research, we know which patients in our hospitals today are likeliest to require ICU admission tomorrow, allowing us to intervene twenty-four hours before it becomes necessary. And because we know which patients are likeliest to return to the ER after discharge, we can monitor their treatments longer before sending them home.

Across the country, only a tiny fraction of hospitals apply advanced data analytics to improve patient care. That's troubling. When researchers have access to comprehensive sets of patient information, they can identify clinical solutions to problems that would otherwise have remained hidden.

For example, a colleague of mine named Dr. Elizabeth Suh-Burgmann (she goes by Betty) recently analyzed the medical records of more than 1,000 women with an ovarian mass, a medical problem that is terrifying to both the patient and the doctor. Her findings, published in the *American Journal of Obstetrics and Gynecology*, demonstrate how data can overcome the gap between faulty perception and medical reality.

Current, intuition-based gynecological practice dictates that women with an ovarian mass should undergo major surgery or, at a minimum, receive lifelong radiological testing. But like so many of our old assumptions and practices, this one has been proven wrong by new data.

Rather than basing her clinical decisions on guesswork or anecdote, Betty looked at what actually happened to these patients. She learned, to her surprise, that less than 1 percent of these ovarian masses were ever cancerous. And most important, Betty found that when a discovered mass doesn't grow over the next year, it *never* turns out to be cancerous. This was a huge finding. Suddenly, science informed by technology (not intuition) was guiding conversations with patients. Now, doctors who discover a mass can simply follow the patient for twelve months and intervene only if they spot a change. No more unnecessary surgeries, no more never-ending tests.

To a greater extent than ever before, data are debunking health care's old assumptions and overthrowing its old approaches. Dr. Carlos Pestana from the University of Texas points out that half of what we know in medicine is wrong. Unfortunately, he reminds us, we just don't know which half. Big data helps us make that determination and decipher which clinical approaches are better than others. Once one approach has been proven superior, all physicians should follow it.

The best medical programs do, and they earn five-star ratings from Medicare Advantage and the NCQA. But will more organizations in the future learn from their expertise and follow their lead, or will they resist change? Time will tell.

Unlocking Electronic Health Records

A Bank of America ATM can figure out who you are and how much money is in your account in seconds. It can spit out cash in virtually any currency from nearly any spot in the world, even if you're a Chase customer. Any ATM, regardless of which company owns it, has the ability to communicate with a central data server. The server contains your bank balance and other pieces of information the bank needs to confirm your identity before it will hand over your cash. The underlying software capability that enables this process is called "interoperability," and it's the reason you can access your funds safely and immediately from anywhere in the world.

So, with a slide of your debit card and the push of a few buttons, presto, you have the money you need for your travels, whether the local currency is euro, peso, or yen. And it accomplishes that feat at the exact exchange rate set by a consortium of international banks through a foreign-exchange market, sometimes located thousands of miles away.

It all sounds far riskier and more problematic than when a doctor exchanges a patient's medical information with a colleague a mile or two away, doesn't it? In health care, connecting doctors with patient data isn't all that technically complicated. It's just financially and politically complicated.

To explain these difficulties, it's helpful to begin by defining the difference between an "electronic health record" and a "comprehensive electronic medical record."

The former includes only the patient information that's entered digitally into a computer system by a single doctor or a hospital staff member. This is better than a paper record, as the information is (1) legible, (2) accessible to the doctor anytime, and (3) comparably formatted for every patient.

But just having the information digitized doesn't significantly improve the quality of the care an individual physician can provide.

Instead, what is needed is comprehensive information, which includes all of the patient information that exists, regardless of how many different doctors the patient saw or whether the care was provided in an office or hospital. It's not hard to see how giving your cardiologist, dermatologist, primary-care doctor, and Emergency Room physicians immediate access to the entirety of your medical information could improve (perhaps even transform) care delivery. A comprehensive electronic medical record is what allowed Christy to save Sarah's life. It could have helped the two hand surgeons avoid the mistakes that led to their patients' deaths. And it is essential to achieving the highest-quality outcomes in the future.

Unfortunately, the manufacturers of the large electronic health records don't want to facilitate the implementation of comprehensive systems, unless the only application used is theirs. They fear what interoperability between systems would mean for their businesses. If health-record vendors allowed third-party developers to access their application program interface (also known as an API, a set of protocols and tools used in new software development), all your medical information could be combined into a single, *comprehensive* system—much like the one you access through an ATM. This would be extremely beneficial for patients and physicians. But doing so would make it much easier for doctors and hospitals to switch from one manufacturer to another, therefore reducing what these powerful companies can charge for their software.

Manufacturers of electronic health records could make their systems compatible. After all, other industries—from airlines to financial institutions—have long since solved the interoperability and data-aggregation problem. They just don't want to. As is too often the case, health care remains an outlier.

Reinventing the House Call

In Chapter 3, we met Emma and Felipe, both of whom had their lives changed by virtual doctor visits. As patients, their problems were not unique.

Any parent who has been woken up in the middle of the night by a sick child would appreciate the ability to access a doctor remotely to help decide whether to go to the Emergency Department right then or wait for the morning. Technology makes it possible, but relatively few patients have access to this option today.

This year, the physicians in Kaiser Permanente in Northern California are on pace to provide upward of 1 million virtual visits each month through a combination of video, secure e-mail, and telephone. By 2018, our organization expects to provide our patients with more virtual visits than in-person office visits. We don't force anyone—doctors or patients—to use this approach. But when it's offered, nearly every patient chooses it. And when they do, patients report higher satisfaction with virtual care, particularly with video, when compared to in-person visits. People want more convenient care. The hardest part for most is finding it.

A recent Nielsen study on behalf of the Council of Accountable Physician Practices revealed that just one in five patients has access to online appointment scheduling with their doctors. Only 15 percent of patients can use e-mail to communicate with their providers. And a scant 2 percent have access to video visits.

The reasons are plentiful. For example, insurers in about thirty states won't pay for video care. Their excuses are ambiguous. Most likely, their concerns revolve around having to pay for the service in the first place and the fear that, once they do, doctors will simply drive up the volume of these services, even when it is not required.

State medical boards are another barrier. In Idaho, a doctor was fined $10,000 for prescribing an antibiotic over the phone.

Meanwhile, physicians are legally prohibited from providing telehealth services "across state lines." Today, it is legal for a doctor in San Diego to treat a patient in Eureka, California, more than 700 miles away, but not for a physician in, say, Chicago to provide a video visit to a patient thirty miles away in Gary, Indiana.

Progress is slow, but signs of life are emerging in some unexpected places. UnitedHealthcare, for example, announced not long ago that it would cover some video-based doctor visits just as it would in-person visits. Likewise, some Blue Cross health plans have also recently adopted telemedicine programs. At some point, this will be the standard for medical care, but that could be years from now.

Disrupting Health Care

Technologically enabled health care will become a reality for more patients. The question still to be answered is: How will the transition occur?

It could start to gain momentum as a low-cost alternative to in-person visits, one that would be especially attractive for people paying their health care expenses out of pocket. Or perhaps it will begin among those living in rural areas, far from the nearest specialist. To them, video would be incredibly valuable.

Both of these scenarios would be consistent with a sequence of broad adoption that Clayton Christensen calls "disruptive innovation." In most industries, consumers shopping on the lower end of the pricing spectrum have been the earliest adopters of disruptive products. For example, look at the emergence of Japanese automotive manufacturer Toyota in the United States.

The company entered the market by offering a cheaper alternative to the least expensive cars manufactured by American automakers. Once Toyota established a foothold, the company introduced progressively more luxurious but relatively lower-priced autos in the midsize range. Then Toyota unveiled the Lexus to compete with the most profitable and premium automobiles.

This progression is one reason Toyota is America's top-selling car brand today. Had the company tried to compete with luxury auto manufacturers from day one, it would have failed.

Video visits could be aimed at those who can't afford an in-person office visit; however, that's not their likeliest path for going mainstream in American health care. The group most attracted to this alternative is likely to be "high-end" consumers, the busiest of corporate executives who don't want to take time away from work to drive to the doctor's office. Knowing they could access medical care from the comfort of their office, without having to leave work, would be a game changer. And as soon as they realized this form of high-quality, convenient medical care costs less, not more, they would want it for their employees, too.

This sequence of disruption would be more consistent with the emergence of the UberX ride-sharing service. Some riders hopped on the bandwagon because it was cheaper, but the deciding factors for many urban professionals were (1) the time UberX saved them over hailing a taxi, (2) the friendlier drivers with cleaner cars, and (3) the convenience of not having to fuss over cash. What turned the taxi model on its head wasn't so much the riders who couldn't afford a traditional cab as it was the individuals who valued the convenience and improved experience UberX offered.

Uber is an exception to most disruptive models, and it's quite possible that health care will follow it. And we're not just talking about video visits. Those with the best coverage and busiest schedules are exactly the kinds of patients who would embrace communicating through secure e-mail, obtaining their diagnoses using digital technology and accessing their personal medical information on mobile devices. The spread of telehealth is likely to follow the opposite trajectory of a traditional disruptive innovation. But whenever and however it happens, those health care providers who are late to the game will join the disrupted ranks of the conventional taxi industry.

Technology will be essential for the future of health care for many reasons. When the Institute for Healthcare Improvement looked at how to make American health care better, it adopted a triple aim: better care for individual patients, increased health of the community, and lower annual cost per person. Technology, both comprehensive electronic health records and mobile solutions, can help our nation achieve all three parts.

Without information and data on care gaps, doctors can't maximize individual health. And without linking computer systems together, the health of communities will improve at a snail's pace, if at all. And without viable alternatives to the physician's office and the hospital, costs will continue accelerating as rapidly in the future as in the past.

The combination of integration, prepayment, and technology prove synergistic in practice. Integration allows comprehensive data entry and distribution of best practices. Prepayment from the insurance company to physicians and hospitals (for a specific population of patients) creates added incentives for providers to help prevent disease, avoid medical complications, and deliver health care in the most effective ways possible. In addition, it provides the motivation to make necessary investments in hardware, software, and training. And technology allows physicians to provide higher-quality care, more rapidly and at a more reasonable cost. This combination is what business schools call a "virtuous cycle." But without the final pillar, none of this will work for the patient.

Pillar 4: Who Will You Trust?

Health care will need to be physician led, which will require greater leadership training and development.

Residents in plastic surgery train for six or seven years after medical school. In my last year of residency, I spent a week providing medical and surgical care to people in a rural village located in the mountains of Mexico. Most of the villagers were sustenance farmers, living off the basic staples they could grow.

Most days, I would come back from an early morning run to a three-room hut where I lived with a host family. There I'd find the matron, a young mother, bent over a small fire, preparing breakfast for her children. Each day, she cooked tortillas from flour, ground by hand, along with beans and a fried vegetable dish she made from a large squash that resembled a green pumpkin.

To harvest this squash, she had to hike for forty-five minutes up the mountain to a small plot of land her family owned. After enjoying a week of the family's hospitality, I felt the least I could do was to help her carry down one of these pumpkin-sized squash. As we got ready to leave, I had an ingenious idea. I would bring my backpack so that I could carry not one but two squashes down the mountain.

I would repay her generosity by teaching her how to double her carrying capacity. As we hiked through the heat, the climb was beautiful but taxing. At our destination, she harvested two squashes. I presumed she would give one to me and carry the other back down herself. I quickly interjected and tried to explain that I could carry both, one in my backpack and one in my arms.

She thanked me, harvested two more and walked over to a tree. With her machete, she cut down two vines. She tied a pair of squashes to the ends of both vines. As we prepared to leave, she draped one vine over each shoulder with a squash at each end. Then she balanced one on her head and placed the final one in her arms. I never felt more foolish. I had climbed up the mountain confident I could teach her how to transport two squashes at a time. She came down carrying three times that many.

As physicians, we often assume we know everything. After all, we can perform remarkable operations with miraculous results. But expertise in one area doesn't automatically translate to another. So physicians who want to lead the future of health care need to be willing to learn.

Fortunately, physician leadership is a skill that—as in every industry—can be taught, honed, and developed.

Grooming Physician Leadership

As a nation, we do a poor job providing the expertise physicians need to take on leadership roles. Jay Conger of Claremont McKenna College jokingly calls our approach the "French school of swim instruction": throw people into the deepest part of the pool, trust that one way or another they will figure out how to reach the other side, and don't worry if they swallow some water in the process. Of course, there are better ways.

In my CEO role, I devote considerable time and effort to supporting the development of physician leadership. More than a decade ago, our medical group established one of the largest leadership training programs in the nation. Creating such an elaborate infrastructure is expensive, and it takes a long time to reap benefits. It also requires role models who are willing to give future physician leaders more than textbooks and presentations from which to learn and grow.

Dr. Sharon Levine, a pediatrician and associate executive director in our medical group, is the kind of leader whose commitment has benefited thousands of physicians and millions of patients. As the first woman member of our executive team, Sharon created a program more than a decade ago to educate and support women in leadership roles. Her program and ability to lead by example explain why nearly half of all physician leadership roles in The Permanente Medical Group today are filled by women.

More recently, Dr. Levine spearheaded our effort to implement the nation's most stringent conflict-of-interest policy. Our doctors are now prohibited from accepting anything, regardless of value, from for-profit drug and medical-device companies. As you might predict, physicians in the past enjoyed the free trips and expensive meals. But Sharon led this crusade so that patients would never have to question the motives of a physician who ordered a certain medication or device. Through her leadership and dedication to our patients, only two of our thousands of physicians left as a result of this policy. Today, it remains the gold standard in health care.

Thanks to Sharon's efforts, no other investment (not in information technology or brick and mortar) has yielded a higher return on investment than our programs to select, train, and develop future leaders.

Over my medical career, I've had the opportunity to observe hundreds of physician leaders—both successful and unsuccessful—and to see their impact on more than 10,000 doctors. As a CEO and faculty member at the Stanford Graduate School of Business, I know the role of the physician leader is different than in other lines of work. But I've found that the best of the best, regardless of their industry or the challenges they face, demonstrate the ability to touch and influence three vital organs of their fellow colleagues: the heart, brain, and guts.

Engaging the Heart

Most physicians are smart and very talented. They're skilled clinicians and technically superb, priding themselves on their analytical thinking. They're trained from the first day of medical school to reach decisions without bias.

But medical practice is inherently intimate and emotional. Being a doctor means being a part of life's most personal experiences, from birth to death. As such, leaders must be comfortable with and capable of engaging the heart.

The heart in this sense is a combination of purpose and mission. It motivates future physicians to spend a decade in training. To engage a physician's heart, leaders must create a vision that is both aspirational and achievable.

Try lecturing physicians on the importance of reducing hospital expenditures, passing an accreditation survey, or lowering the rates of hospital-acquired infections, and they will hardly pay attention. But bring in the family of a patient who died from a hospital-acquired infection and watch everyone lean forward in their chairs.

It's true that most physicians care deeply about the lives they affect. It's also true that the day-to-day grind of modern medicine can wear down a doctor's compassion and empathy for both patients and fellow colleagues alike.

I advise emerging physician leaders that how they treat people matters. When I'm selecting a leader, I've learned that a great place to start is by asking nursing assistants or departmental secretaries for their opinion. They're usually right. The physician leader who cares enough to learn the name of the receptionist's daughter is usually a more successful leader than the one who sees no value in getting to know staff with "lower status." The bigger the heart, the greater the impact.

Stimulating the Brain

Presented with a vision for the future, most physicians worry that they'll be asked to do the impossible to achieve it. Leaders address this fear by explaining the specific changes in behavior needed, the context for the change, and how success will be measured.

Behaviors are specific and observable actions. Examples include washing your hands every time you walk in and out of a patient's room or ordering a mammogram every time you see a woman like Sarah who hasn't had one in the past two years. No one can determine exactly what motivates other people, but we can observe their actions. Once physicians know exactly what they are being asked to do, they are likely to realize that the magnitude of change is less than they originally feared.

Physicians also want to understand the reasons and context for change. They won't move forward until they understand the "why."

Data on physician performance, when used appropriately, have a powerful impact. Successful leaders distribute data to show variations in results and what the highest performing physicians are able to accomplish. Often, the first step in the change process is to help everyone recognize that what seems impossible, isn't. After all, someone is likely already achieving the desired outcome.

Knowing When to Trust Your Gut

Physicians will take action and propel change only if they trust their leaders. Trust is described as a "gut feeling," even if the label is physiologically incorrect. Leaders who want to earn that trust can't just send memos. They must engage with physicians individually and in small groups, look them in the eye, tell the truth, and lead.

Success requires leaders to model the behaviors they wish to inspire. Colleagues understand that new physician leaders have many responsibilities and can no longer be on call as often or take on as much clinical work as before. But when a crisis develops and help is requested, the only answer that preserves the credibility of the leader is "yes."

Being a leader is not only a responsibility but also a privilege. No one will or should care more about the success of an organization or work harder than its leaders. If they are unwilling to make the commitment required, they'll never succeed in influencing hearts, engaging minds, or earning the trust of those around them.

Human beings have finely honed mechanisms for reading body language and unspoken messages. Malcolm Gladwell describes this intuition as our ability to "thin-slice" the decision-making process. As humans evolved, their lives often depended on their ability to follow the right leaders. That same instinct persists today. Our "guts" are wired to tell us who is safe to follow and whom we should abandon. And as a result, leaders who deceive others can sometimes get away with it once, but rarely twice.

Leaders who want to inspire trust must also be willing to take risks. For physicians, nearly every decision involves a level of uncertainty, both for themselves and for the organization. Managing risk is essential for keeping an organization on the cutting edge. Making difficult decisions and taking chances require courage. Leaders can't be foolhardy. But those without the bravery needed to address performance issues or make a clear decision despite certain risk will not just underperform themselves, they'll lose the confidence and trust of those around them.

Each of the elements described above is essential for developing the kind of leadership that will succeed in transforming health care. Leaders who want to get the job done can't take shortcuts, cherry-pick the easy approaches, or ignore difficult conversations. They need to provide an aspirational vision, detail the behaviors expected, present context and data, and engage in authentic ways with the people they hope will follow them. With sincerity and skill, leaders can inspire physicians, nurses, and staff to accomplish more than they ever dreamed possible.

What Happens if Physicians and Hospitals Refuse to Change?

Ask him what he does, and Dr. Devi Shetty will tell you that he sets the price of a human life.

"Each morning that I come to the hospital there is a line of mothers, each with a child in her arms," says the US-trained cardiovascular surgeon who currently practices in India. "All have been well worked up and each would benefit from surgery. When I tell them the cost of the procedure, they understand that they will need to borrow this money. When they can, the child lives. When they can't, they take their children home to die."

Today, he and his team perform complex heart surgeries at $1,800 a case, a fraction of what such a procedure costs in the United States and with results equal to the best American hospitals.

Devi knows that if he can get that price down to $1,500, many more children will live. He knows that if we truly valued the lives of children, none of them would die unnecessarily. Therefore, his goal is to lower the cost of heart surgery to $800 a case by 2020.

As a former personal physician to Mother Teresa, Devi shares her commitment for helping the poor. Every day, he and his colleagues provide no-cost surgeries to as many patients as possible who can't borrow the rupees needed to pay the hospital fee. But there are always more patients than resources. He laments that "charity is not scalable," and at the end of the week, he needs to pay his staff and his hospital bills.

Despite the challenge he faces, Devi is constantly looking for ways to double the number of lives he can save. Both a visionary and a humanitarian, he is also one of the best operational leaders I have seen. He understands that "operational excellence" requires a razor-sharp focus on every detail. When the cost of surgical gowns in India went up, he contracted with young entrepreneurs from a local clothing company, using their sewing skills to create disposable gowns and drapes at half the price of traditional suppliers.

Some of his successes have come by way of reduced labor expenses in India. Many more have come by way of technological advancements.

He has implemented one of the world's most sophisticated information-technology systems. By noon each day, all managers in his hospitals know the profit/loss from the day before. This allows them to immediately offset waste and correct inefficiencies. It also helps them figure out how many free surgeries they can offer the following day. Every morning, he reviews how long it took physicians the night before to respond to a major deterioration in the clinical status of a patient. His average time delay is under ten minutes, less than one-third of the delay in a typical US hospital.

Devi's vision doesn't end within his hospital walls. He developed an insurance program for more than 1 million poor farmers. With it, they pay less than $1 a month to obtain coverage for whatever surgical procedure they may need. The program affords access to a variety of procedures for patients who would otherwise be denied his services. Even sophisticated procedures such as implementation of left-ventricular-assist devices (mechanical heart pumps) are included.

He invests in India's next generation by hiring impoverished women for most of the jobs in his hospitals. He explains that men will spend half their salary on themselves, whereas women will use more than 90 percent of their income to support and educate their children, a step toward improving the nation's future.

Three years ago, Devi opened a hospital in the Grand Cayman Islands, less than one hour by plane from Florida. The island is beautiful, a vacation destination for many. The nation is renowned for its tourist culture, its outstanding service and safety. The people on the island speak English as their first language, and wages are similar to those in the United States.

His hospital, which boasts superb clinical outcomes, can't yet offer heart surgery for $1,800 a case, but the facility can do it for $10,000. That's still one-fifth of what the procedure costs in the United States.

Although the hospital is modestly sized and serves mainly patients from the Caribbean, Devi has been granted authorization to build a 2,000-bed hospital on the island of 50,000 citizens. Most likely, his goal is to fill the majority of those beds with American patients who are tired of paying too much for outcomes that have fallen behind the best hospitals in the world.

For American doctors and hospitals, Devi's success should serve as a call to action. Whether patients in the United States put their lives in the hands of their local physicians or go to Dr. Shetty's new center will depend on the ability of America to transform and improve its health care system. There is no way to predict how President Trump would view this type of medical tourism. On the one hand, he could see it as a threat to American health care jobs. On the other hand, if the approach lowers health care costs for employers, they can add more jobs and raise wages faster than today.

We can't rebuild American health care from scratch. But as the four pillars of transformation demonstrate, we can and must do better as a nation in the future. I hope that President Trump, as both a businessman and a leader who is committed to improving our economy, will encourage legislation that leads to the implementation of these four pillars, supporting the edifice we call American health care.

Chapter Eight

WHAT PATIENTS WANT AND NEED

Throughout his life, A. Bartlett Giamatti was many things. He was a professor of English Renaissance literature. He was the youngest president of Yale University. He was the seventh commissioner of Major League Baseball (MLB). Giamatti had many passions and professions, but that last one in particular topped them all. He adored baseball. And in "The Green Fields of the Mind," a *Yale Alumni Magazine* article he wrote forty years ago, he left no doubt.

> It breaks your heart. It is designed to break your heart. The game begins in the spring, when everything else begins again, and it blossoms in the summer, filling the afternoons and evenings, and then as soon as the chill rains come, it stops and leaves you to face the fall all alone.

These words perfectly capture the emotions of being a die-hard baseball fan. And they apply just as well to life's journey, from the joys of birth to the inevitability of death.

As a fellow baseball fanatic, and as a Yale School of Medicine graduate, I have followed Bart Giamatti's career closely. I cherish the simplicity and significance of his words as much as any I have read. And given a similar choice between being the CEO of the nation's largest medical group and manning the top post in all of baseball, I wouldn't hesitate to serve as the sport's eleventh commissioner.

Like Giamatti, my infatuation with baseball started at an early age. My father grew up in the Bronx, home of the feared New York Yankees. My mother lived in the birthplace of the Brooklyn Dodgers, a team affectionately referred to as "Dem Bums." But my parents, hailing from two storied baseball boroughs, somehow both proudly declared themselves New York Giants fans. Note, they rooted for the former *baseball* Giants, not the New York *football* Giants (that team actually plays in New Jersey).

Like religion, baseball attachments are handed down from one generation to the next. My father and I would talk baseball at dinner, in the car, or while playing catch in the yard. Together, we celebrated the heroics of Mel Ott, Christy Mathewson, and of course, Willie Mays, the "Say Hey Kid." I am sure I have watched Mays's dramatic over-the-shoulder catch from 1954 (also known as "The Catch") thousands of times, never losing my appreciation for his speed in running down that fly ball or of his miraculous quick-turn throw back to the infield, preventing the runners from advancing.

Growing up, I was an avid baseball-card collector, always trying to assemble a full roster of Giants. I can remember placing the cards of our hated rivals such as Mickey Mantle in the spokes of my bike, reveling in the clatter as they were ripped to shreds with each crank of the pedal. In retrospect, I probably destroyed thousands of dollars of memorabilia.

Throughout my childhood, the highlight of each year came when one of my father's longtime patients brought him tickets to see the Giants. I can't be sure, but I suspect my dad scheduled this man's dental checkups and cleanings during home-game stretches.

With tickets in hand, my father would race home early in preparation for the game. The drive to the stadium was always filled with excitement. I brought my baseball glove with me in the hopes of catching a foul ball. During the game, I would dutifully record every play on my scorecard. And between innings, the Nathan's hot dogs and freshly roasted peanuts we ate tasted as wonderful as any meal I've ever had.

Even when the Giants lost, I left the ballpark happy, although not nearly as happy as when they won. Looking back, all that mattered was that magnificent feeling of being at the game with my father, both of us getting lost in the energy of our national pastime.

I remember one particular game in September that ran deep into extra innings. The teams must have played at least thirteen before the Giants won and the stadium emptied out into the afterglow of Manhattan at night. Although it was well past my bedtime, I stayed wide awake the whole way home, talking with my father about the Giants and life and my dreams of someday playing pro baseball. I was grateful when my mother called the principal's office the next morning, excusing my absence from school. As I lazed in bed, I replayed the night's events in my mind, from the first pitch to the ride home. Although I have many wonderful memories of my father, none were as magical as those summer nights at the Polo Grounds in New York City.

On Care and Competition

Having played athletics my whole life, I enjoy and value competition. In golf and track, there is a personal score or a time. You compete against yourself as much as others. I enjoyed both of these sports growing up. But I found team sports most fulfilling, and baseball more than any other, hands down.

Baseball is one of the few sports where no one person—not even an all-star—can consistently win or lose a game. Several pitchers have thrown no-hitters only to find the score knotted at zero after nine complete innings. It's not like basketball, where one player can take most of the shots, score forty points a night, and singlehandedly take his team to the playoffs. In baseball, winning requires the contributions of every player on the field.

No one body type dominates in baseball, either. From the huge power-hitting catcher to the scrawny yet speedy middle infielder, there's beauty in the physical diversity of a baseball roster. In many ways, a baseball team is like the human body. Every organ contributes in its own important way to the beautiful harmony of life.

This idea of being part of something bigger than oneself is the essence of baseball. It's the same idea that motivated me to pursue a career as a surgeon. In the best operating rooms, the entire team works as one, every person doing his or her part with one focus: the patient. And this attraction to being part of a team is why I decided to practice in a large medical group when I completed my residency. It is why, years later, I continue to believe it's the best model for our nation. In health care as in baseball, the best results come not just from talented individuals but from the strength of the collective unit—the team.

Baseball and health care have followed parallel paths over the years, and I worry that each has veered off course in similar ways. There was a time when baseball was as much of a sport as a business. Similarly, for most of history, American medicine was a calling and a profession, not a trillion-dollar industry.

Of course, owners have always needed to turn a profit. Likewise, doctors have always deserved an adequate income, and for hospitals, an appropriate return on capital investments. But over the past couple of decades, both health care and baseball have become ever-bigger businesses. Each has lost some of the magic that comes with being a pastime, a passion, and a calling.

Baseball franchises today are worth billions. The average pro now earns $4 million a year as fans are being priced out of the ballpark experience.

Health care, too, is a booming enterprise, particularly among multibillion-dollar insurance companies and drug manufacturers. Just turn on the television, and along with a series of beer and car commercials, you'll encounter plenty of ads for the most expensive medications and even procedures, something unimaginable twenty years ago.

As a health care leader and continued baseball devotee, I worry that the pleasure and fulfillment that once defined these two great traditions is slipping away. And though I may be romanticizing the past a little, the idea of paying a mediocre pitcher millions of dollars troubles me in much the same way as paying a drug company $100,000 for a single course of treatment. In each case, it's a calculation of what the market will bear, not a benchmark for what's reasonable or appropriate. And both will stay that way unless Congress revokes baseball's antitrust exemption and reins in the predatory pricing of the pharmaceutical world.

I'm not naive about reality. We can't turn back the clock. Free agency in baseball was the right thing for the players and was legally upheld by the courts. Similarly, I would not wish to return to the ineffective medical treatments of the past. The advances of medicine have improved clinical care and extended life significantly. The team owners, like drug-company shareholders, need to earn an appropriate profit for the size of their investments and the risks they take. But the economic pendulum has swung too far, and the ones paying for these excesses are the American people. If nothing is done to restore the balance, the prices of both baseball and high-quality medical care will stretch beyond the reaches of the middle class.

I have many ideas about how to solve the challenges of baseball, but they'll need to wait for another book. For now, my focus is on fixing the perverse incentives of health care. The rising costs are not happenstance. Instead, they reflect a growing set of imbalances: between specialty and primary-care salaries, between drug prices and drug innovations, between a focus on intervention and prevention, between doing more to patients and doing right by them.

One might assume many of these imbalances would favor the doctors and that their satisfaction would be at an all-time high. That's not the case. The personal and professional satisfaction among physicians has sunk to an all-time low. Thirty percent of medical students and residents are depressed, and over half of doctors feel burned out. Every year, four hundred doctors commit suicide. Their unhappiness is a result of the growing demands of medical practice and their sense of powerlessness. You can hear their frustration in the words they use to describe themselves, their patients, and their colleagues.

Fighting Words

On stage at a recent health care conference in New York City, one prominent speaker offered her thoughts on improving clinical practice through innovation and change. I didn't agree with all the ideas she presented, but they were certainly a good start. I looked forward to hearing what the audience thought.

As soon as the microphone opened for Q&A, a physician seated in the front row began his question with, "As a front-line physician . . . "

Then another asked his question as someone "in the trenches." And yet a third wondered how doctors can provide medical care when they're getting "bombarded" by so many mandates.

As I travel the country speaking to doctors, I hear these same words with accumulating frequency and from every specialty. These same military metaphors are used across society, but their presence in health care is disturbing. They aren't words of purpose, mission, and compassion, and they don't speak to our intrinsic desire to care for patients.

These are fighting words. Specifically, they derive from World War I, one of the bloodiest and most devastating wars in history, a conflict defined by trench warfare. Language is a powerful force in shaping how we view the world and the options we're open to considering. The words, images, and metaphors we use create context and influence our perceptions.

There was a time when physicians and patients saw disease as the common enemy, describing their efforts as "fighting" polio or "battling" heart disease. Together, they spoke like two friends plotting to take down a bully. The language physicians use today is different. Doctors who describe themselves as "in the trenches" or "on the front line" evoke images of men and women under siege, powerless to defend themselves. When the medical community uses these words of war, we can imagine doctors steeling themselves against an onslaught of patients with irrational expectations. Rather than attacking disease, doctors appear focused on hunkering down and protecting themselves.

The more these battlefield expressions enter the physician's dialogue, the more they corrode the mission-driven spirit of the profession. Taken together, these metaphors portray doctors as helpless victims; their only option is to dig deeper trenches and put up higher walls.

Attempts at humor and sarcasm evoke similarly destructive images. Doctors in fee-for-service medicine commonly use the phrase "you eat what you kill," the idea being that a physician's personal income is dependent on enticing patients into their offices and getting them to agree to remunerative procedures and services. There may be aspects of the fee-for-service world that resonate with this metaphor, but the words undermine what is best about medicine. The word "kill" contradicts our vision of physicians as healers. It undermines the reason physicians chose medicine as their profession.

Doctors today have much they can do to improve American health care, but nothing will change unless they see and talk about their mission as working together on behalf of patients.

None of my criticism denies the difficulty of practicing medicine today or the growing demands of an aging and ever-sicker population of

Americans. Instead, it represents my hope that physicians will lead positive change through innovation, collaboration, and commitment. They are the individuals best equipped to do so.

In the fourteenth century, the Black Plague swept the Middle East and Europe. We now know that the disease was caused by a bacterium, *Yersinia pestis*, transmitted by a combination of fleas and rats. In total, the plague killed upward of 100 million people, more than half the population of Europe. People at the time were ignorant of the true cause of so much death. The fear was extreme. But in spite of the personal risk, doctors went into the streets to care for the suffering. Physicians were no more immune to the disease than their patients, but they embraced their mission to heal.

That same dedication to healing was evident in West Africa following the 2014 Ebola outbreak. Once again, medical professionals were uncertain about the pathogenesis and transmission of the virus. Again, the fear ran deep. And as *Time* editor Nancy Gibbs wrote, "Anyone willing to treat Ebola victims [runs] the risk of becoming one." The World Health Organization estimated that over 11,000 people died in a relatively small geographic area.

Indeed, these Ebola fighters, those risking their lives to care for the African communities affected by this disease, did so with a commitment and sense of duty that has defined the profession for centuries and will continue for centuries more. Colleagues of mine volunteered to go there and treat the sick, often not just once, but two and three times. Not all doctors are so brave. But there is in most physicians an implicit motivation, one that is furthered by their medical training, which inspires this same dedication to helping others. Even if doctors don't volunteer in epidemic zones, those who approach medicine as a calling find increased fulfillment in their professional lives. As a nation, we can't allow this spirit to languish if we are to solve our greatest health care challenges.

Medicine should be the most humanistic of professions. The language of war contrasts with the values of the profession and, left unchecked, will ultimately undermine the power of the doctor-patient relationship.

If Bart Giamatti were appointed the imaginary position of "Commissioner of Health Care," he might describe obstetricians and pediatricians as starting pitchers for their important role in the beginning of life. Perhaps he would call gerontologists and cardiac surgeons the closers, each wanting to earn a "save" toward the end of a patient's life.

Emergency-medicine physicians could be the pinch hitters, entering a person's life at a crucial moment, needing to deliver in the clutch.

As commissioner, he would instruct everyone on the team, including physicians, insurers, and hospital administrators, to always put the patient first, reminding them that the patient, like the fan, pays their salaries and deserves their respect. And through the power of his words, he would elevate the practice of medicine to that of a true calling, ensuring that for decades to come, the best and brightest, those most dedicated to the values and mission of the medical profession, would continue to choose health care for their career. And rather than alluding to death and destruction in the trenches, Giamatti would celebrate the beauty, the purpose, and the teamwork intrinsic to health care, our nation's other greatest pastime.

A Part of Life

Together, physicians and their patients share some of life's most intimate and heart-wrenching moments. Death is one of those moments. As Bart Giamatti reminded us, all seasons come to an end. People die. We are designed to die.

Giamatti's own life came to an end sooner than it should have. Despite his brilliance, he was a heavy smoker. And though he knew the risks associated with this behavior, he died from his cigarette habit at the young age of fifty-one. A little over one year into his tenure as MLB commissioner, during what should have been a relaxing family vacation with his wife and son on Martha's Vineyard, Giamatti collapsed from an apparent heart attack. Doctors tried for more than an hour to resuscitate him before he was pronounced dead at a nearby hospital.

Death is difficult, even when it offers relief from pain and suffering. But not all deaths are the same. For a physician, one of the most painful experiences you can have is harming a patient. Nothing affects you more than when you bear some responsibility for a person's death. The loss stays with you forever.

In my career as a reconstructive plastic surgeon, I would estimate that I have saved the lives of several hundred patients. Some had cancer of the head and neck. Others were diagnosed with melanoma. Some were children with major infections that began in their feet or hands, requiring radical surgery to prevent spread to the rest of their body. A few of the lives I saved were of infants with severe congenital anomalies that affected their ability to breathe.

I still receive thank-you notes from families and pictures of former patients celebrating birthdays, graduations, and weddings. I cherish these kind gestures and fond memories more than they know.

But the medical success stories are not what I think about the most. Instead, my clearest memories are of the role I played in the deaths of two patients who should not have died so soon.

Laura

Three months before she was born, the ultrasound revealed her sex and her parents named her Laura. The same ultrasound revealed her congenital problem, a severe bilateral cleft lip and palate. I met Laura, along with her parents, an hour after she came into the world. Her mom and dad listened intently as I outlined the six operations their daughter would need over the next eighteen years of her life.

The first procedure would come in three months, and when the day arrived, our team closed two holes in Laura's upper lip and performed the first stage of reconstructing her nose. The improvement in her appearance was wonderful, and the look of elation on her mother's face made what happened later even more painful.

Laura's second surgery was scheduled for six months later. We repaired the gaping hole in her palate so that she could eat and swallow more easily, and one day speak more normally than she would have without surgery.

There is a particular part in the back of the palate called the uvula, which moves toward the throat when you say "ahh" in the doctor's office. When you eat, it ensures food goes down into your stomach, not up into your nose. And when you speak, the associated muscles close off the nasal passage so you can make a variety of "hard" sounds like *p*, *d*, or *k*. In children born with a severe cleft of the palate, the musculature in this area is often weak.

There are a variety of options to strengthen the palate, but in the most severe cases, when the child's speech remains unintelligible, surgeons perform an operation called a pharyngeal flap. The procedure helps compensate for the muscle's inability to pull the uvula all the way to the back of the throat. If successful, the operation makes the child's speech dramatically more understandable.

By the age of three, Laura was old enough to have her speech evaluated. The speech pathologist documented the debilitating problems caused by her poorly functioning palate. Looking down through Laura's nose, it was obvious that her palatal muscles weren't functioning as they needed to and that in spite of her trying, she could not close off the space in the back of her throat.

Laura's operation went smoothly, with minimal bleeding and no complications. The pharyngeal flap surgery connected her palate to the back of her throat, sealing off most of the airway but leaving two narrow passageways on each side for air to pass.

That evening, the nurses on the pediatric ward reported that Laura was having trouble breathing in her sleep. We evaluated her immediately and kept a close eye on our patient throughout the night. Because the operation intentionally narrows the air passage, it's not uncommon for children like Laura to have some difficulty breathing right after surgery. But the young girl was having more difficulty than was normal. So we kept her in the hospital for a couple more days to monitor her progress.

The medical team debated what to do next. We spoke with the parents and explained the three options available. We could continue to watch their child in the hospital to see if her condition improved. We could separate the flap from the palate and reopen space in her airway, though we cautioned this would re-create much of Laura's speech problem. Lastly, we told Laura's parents they could take their daughter home with them. After thinking over the options, they decided to bring Laura home. Three days later, she died in her sleep.

I look back now and rethink these options, weighing them over in my mind. All were reasonable and each had its own set of difficulties. Medicine is not an exact science. It's a probability profession. Every surgery comes with odds for a major complication, and every decision bears consequences.

This is the reality of being a physician. Care for so many lives, do enough surgical operations, and eventually something bad will happen. When the procedure you perform requires you to narrow the airway of small children, you risk becoming a part of someone's death. Doctors think about these types of consequences frequently, and when something does go wrong, they never forget the experience.

Laura would be in college today. I would have performed her sixth and final operation by now. I wonder what she would have been like, what she would be studying, what path her life would have taken if we had kept her in the hospital and reopened her air passage. I think about her parents often. I know they ponder these same questions every day.

Steven

A young man in his twenties, Steven had just been involved in a severe motorcycle accident, slamming into a tree and breaking nearly every bone in his face. He needed complex surgery to replace his crushed facial bones with others taken from different parts of his body.

By the time we were done, we had aligned his remaining teeth, repositioned his eyes, and brought his nose back to the midline. The procedure was long, but the results were excellent.

Six weeks later, we brought Steven back to the Operating Room for a much simpler procedure. We removed the metal bars wired to his teeth and tidied up a few of his wounds. The operation went without any problem. At the end of the procedure, I removed my gloves and sat down to write Steven's postoperative orders.

As I was writing, the anesthesiologist asked if he could suction the blood out of the patient's stomach to prevent vomiting. Without looking up, I said yes. My assumption was that he would pass the flexible suction tube through Steven's mouth. Instead, he passed it through Steven's nose.

In normal situations, the bone that separates the nose from the brain would turn the tube down toward the stomach. What the anesthesiologist did not know was that this bone was severely damaged in the accident. So, rather than the tube turning down, it went up, carrying bacteria from the nose into Steven's cranial cavity, causing an infection in his brain that took his life in less than a week.

In Steven's case as in Laura's, I keep replaying the "what-ifs" even decades later.

At most jobs, failure to communicate is a daily occurrence with minor or moderate consequences. In medicine, that same failure can be deadly. Many of the nearly 200,000 people who die each year from medical error would have lived if their physicians had communicated effectively.

I thought the anesthesiologist was asking whether or not I had a problem with his suctioning the blood from Steven's stomach. In retrospect, he was asking whether there was a problem with his passing the suction tube through Steven's nose. Sometimes doctors make mistakes, and most of the time they're lucky. If there had not been the damage to the bone separating the nose from the brain, the error in communication might have disrupted the soft tissue repair I had just done, but nothing more. In the parlance of safety experts, it would have been a "near miss." But when luck runs out, lives are lost and families are ruined. As a doctor, that's something you can never forget.

Death is universal, but some deaths are perceived as more tragic than others. In general, we find it sadder when a younger person dies rather than someone older, or when a healthier person dies rather than a sicker one. And of course, it's always harder when those closest to us pass away. As a nation, we perceive death after intervention as worse than death from omission. With all of these losses, the hardest part for any doctor is personally contributing to a patient's demise. There is little you can do except tell the patient's family what happened, tell them as compassionately as possible, and apologize.

Opening Our Eyes

Most health care professionals work hard to do what's right for their patients. They want nothing more than to improve and maximize the health of those they serve.

This is the prevailing mindset of American medicine. And though it must be acknowledged that a few individuals in health care do not share this mentality, be they greedy or sinister or consciously using their authority and position to the detriment of others, they stand on the fringes. They are the exceptions. Poorly trained doctors, underhanded administrators, and seedy pharmaceutical executives do exist. And we need to address these threats. But they do not account for most of the poor clinical quality that Americans experience.

Mistreated has focused on the ability of context to sway perception and affect behavior. As you have read throughout this book, the environment in which health care is administered has a far greater influence on our nation's clinical quality than any one person ever could.

But if you have any lingering doubt about an environment's command over your behavior, I invite you to examine the works of Chen-Bo Zhong and his colleagues at the University of Toronto.

In one experiment, Professor Zhong and his cohorts took eighty-four students and randomly divided them into two groups, placing half in a well-lit room and the other half in a dimly lit one. The students were given a series of mathematical problems and an envelope filled with $10 in fifty-cent pieces. Once finished, the researchers left it up to the students to score their own work, keep fifty cents for each of the twenty answers they got right, and drop their test (along with any money they didn't earn) in a box on their way out.

In the brightly lit room, students reported getting fewer than eight answers right on average, whereas those in the dimly lit room reported getting almost twelve answers correct on average. Simply darkening the room increased cheating by 50 percent.

In a related experiment, Zhong's researchers invited fifty new students into equally well-lit rooms, giving half of them sunglasses and the other half clear glasses. This time, students were asked to sit at a computer and divide $6 between themselves and a stranger on the other end whom they couldn't see but could interact with electronically (this person was an experimenter). The students were assured they'd never meet face-to-face with the person on the other end. With anonymity guaranteed, whether students wore sunglasses or clear glasses should not have altered the amount they offered the stranger. But it made a huge difference.

Those with clear lenses divided the money almost equally, keeping $3.29 for themselves and sharing $2.71 with the stranger on the other end. Those with sunglasses (who *felt* more anonymous) gave an average of $1.81, keeping $4.19.

None of this makes sense from a logical standpoint. But perception is not rational and, as we have seen, is shaped by the context of one's environment. When individuals wear sunglasses or find themselves in a dark room, they feel more anonymous and their behaviors change. The impact of context may not be conscious, but it's very real. We see the same outcomes in health care environments.

Every year, I teach a course through the Stanford Department of Plastic Surgery for physicians about to take the oral part of their boards. This is a high-stakes examination, as hospitals increasingly require board certification before granting privileges. The weeklong course focuses on complex clinical problems and the best operative solutions to each. As part of the examination itself, the candidates must bring all of their records on five patient cases that they completed over the previous twelve months.

A major reason some individuals fail this examination is because of inappropriate coding and billing for the operations they performed. Integrity is an important part of the certification process, and this is one of the ways national examiners assess the ethics of the examinees. Invariably, when participants realize they are about to fail the examination, they ask what they can do to reverse the errors in coding and billing they made. At this point, I tell them nothing can be done. I often ask them why they overcharged for their procedures in the first place. The story is almost always the same.

"I joined a practice," they say. "That's how the senior members of the group did it. I just signed the forms prepared by the billing staff."

All of them logically should have known that what they were doing was wrong, just like the subjects who put on the sunglasses or took their exams in the dimly lit rooms. But in the context of working among associates who did the same thing, the surgeons' perception shifted. Maybe if they had to fill the forms out themselves, they would have completed them correctly. Maybe if they had different senior partners, they would have been more honest. But once perception shifts, so does behavior.

What's It Worth to You?

If you're still not a believer in the subtle power of context, meet Avni Shah. As a doctoral student at Duke University, she wanted to compare how a buyer felt when purchasing something with cash versus credit card. So she went around selling coffee mugs with the university's logo to faculty and staff at the promotional price of $2. In this well-designed experiment, all but one variable was held constant. Half of the time, she said she could only take cash. For the other half, she'd only accept plastic.

Two hours later, she returned to each office, explaining that she was unable to complete the sale and would need to buy back the mugs. Although disappointed, the subjects were assured they'd be compensated for the inconvenience. Shah asked them to name their price.

You might expect that the people most perturbed by this would be the credit-card payers. They might worry about getting charged twice or being penalized by the credit-card company. They might be annoyed about having to check their statements repeatedly to make sure the refund actually went through. With cash, on the other hand, the transaction was simple. Fork it over, hand it back.

But it turned out that Shah's subjects were much more attached to their cash. Those who paid by credit card demanded an average of only $3.83 for their troubles. Cash payers expected an average of $6.71 in return.

Why was the same mug worth more than triple the asking price to those who paid cash? As Shah explained to *Forbes,* it's all about perception. Handing over cash is immediate and tangible. Not so with credit and debit. Your bill won't arrive for a month. There is not the same perception of loss among credit-card users.

The same distortion is magnified in health care through insurance. Patients with prescription coverage, for example, rarely think about the impact of the transaction when picking up their medications. The bottle of name-brand pills is perceived to cost little or nothing.

But they are paying more for it than the number on the cash register indicates. Americans are paying for that expensive bottle through lost wages, higher premiums, and the collective transition of wealth from patients to pharmaceutical-company executives and their shareholders.

Of all the things that distort perception, money is most powerful. It's a fact that reveals itself often in health care, even in some university research laboratories.

A Complicated Mess

The economics of health care are extremely complicated, contradictory, and distinct from any other industry. The traditional lines between supply and demand are blurred.

Part of the reason is that physicians determine both the demand for a procedure and the price. Increase the supply of doctors or hospitals, and costs for care should drop. They don't, because doctors and hospitals subconsciously lower the indications for procedures, increase the volume performed, and continue to charge their "usual and customary fees." Patients have few options but to pay. Raise the prices for drugs by a factor of five, and sales should crash. But they don't, not when the product is a necessity and competition is nullified through patent protections.

You might think the only area of health care saved from this distortion would be academic medical research: objective and pragmatic analysis of a drug or device. But even the hallowed halls of university medical centers aren't protected from these influences. And because of that, patients suffer.

When treating patients with an open wound, one of the newer techniques available involves placing a suction-type device over the wound, which creates a vacuum. No one is exactly sure why, but this practice has been shown to accelerate healing. It's possible the suction cleans the wound by constantly extracting the overlying fluid and associated bacteria. Maybe it speeds up healing by pulling the tissues toward each other, or perhaps the negative pressure brings healing cells from the blood vessels to the damaged tissues. Regardless of the exact science, it works.

Today, there are two types of suction devices available on the market and, as you might assume, tremendous competition between the two companies that make them.

No business in health care likes to compete on lower prices. So, to justify higher prices and convince more surgeons to use their device, these two suction companies are motivated to demonstrate that their product is better.

In medicine, peer-reviewed journals are the gold standard for proving a product's worth. Doctors assume the information in them is accurate, and editors insist the results be bias free. But as you've no doubt already guessed, that's not always the case.

Perhaps the most damning evidence of bias came by way of a literature review in *Plastic and Reconstructive Surgery*. The authors began by identifying twenty-four published peer-reviewed studies that compared these two types of suction devices. They then asked five independent surgeons to read all twenty-four papers and decide whether the results favored suction device A or B, or neither. The researchers than compared the device that was judged superior in the published article with the company that funded the project.

Of the twenty-four studies, five did not receive funding from either company. Among the nineteen that were funded, some of the studies favored one device and a similar number favored the other. But the correlation between a positive review and the funding source was far from random.

Those studies that concluded that company A's product was better were funded by company A. Those research studies that found company B's product superior were funded by company B. In only one case did the researchers not conclude the funding company's product was better, and in that article the independent surgeons were split as to which product rated higher.

In every case, the funding company's product came out as good as, and usually better than, the alternative.

The odds of this happening by pure chance are miniscule. This result is the equivalent of flipping nineteen coins and having them come up heads each time: not impossible, but not very likely. We might expect that because the two suction devices were relatively equal, the product sold by the nonfunding company should have been judged as better (or at least equal to its counterpart) about half the time. And if one was really better than the other, we would have expected every paper, regardless of whatever company funded the work, to reach that conclusion.

But to have no study go against the funding company would be a total anomaly. From a statistical perspective, there's a one in 262,144 chance of that happening.

There is no way to interpret these results other than to assume the researchers themselves were biased by the company that paid for the work. Not consciously biased, mind you, but influenced greatly by the dollars the device companies paid researchers to fund the projects. Of course, if you accused the researchers of not being objective, they would deny it and probably become incensed. Dishonest research is a career destroyer for academic physicians pursuing tenure. Every journal would reject their subsequent submissions and question their findings.

We can also assume that no drug or device manufacturer would be foolish enough to demand outright that investigators reach a specific conclusion. Discovery of such a quid pro quo would result in a major scandal and taint the reputation of both the funding company and the university itself. And yet in the case of the suction study, there's a 99.99 percent probability that bias happened and that money was the root cause.

The use of context to alter doctors' perceptions and influence their behaviors spills over into offices and hospitals across the country. Drug and device companies are experts at manipulating doctors. To do so, their representatives use "food, flattery, and friendship," commonly referred to as the three F's.

The process begins when a friendly rep comes to a hospital and offers free bagels and donuts. Having been invited in, she becomes friends with the doctors and asks if she can visit them in their offices. They exchange niceties as the rep gushes over the doctors' family photos. She offers free samples or leaves a coffee mug embossed with the name of the company's most expensive drug on the front.

Drug and device companies monitor closely who is using and prescribing their most expensive products. Once doctors become top customers of the drug or device manufacturer, they're invited to participate on panels where they're introduced as experts (even though the only expertise the drug companies evaluate is how effectively the doctors tout the products to their colleagues), and they are paid well for their time.

In a laboratory setting, the three F's are only slightly different. The food takes the shape of grant money. The friendship comes in the form of visits from company representatives to check on the progress and results of the study. And for the researchers who deliver positive findings, there are "advisory councils" where they spend a weekend at a luxury resort and provide keynote speeches with a nice stipend. None of this is illegal. All of it is calculated. And in the end, none of it helps improve the health of Americans.

What Patients Want

The latter chapters of this book have examined solutions for health care's toughest problems from a variety of angles. They have dissected the 1,000-page Affordable Care Act and its key provisions. They have examined health care's flawed economics and looked for ways to reconcile the system's $3 trillion price tag. They have focused on health care's structure and payment model, along with its lack of technology and leadership, as opportunities to transform the current system. They have looked at different approaches to implementing change through the lens of two very different American presidents. And they have offered solutions that represent a step in the right direction. However, the change required is massive. It will take the commitment and courage of both doctors and patients.

It will require us to recognize that our health care decisions have consequences for ourselves, our families, and our communities.

When people choose to receive care from fragmented providers who are unsupported by modern technology, they're risking their health and that of their family. When most people receive care in this way, costs rise more rapidly than the nation's ability to pay, and millions of Americans face the possibility of bankruptcy. Conversely, when they demand from their health care the same convenience and use of technology they would expect to receive anywhere else, they accelerate the process of transformation needed to solve the challenges of American health care.

What most Americans want is reasonable and possible. They would like affordable coverage, limited out-of-pocket expenses, and convenient access to medical care. They want clinically excellent doctors who understand the Golden Rule, treating their patients in the same way they would a family member or dear friend. Patients would like their doctors to avail themselves of the latest in information technologies and coordinate the medical treatment they provide. Finally, all of us want compassionate physicians who respect our wishes and tell us the truth about our medical problems.

Together, these expectations can be thought of as the four C's: *cost, clinical excellence, coordination, and compassion.* If the American health care system can address each of the four C's, we will improve the patient experience in powerful and important ways. Through this lens, providing great medical care doesn't seem that complex or difficult.

Cost: Make Health Care Affordable

For most of his adult life after college, Sean Casey was a software engineer. The job paid well, though the hours were long and the work demanding. After twenty-eight years of rolling up his sleeves and solving complex problems, Sean was starting to burn out—a feeling punctuated by concerns over his mother's worsening dementia.

Although his choices were difficult, Sean did what he needed to do. He walked away from his company to take care of his ailing mother.

With a wife and two kids, Sean was mindful that his former company's health benefits were the cornerstone of his family's well-being. Through COBRA coverage—a government program that ensures continuing coverage after certain life events—Sean had some extended peace of mind. That is, while the coverage lasted. After about eighteen months of unemployment, as his COBRA coverage was set to expire, Sean grew anxious.

For the first time in his life, he found himself shopping for private insurance. Although it was somewhat more expensive, he was able to find a carrier that offered him and his family what they needed.

In time, Sean was able to find a safe, around-the-clock care facility for his mother. Knowing she would be taken care of, he went back to work, dropped his private insurer, and again joined the company's health plan. Sean preferred the company's coverage but didn't care much for changes happening inside the company itself. So, he resigned.

Soon, he was back on COBRA for a few months before once again researching private insurers. All this hopscotching between plans was time-consuming and vexing, but manageable. That is, until Sean received some discouraging news.

"When I came off COBRA a second time, I applied to all the same insurance companies as before and got turned down by all of them," he told me.

Why was that? Sean had been involved in a serious bicycling accident that left him with broken bones and $100,000 in hospital bills, costs that were largely covered by his previous health plan.

At the time, not long after the passage of the Affordable Care Act, Sean had the distinct feeling the insurance companies—not knowing how the implementation of the ACA would play out—were turning down anyone with an expensive medical history. Although he had made a full recovery, and his health was just the same as before (with the same prescriptions and everything), the private insurers turned him down flat.

Fortunately, there was one health-insurance option out there that would cover Sean with his "preexisting medical conditions." The solution came courtesy of former president Bill Clinton, who in 1996 signed into law the Health Insurance Portability and Accountability Act (HIPAA). The law was the first of its kind to ensure health benefits for Americans who were out of work and needed protection against discriminatory health plans.

But between Sean's HIPAA coverage and private health insurance for his son and daughter, the Casey family's total premiums added up to $32,000 a year.

"Thankfully, the year my wife and I were using HIPAA was the year before the full implementation of the Affordable Care Act," Sean said. "So, I was monitoring Covered California (the state's online health insurance exchange) and called their customer service numerous times as the sign-up period approached."

Sean had heard rumblings in the media about the federal insurance exchanges not working, bugs and crashes galore. But as a "semi-retired" software engineer, Sean felt confident that Californians on the state-based exchange wouldn't have those same issues. So he decided to send President Obama an e-mail.

"I figured he'd like to hear something positive for a change. So I told him about my confidence in the ACA and how much I enjoyed the experience. When our benefits kicked in, the savings were almost enough to offset my daughter's first year in college. For me, that was a big deal."

On April Fool's Day of 2014, about seven months after he hit send on his e-mail to the president, Sean got a pleasant surprise. It was the surprise of a lifetime, actually. He was taking his lunch break while serving jury duty about thirty miles from his home. On the television in the jury room, Sean stood and listened as Barack Obama delivered a speech from the Rose Garden of the White House. Just a few minutes into the president's address, Sean heard him say this:

> Let me give you a sense of what this change has meant for millions of our fellow Americans. Sean Casey, from Solana Beach, California, always made sure to cover his family on the private market. But preexisting medical conditions meant his annual tab was over $30,000. The Affordable Care Act changed that. See, if you have a preexisting condition . . . you can no longer be charged more than anybody else. So this year, the Casey family's premiums will fall from over $30,000 to under $9,000.

This was no joke. The president of the United States was talking about him, and highlighting his concerns over the rising cost of health care. Sean's fears were shared by tens of millions of Americans. They still are.

"Having coverage through the ACA has saved me and my family a lot of money," he told me about three years after the president's speech. "It ensured that I could continue to get health insurance and the benefits that come with it. It meant that no one could turn me down and that I could pay a reasonable price for peace of mind."

It's not a perfect law, Sean says, but his Covered California health plan did what he needed it to do.

"It was a little more online and a little more efficient. But the main thing for me was that I needed health insurance. And I was willing to pay a fair price for that."

Since the ACA rolled out, much attention has been paid to the macroeconomics of health care, from the percentage of the population now insured to America's cumulative spending for medical services, doctors, drugs, and devices. In news coverage, we see dollar signs in front of costs that end in "billion" and "trillion." Lost in this focus on health care's colossal price tag is what the former president's law did for the pocketbooks of people like Sean and his family.

Most patients aren't concerned with the total cost of our nation's medical care. Like Sean, they're concerned about whether an unforeseen injury or serious complication will empty their savings account or bankrupt their families.

If Sean had suffered a bicycling accident without insurance, he would have been on the hook for $25,000 to $35,000 in "trauma alert" charges alone before receiving even a single ounce of care at the hospital. Add in costs for surgery, medications, and a few days in a hospital bed—to say nothing of lost wages and follow-up care—and he would have accumulated a medical bill very few American families could afford to pay without insurance. For most, declaring bankruptcy would be the only option.

Thanks to the Affordable Care Act, insurers could no longer discriminate against people with preexisting conditions, or drop them from coverage, or deny their claims. That meant more Americans could enjoy the financial security they want and deserve.

Based on comments made in late 2016 by then president-elect Trump, this part of the legislation is likely to remain. But unless the cost escalation slows, prices will become unaffordable for most. For the past decade, the solution for health care inflation has been to transfer year-over-year cost increases onto patients through increased deductibles and out-of-pocket expenses. In 2010, one-fourth of all workers had a high-deductible plan. That number is now 40 percent. It explains why the average middle-class family is reaching its limit and can't take much more.

Unless we can better manage costs, the price for care will continue to escalate faster than wages, and our nation will slide into a two-tier class system. Already, those who remain uninsured or who live in states with low Medicaid reimbursements have difficulty accessing care. In the future, at the current rate of rising costs, those in the middle class (particularly seniors on Medicare) will find themselves in the same position—with coverage but without access. As a result, they will be forced to delay their treatments or go without, and their health status will erode.

Doctors and hospitals don't see reducing the costs of health care as their responsibility. In fact, when they're reimbursed based on the amount of care they provide, they perceive their job as providing more care, not more efficient and effective medical care. Faced with the demands and time constraints of daily practice, doctors see their approaches to medical care as appropriate. They have trouble recognizing the long-term consequences of their actions.

In the early nineteenth century, the English economist William Forster Lloyd wrote of cattle herders who shared common land on which their cows grazed. What would happen, he asked, if one of the herders got greedy and allowed more cattle to graze upon the open land? Certainly the cows would fatten and that would be a good thing for him. But what if all herders followed his example? Soon, the grounds of the commons would go bare, the land wasted, and all would suffer. It was a hypothetical example intended to warn readers that individually beneficial decisions can negatively affect a community. This came to be known as the "tragedy of the commons," an economic theory that is playing out in American health care right now.

In the last century, back when people paid directly for their care, doctors were cognizant of what their patients could afford. In contrast, the current approach to health coverage separates the expense of providing care from the cost of buying insurance.

As a result, doctors can't see how the inefficiencies of their practice undermine patient quality and make coverage increasingly unaffordable. But it does, and it will until doctors embrace the changes necessary to improve quality outcomes and drive down the costs of care.

Clinical Excellence: Treat Patients Like People

Doctors and patients judge competency in health care quite differently. A hospital administrator or departmental chairman looking to add a new physician to the staff will ask about the candidate's medical school, residency, and published peer-reviewed articles.

Although some patients may pay attention to the diplomas, certificates, and awards hanging on the walls of their doctor's office, they tend to evaluate the doctor with more subjective criteria. They expect their physicians to be well trained and technically excellent. But they also want their doctors to possess people skills. I first learned this lesson many years ago from a patient of mine, a young surfer girl.

Samantha—Sam, as she preferred to be called—was recovering from a terrible car accident. One night, on a winding road leading to her home in the hills of Santa Cruz, Sam's vehicle careened off course, and she fractured a dozen bones in her arms, legs, back, and pelvis.

I met Sam when I was a second-year resident at Stanford University, rotating through the orthopedic service. She was athletic, with a deep-bronze tan and straw-colored hair. Her attitude was at once carefree and recalcitrant. Unaffected and unimpressed by our white coats and rapid-fire medical observations, Sam wasn't concerned about the contents of my clipboard or interested in where I trained. She just wanted to get back on the waves as soon as possible.

Of course, soon wasn't possible. Sam needed surgery to put her bones back in place. And she needed traction for the ones that couldn't be safely realigned, a process that involved inserting stainless steel pins through the broken bones, attaching those pins to a series of weights and pulleys, and keeping her in the hospital on strict bed rest for three weeks. Not until the constant tugging of weights moved the bones back into their original anatomical positions would Sam be fitted in a full body cast and sent on her way. Until then, she'd need to wait.

Our team came to visit Sam every morning during rounds, which began at 6:00 a.m. and had to be completed by 7:30 a.m., when surgery commenced in the Operating Room. With twenty patients to see each day, speed and efficiency were essential. Most of our time was devoted to the sickest patients, the ones who had recently undergone surgery or suffered the most serious complications such as pneumonia, wound infection, or major bleeding. By default, all others received only a brief visit.

After just a week in the hospital, Sam was both medically and surgically stable. So, our team of doctors rarely stayed with her for more than a minute or two during rounds. Each morning, six or seven of us—the attending physician, residents, and medical students—would walk into her room in unison, standing halfway between the door and her bed as one of the students read aloud from Sam's medical chart.

"The patient has no fever, most recent X-rays are good, and the bony fragments are realigning nicely." Next, the resident responsible would turn to her with a big smile and say, "Everything is going great!"

Sam would roll her eyes or flash a sarcastic smile back our way. Then, as though we had choreographed the movement, we would turn as one and leave.

After another week of cursory daily rounds, Sam surprised us. Just as we turned to leave, she told us, "There's moss growing under my leg cast."

With that, she had our undivided attention. We quickly huddled around her bed, pulled back the sheets and began peppering her with questions. "When did you first notice it?" "Are you having any pain?" "Does it itch or burn?"

As we peered closer under the cast, however, we could see that the moss wasn't actually growing there. Sam sighed and fessed up. She had asked her younger sister to go into the forest near their home and bring a piece of moss to her hospital bed. Earlier that morning, she inserted the green patch under the edge of her cast. Sam did it to teach us a lesson.

"You stopped asking me how I was doing and what I was feeling," she said. "I didn't know any other way to get your attention."

From that day forward, each of us made certain to say good morning to every patient on our service and ask how they were doing. After that day, I always asked each patient before I left the room, whether in the hospital or the office, if there was anything else that patient wanted to tell me.

Those few extra minutes I spent listening to my patients have paid remarkable dividends over the years. Dozens of times, I have diagnosed problems that I would otherwise have missed, often spotting them long before the issue could become more serious.

Most physicians are well trained and technically skilled. But patients expect more than that when it comes to clinical excellence. The ability to reposition bones is only half the equation. There is a common adage in medicine that "no one cares how much you know, until they know how much you care." To doctors, this kind of intimacy and connection with patients can sometimes seem impossible, or at least, too effortful to be realistic. In health care, however, clinical excellence extends beyond the Operating Room and requires that doctors show concern, listen, and demonstrate that they care, a lesson Sam taught our whole team.

Coordination: Reduce the Stresses of Medical Care

Most people are confident in their medical care, knowing that each of their doctors is well trained. That is, until they become really sick and realize how dangerously fragmented medical care can be. Patients assume the doctors who take care of them communicate and coordinate with each other regularly and intuitively. That's rarely the case.

When patients require hospitalization, for example, they see a variety of specialists each morning, few of whom ever converse with each other directly. All their coordination takes place in the form of notes buried in the patient's record. Each specialist focuses on his or her own area of expertise, rather than on working as a team to maximize the total health of the patient.

The nephrologist addresses the kidneys, the hematologist addresses the blood, and the cardiologist, the heart. That works until the kidneys affect the heart or the heart medication prescribed has hematological consequences. Not surprisingly, this happens all the time.

Uncoordinated care is the norm in American medicine today. But there are rays of hope, success stories we can point to that might inspire patients to ask why their own care providers don't employ the same degree of coordination. We can learn a lot by studying some of the more successful existing models.

The story of Karen Skoog from Maple Grove, Minnesota, shows us what can happen when doctors work together for the betterment of patients.

Karen and Jerry have been married for forty-eight years. They have a son and a daughter, and two energetic grandchildren. Karen is a very active woman, and has been her whole life. She was an active mom when raising her two kids, and now, her children say, she's extremely active with her grandkids, despite her illness.

Ten years ago, just three months before her first grandchild was born, Karen was diagnosed with late-stage ovarian cancer. "I was a stage three," Karen said, "so I was in the heavier part of the cancer and its treatment. I was sad because I wanted to be a part of my grandson's life. I wanted to continue to live for my family and for myself, because I love life and I still have a lot to teach these kids."

Cancer treatment is very hard. It's painful, ongoing, and complicated. Karen needed to see a number of clinicians in quick succession. And, in the world of cancer treatment, doing the right thing at the right time can mean life or death for patients like her.

Karen was fortunate to get her medical care through a multispecialty medical group, Park Nicollet Health Services, just outside of Minneapolis. Dr. Brian Rank, co-executive medical director, is proud of what is possible at his facility today.

"We're finally at a time when we can link clinicians, patients, and knowledge to create a more perfect version of care then we ever could have before," he said.

In Karen's case, the right care meant having a series of doctors working closely together, as a single team, overseeing every aspect of her treatment.

Most people living with cancer need to schedule a number of different appointments at different locations with several doctors, all of them working on very different schedules. That means getting chemotherapy on one side of town and radiation on the other. It requires seeing a primary-care physician for regular checkups and coordinating multiple visits with surgical specialists.

"We are very cognizant today of the burden that illness places on patients," said Dr. Rank. "They shouldn't be responsible for having to do the coordination of their care themselves."

So Dr. Rank and his colleagues at Park Nicollet helped Karen manage her appointments. They organized a team of providers to develop a game plan for her, making sure that Karen's appointments happened on time with as little travel and time out of her schedule as possible.

And through the health system's comprehensive electronic medical-record system, Karen could see her test results almost instantly and connect with all of her doctors whenever she needed to. For her, having that information available, along with the ability to conveniently communicate with her physicians, gave her more control over her cancer and her life.

It hasn't all been a smooth road for Karen. She has had recurrences. Not long ago, the cancer spread to her lungs. The pain is taxing and the appointments seem never-ending. But Karen says that when it comes to her medical treatment, she is confident in the quality and grateful that the care is coordinated and convenient.

"I needed this team and, if I didn't have this team, I don't think I would be standing here today, a ten-year cancer survivor."

Today, Karen remains active and fulfilled. She volunteers in the cancer center at Park Nicollet and enjoys being able to watch her grandkids grow.

If physicians were to ask themselves how they'd like their own care to be provided, they'd want it to be convenient, personal, and coordinated. If they had to experience what most patients do, they would realize how difficult and frustrating it is to chase down appointments and manage their care from start to finish. And if physicians were to suffer the same types of medical problems Karen has, they might realize how scary the whole experience is when the doctors providing treatment aren't connected with each other.

It's not that doctors aren't aware of what is happening. It's just that they view the wait times and the inconveniences as normal. If you are admitted to a hospital and need a routine procedure or complex test that can wait until Monday morning, you are often expected to do so. Ask your doctors about the delay, and they will tell you it is harmless. That is, until they are the patient tossing sleeplessly in a hospital bed for forty-eight long hours, waiting for their "non-emergent" problem to be addressed.

Similarly, when doctors are paid on a fee-for-service basis, they perceive that the best care happens in their office, even when these office visits force patients to put their busy lives on hold.

In retail stores, clerks are taught to explain to customers not just the features of the products they sell but the benefits, too. For example, you don't tell the customer the jeans are double stitched, you explain that double stitching will make the jeans more durable and longer lasting, and that they'll save the customer from having to buy a new pair in three months.

Using that same construct in health care, features such as improved integration and technology mean that patients like Karen can spend more time with their families and less time worrying about getting test results, scheduling appointments, or traveling from doctor's office to doctor's office. The benefits of integration, advanced information technology, and prepayment should be clear to everyone. Often, however, "health care customers" don't understand the benefits of better care until they become sick. And by then it's too late.

Compassion: Make Health Care More Personal

The advances in medical technology over the past two decades have increased our dependence on machines and turned the physical exam into an overlooked skill.

And though there's a clear place and purpose for sophisticated diagnostic technologies, the human touch remains as powerful in medicine now as in the past. As the rituals once so vital to establishing trust in the doctor-patient relationship fade away, and as specialization in medical practice diffuses accountability, compassion has become a lost art.

For medicine to be great, it must be both "high tech" and "high touch," a lesson I've been reminded of many times in my career, and one that I first learned from a very special patient.

Paul was an artist like my father. In fact, he was like my father in many ways. He was funny and charming and kind. Paul had recently gotten married and was soon to become a father himself, with the couple's first child on the way.

He came to see me with a dark, pigmented spot on his shoulder. His primary-care physician worried it might be a melanoma. So, to determine the diagnosis, I explained to him the relatively minor procedure I would need to perform. Paul told me the word *melanoma* terrified him and asked whether I thought that would be the diagnosis. I told him I couldn't be sure until the pathologist had the chance to do the necessary microscopic evaluation.

But I knew Paul would spend three or four sleepless nights worrying until he got his answer. So I promised I would call him as soon as I received the results.

When the pathology report came back, the diagnosis confirmed Paul's fears. The melanoma was relatively thick and his prognosis poor. For most cancers, the mortality rate depends on how far the tumor has spread. Physicians can predict the chances of death from melanoma based on the thickness or depth of the lesion.

I explained to Paul that the surgical procedure would require a wide excision, skin grafting to close the wound, and removal of the lymph glands under the arm, the first place the tumor cells would spread.

Paul joked that he was glad he had a left-sided cancer, since he painted with his right hand. And he was glad that no matter how debilitating the surgery, it would not interfere with his art. Of course, he understood there was nothing funny about his situation, but his humor in the face of such overwhelming news was my first clue to his resiliency. I warmed up quickly to Paul, and he warmed up to me.

In most cases, the doctor-patient relationship stays professional. But sometimes it becomes personal. Paul and I looked forward to our conversations in the office. I would always reserve extra time, knowing that after we addressed his medical issues, we would chat for at least another fifteen minutes about life, family, and our hopes for the future.

Shortly after the birth of his son, I had to inform Paul that the cancer had spread to his lung. I told him that chemotherapy would slow its progression but that a cure was impossible. As he always did, Paul understood and accepted the facts. And he maintained his optimism, further proof of his resiliency.

For the next several months, Paul's oncologist provided most of his care. I rarely saw him as a patient after that, but he always sought me out and updated me on his family. We shared an interest in growing fruits and vegetables in our yards, and he would always bring me a juicy tomato or peach.

I was saddened to see the tumor spread as his condition worsened. One day, he came to my office and asked to talk. He had brought me a present, a self-portrait he had sketched in charcoal. On the back he wrote, "Life ends and we should enjoy each day." And in his familiar joking style, Paul added, "You will never be a good farmer, but if you work hard at it, you might become a great physician."

I hugged him and thanked him for the beautiful picture and for the inspiration he had given me. His kindness overwhelmed me.

Sometimes, the most difficult part of being a physician is accepting our limitations and letting go. And when there is nothing more we can do for our patients by way of medical treatment, the most important skill we possess is our ability to show compassion, especially at the end of a patient's life. Paul has been gone for many years now, leaving behind his wife and son. I carry our friendship in my heart and will always remember the lesson he taught me about the importance of compassion.

Having treated thousands of patients, I know most are respectful of physicians and grateful for the care we provide. Most people don't expect the impossible, only that we do our best. To me, that means treating them as we would a family member or friend.

That's why, starting early in my practice, I would give patients my home phone number after outpatient surgery. I would tell them to call if they had a problem that night. My colleagues thought I was crazy, thinking that my phone would ring at all hours of the night.

In more than twenty years of practice, I received a total of three calls, two of which were problems that required immediate attention. Both were solved the same night I received the call after meeting those patients in the Emergency Department. The third call was inappropriate but a very small price to pay for the gratitude of thousands of other patients. It's remarkable to me how often doctors try to protect themselves from the 1 percent of patients who will abuse a privilege. Little do they realize that in doing so, they project their distrust onto the other 99 percent, compromising their relationships with their patients and the quality of their medical care in the process.

What Health Care Needs

The four C's (cost, clinical excellence, coordination, and compassion) are all individually important. The best health care, however, will happen when we achieve all four at once. We won't be able to address the economic fears of individual patients unless we can improve the health of the entire nation. And this won't happen until physicians work together to address chronic illnesses, reduce medical error, and improve the coordination of care they provide.

Doing this will demand that physicians learn from their colleagues, share patient data through modern information technology systems, and focus as much on avoiding health problems as on correcting them. Once these pieces are in place, physicians and elected officials can focus on new ways to address social determinants of disease and implement programs to decrease the disparities in health outcomes.

In moving from fee-for-service to prepayment, whether through capitation or bundled payments, insurance companies will have the opportunity to unclutter the practice of medicine and stop demanding that physicians obtain authorization to do the right things for their patients.

As each opportunity is embraced, the improvements in medical care will build greater and greater momentum, creating a virtuous cycle.

When all of this happens, the rate of health care inflation will flatten and quality will improve, as will access to the best medical care available. This is the future the four pillars offer for American health care and the American people.

The Destination

Yogi Berra, the late New York Yankees catcher and former manager of the New York Mets, was known as much for his "Yogi-isms" as he was for his hall-of-fame playing career. One of the old truisms sometimes attributed to him goes like this: "It's tough to make predictions, especially about the future."

That's particularly applicable to health care. No physician has a crystal ball, but two specific predictions about health care's future seem probable.

First, the practice of medicine is and will always be a great profession. In spite of the demands placed on physicians, it's an honor to improve lives and help those who need medical care.

Second, over the next decade, doctors will be forced to change their ways before they're ready. Most likely, they will be able to practice under the current model for a while longer. But at some point, industry-wide disruption will begin. It has to.

This reality has doctors in private practice doing the calculus, deciding whether to embrace change quickly, dig in their heels, or abandon ship. They see more and more newly trained doctors joining medical groups and taking jobs in hospitals. To physicians in solo practices, the thought of giving up their autonomy and control is scary. They are caught in a quandary.

These doctors understand that providing patients with access to their medical information online will make their lives simpler. But these same physicians worry it will open the door to greater malpractice risk and force them to modify what they enter in the medical record. Offering video visits to their patients would make medical care more convenient, but doctors worry they will not be paid for these services. And they know e-mail would make it easier to connect with patients, but they can envision their inbox overflowing the moment they offer it.

Many physicians nearing retirement are ready to give up. I hope they don't. We need their expertise. I know they see the downside of what is happening, but I hope they can recognize the opportunities before them as well. Technology can be a friend, not just a burden. Embracing scientifically proven best practices can improve patient care and help physicians avoid the horrific pain they feel when something goes wrong. Lowering the cost of care doesn't have to start with reductions in reimbursement. It can be achieved through increased teamwork and decreased medical error.

This is a challenging time in American health care, but it is also one of the most exciting. Change always feels uncomfortable at first. That is its nature. And amid rapid change, it's tempting to feel like a victim and cling to the past. It feels safer. But embracing the future usually proves most rewarding. The gratitude of patients, the satisfaction that emerges through the doctor-patient relationship, and the sense of accomplishment that accompanies innovation all align perfectly with the mission and purpose of medicine. If together we can provide patients with each of the four C's, I believe we can restore the fulfillment of our profession and make health care a rewarding career for the next generation of physicians.

Two Paths

As medical school begins all across our country, new students line up to participate in the heartwarming "white coat ceremony," one of the first rituals in becoming a physician. The event typically includes a reading of the Hippocratic Oath or one of its newer versions, after which future doctors receive the stethoscopes they will use for decades to come. Parents walk onto the stage with their adult children and help them put on their white coat for the first time. This is a moment of great pride, a time to reflect on the hard work and academic successes that brought them this far. But most important, it is a passing on of the values, mission, and responsibilities of becoming a doctor, a moment made possible not just by the school and the parents, but by 5,000 years of doctors who came before.

Still aglow in the newness of their path toward becoming a doctor, students are filled with enthusiasm. For many, however, this sense of fulfillment dissipates over the course of their training. The seemingly endless grind of rote learning, testing, and sleep deprivation combines with the sometimes dehumanizing aspects of practicing medicine to drain the joy they felt the day they tried on their first white coat.

And even once you become a doctor, your enthusiasm and pride have a tendency to get lost in the demands of running an office, battling insurance companies, and facing the threat of being sued. But it doesn't have to remain this bleak. Like the grass under the snow, the doctor's passion can be reborn. It must be reborn.

In President Obama's reflections on ACA in his *Journal of the American Medical Association* article, he rated the advances in coverage highly and was proud of the millions of Americans who could now obtain medical care without suffering personal financial hardship. But he lamented the slow pace of delivery-system change, the compromised quality patients endure, and the high cost of medical care that persists.

Achieving delivery-system improvement is the fundamental challenge our nation faces. Without a reduction in the cost of spending, we will have no choice but to ration health care, depriving large segments of our population of the care that people want and deserve. If that happens, we will be sorry that we didn't change sooner. Unlike most health care predictions, this one is not an opinion but a matter of mathematics and time.

What My Father Deserved

Last year, I had the chance to speak at a meeting in Washington, DC, about the opportunities and challenges of providing care to patients with complex, chronic illnesses. The program was designed to bring together the voices of physicians and patients so that they could learn from each other's perspective.

I began by telling those in the room that I would have liked nothing more than to bring my father on stage with me.

As I told them the story of his life and death, I explained how thrilled my father would have been to hear so many people thinking and talking about ways to improve patient care. He had such affection for those who meant well, those who wanted to do the right thing. My dad put so much trust in the physicians who tried to put him back together and always spoke highly of them.

Although my father was a gentle man, he also had no tolerance for those who mistreated others. During his recovery, as we sat together reading the *New York Times* each Sunday, I remember how angry he would get at the politicians he believed were putting their own self-interest before their concern for others. He would shake his head and raise his voice at their decisions, especially when they negatively affected those who had so little. Even when I was the only one listening, my father felt an imperative to speak out and confront the wrongdoings of the world.

As I spoke to the audience at that meeting, I imagined my father standing beside me on stage, the hardworking man who believed that when you identify a problem, it's your job to fix it. I knew that if he could be there, he would want to know if our health care system had gotten any better since his death. I'm sure he'd ask me whether we as a nation have succeeded in bringing doctors together so they could more effectively care for their patients and reduce medical error. And I would have to tell my father the truth. No, not yet.

He would inquire whether all physicians in the United States were using electronic health records and other technologies that could help other families avoid the same problems ours had experienced. And again, I would need to disappoint him.

He would wonder whether doctors were consistently telling the truth to families at the end of a patient's life. He would ask if they were any better at showing compassion to patients during their most vulnerable moments. Again, I would confess that our health care system is failing to meet its potential.

At some point, realizing how little had changed over the past decade, my father would become angry and frustrated—the way he always did when he confronted ineptitude and injustice. If he had been standing on stage with me at that moment, I am sure that he would have placed his hand on my shoulder, looked in my eyes, and said in front of the entire audience, "Robbie, what are you going to do about it? How are you going to fix it?"

As I spoke that day, I was overwhelmed with sadness. More than a decade after his passing, it is difficult for me to think about him without my eyes welling up. Of course, he wasn't there. But I knew from our many years together what he would have said next: "Why don't you tell others my story, so that no one else will have to suffer the way I did?"

I'm often asked if I'm still angry or resentful about what happened to my father. I admit that I was, for close to a year. For the first few months after my father's death, I went through the classic stages of grief, beginning with denial, followed by anger. On some days, I couldn't believe he was gone. Other days, I was furious about what had happened.

I remember spending weeks on the phone after his death, calling the offices of the doctors who cared for him, growing frustrated as I realized what little information they had and how many opportunities they missed to prevent his medical problems. Eventually, I was able to accept what happened. But it has taken me much longer to accept the lack of compassion that accompanied my father's final days.

I realize now that each of the dozen or so physicians who cared for my father during the final decade of his life was as clinically excellent and dedicated as my colleagues and me. They were well trained and hardworking. Most likely, they arrived at medical school just as I did, filled with drive, enthusiasm, and the desire to provide patients with the best medical care possible.

My father didn't die at the hands of bad or callous doctors. Although every one of them knew he needed the pneumococcal vaccine that could have saved his life, they didn't fail to administer it because they wanted to hurt him. They weren't careless or incompetent. No matter how angry I wanted to be or how much I wanted to blame them, I ultimately accepted that his death wasn't their fault.

My father died because his doctors were disconnected from each other, practicing in offices that lacked the latest information technology or the ability to coordinate his care effectively. They were practicing in a culture that tolerated errors of omission much more than errors committed during procedures. And they were paid only for the tests they ordered and the procedures they performed, not for the compassion they could have shown. They simply lacked the tools, the incentives, and the systems to do the right thing. None of them wanted to hurt my father or our family. Mistreatment wasn't their intent. It was simply the consequence of the health care system in which they practiced.

In time, acceptance replaced my anger. But even now, after all the time that has passed since my father's death, I miss him every day. This book is for him, written with the hope and belief that once we—all of us, physicians, politicians, insurance and drug-company executives, and most important, patients—understand the failings of our current health care system, we can and will do something about it. And when we do, a better health care system will replace the one we have today, and my father's death will have served a purpose.

ACKNOWLEDGMENTS

Every page of this book was inspired by my parents and my patients. I have learned the most important lessons in life from both.

Illness can be difficult, fear-provoking, and painful. It can bring out the best in American doctors and hospitals. It can also expose us to a health care system that lacks compassion and tolerates medical errors. My father experienced the latter not long before his death, which came far too soon and left a great void in my life. My mother passed away before him, although her illness was shorter in duration and her care more satisfying. Every year, my brother, Ron, and sister, Karen, take time to connect on the anniversaries of our parents' deaths. Doing so reminds me how grateful I am for the love and emotional support of my siblings.

Mistreated was made possible with the help of many people. The words and stories in this book were made better through the contributions of my editing partner, Ben Lincoln, an exceptional and hardworking writer. The book's structure and clarity were greatly improved through our collaboration. To Anya Greenberg, my colleague and friend, your commitment to helping me complete this book was invaluable. Thank you, Ben and Anya, for your talent and honest feedback. Without your support, *Mistreated* would be incomplete.

I would also like to thank Ben Adams and the team at Perseus Books for lending their publishing expertise, and for encouraging a first-time author to aim high. John Maas at Sterling Lord Literistic was equally supportive and tremendously helpful in the early stages of this book's development.

To my dear friend and colleague George York, thank you for your contributions to the field of neurobiology and to my now-better understanding of its impact on American health care. To the nearly 10,000 other physicians in The Permanente Medical Group and The Mid-Atlantic Permanente Medical Group, I offer my sincerest thanks for your confidence in me as CEO, and for the hundreds of incredible and innovative ideas you have shared with me over the past eighteen years. Thank you to my brilliant and demanding teachers at the Yale University School of Medicine, where I first learned the fundamentals of medicine, and at the Stanford University Medical Center, where I gained the confidence and skill to practice surgery.

I wish to thank the Council of Accountable Physician Practices for allowing me to serve as your chairman, and for sharing the stories of patients and doctors who demonstrate what is possible in medical practice.

Most important, I thank all of the individuals whose personal stories fill these pages. You have been the best teachers. I am optimistic that the lessons you have taught me will further advance our nation's health and well-being.

BIBLIOGRAPHY

The following bibliography is not designed to be comprehensive but rather to offer additional resources for readers wanting to know more about topics such as the Stanford Prison Experiment, the Affordable Care Act, or the origins of direct-to-consumer pharmaceutical advertising. It also includes references for some of the most controversial statistics and conclusions in the book. Finally, it includes a few of the *Forbes* articles I have written, intended to provide a deeper perspective on some of the themes addressed throughout the book. These articles are not meant to serve as source material.

CHAPTER ONE
Analyzing the Symptoms
"NHE Fact Sheet." Centers for Medicare and Medicaid Services, August 10, 2016. http://www.cms.gov/Research-Statistics-Data-and-Systems/Statistics-Trends-and -Reports/NationalHealthExpendData/NHE-Fact-Sheet.html.

Woolf, Steven H., and Laudan Y. Aron. *U.S. Health in International Perspective: Shorter Lives, Poorer Health.* Washington, DC: National Academies Press, 2013.

"Majority of Americans Don't Use Digital Technology to Access Doctors." Survey conducted by Nielsen Strategic Health Perspectives on behalf of the Council of Accountable Physician Practices (CAPP), November 4, 2015. http://accountablecaredoctors .org/health-information-technology/majority-of-americans-dont-use-digital -technology-to-access-doctors.

"Nielsen Survey Shows Gaps in How Patients Are Experiencing Accountable Care." Survey conducted by Nielsen Strategic Health Perspectives on behalf of the Council of Accountable Physician Practices (CAPP), June 15, 2016. http:// accountablecaredoctors.org/capp-in-the-news/nielsen-survey-shows-gaps-patients -experiencing-accountable-care.

Ginsburg, Paul B., and Richard Amerling. "Should the U.S. Move Away from Fee-for-Service Medicine?" *Wall Street Journal*, March 22, 2015. http://www.wsj.com /articles/should-the-u-s-move-away-from-fee-for-service-medicine-1427079653.

"2015 National Healthcare Quality and Disparities Report and 5th Anniversary Update on the National Quality Strategy." Rockville, MD: Agency for Healthcare Research

and Quality (AHRQ), April 2016. http://www.ahrq.gov/research/findings/nhqrdr
/nhqdr15/index.html.

Palo Alto, 1971
Zimbardo, Philip G. *The Lucifer Effect: Understanding How Good People Turn Evil.* New
York: Random House, 2007.
The Stanford Prison Experiment. Directed by Kyle Patrick Alvarez. USA: IFC Films,
2015. Film.
Zimbardo, Philip G. "Stanford Prison Experiment." http://www.prisonexp.org.

Widow-Makers
Feng, Violet. "Unhealthy Diagnosis." In *60 Minutes*. CBS. July 17, 2003.
Pollack, Andrew. "California Patients Talk of Needless Heart Surgery." *New York Times*,
November 4, 2002.
Klaidman, Stephen. *Coronary: A True Story of Medicine Gone Awry.* New York: Scribner,
2008.
Milgram, Stanley. "Behavioral Study of Obedience." *Journal of Abnormal and Social
Psychology*, October 1963. doi:10.1037/h0040525.
Milgram, Stanley. "The Perils of Obedience." *Harper's Magazine*, December 1973.
Kerckhoff, Alan C., and Kurt W. Back. *The June Bug: A Study of Hysterical Contagion.*
New York: Appleton-Century-Crofts, 1968.
"Teenagers Hit by Soap Opera Virus." *Reuters*, May 19, 2006. http://www.news18.com
/news/india/teenagers-hit-by-soap-opera-virus-236423.html.

The Perception Problem
Gawande, Atul. "On Washing Hands." *New England Journal of Medicine*, March 25,
2004.
"Nearly Half a Million Americans Suffered from *Clostridium difficile* Infections in a
Single Year." Centers for Disease Control and Prevention (news release), February
25, 2015. http://www.cdc.gov/media/releases/2015/p0225-clostridium-difficile.html.
Hartocollis, Anemona. "With Money at Risk, Hospitals Push Staff to Wash Hands."
New York Times, May 28, 2013. http://www.nytimes.com/2013/05/29/nyregion
/hospitals-struggle-to-get-workers-to-wash-their-hands.html?pagewanted=all.

The Duality of Doctors
"Emergency Response After the Haiti Earthquake: Choices, Obstacles, Activities and
Finance." Doctors Without Borders, July 2010. http://www.doctorswithoutborders
.org/news-stories/special-report/emergency-response-after-haiti-earthquake-choices
-obstacles-activities-0.
Kohn, Linda T., Janet Corrigan, and Molla S. Donaldson. *To Err Is Human: Building a
Safer Health System.* Washington, DC: National Academy Press, 2000.
James, John T. "A New, Evidence-Based Estimate of Patient Harms Associated with
Hospital Care." *Journal of Patient Safety*, September 2013. doi:10.1097/pts.0b013e
3182948a69.

CHAPTER TWO
Mukherjee, Siddhartha. *The Emperor of All Maladies: A Biography of Cancer.* New York:
Scribner, 2010.

Drawing Blood

Kazak, Don (a friend and reporter for the *Palo Alto Weekly*). Subject matter appearing in this section ("Drawing Blood") was written in collaboration with Kazak in June 2011. Kazak conducted interviews and research, then partnered with me in the telling of these stories.

A Powerful Killer

Funk, Duane J., Joseph E. Parrillo, and Anand Kumar. "Sepsis and Septic Shock: A History." Critical Care Clinics, January 2009. doi:10.1016/j.ccc.2008.12.003.

Rivers, Emanuel P., and Bryant Nguyen. "Early Goal-Directed Therapy in Severe Sepsis and Septic Shock." *New England Journal of Medicine*, November 8, 2001. doi:10.1056/NEJMoa010307.

Physicians and Fear

Tversky, Amos, and Daniel Kahneman. "The Framing of Decisions and the Psychology of Choice." *Science*, January 30, 1981. doi:10.1126/science.7455683.

The Conformity of Fear

Heath, Chip, and Dan Heath. *Decisive: How to Make Better Choices in Life and Work.* New York: Crown Business, 2013.

"Governor Cuomo Announces New York State to Lead the Nation in Fighting Sepsis, the #1 Killer in Hospitals, and Make Major Improvements in Pediatric Care Through 'Rory's Regulations.'" New York State Department of Health (news release), January 29, 2013.

Dwyer, Jim. "Death of Boy Prompts New Medical Efforts Nationwide." *New York Times*, October 25, 2012. http://www.nytimes.com/2012/10/26/nyregion/tale-of-rory-stauntons-death-prompts-new-medical-efforts-nationwide.html.

Medicine: An Art or a Science?

Jaffe, Marc G., Grace A. Lee, Joseph D. Young, Stephen Sidney, and Alan S. Go. "Improved Blood Pressure Control Associated with a Large-Scale Hypertension Program." *Journal of the American Medical Association* (hereafter *JAMA*), August 21, 2013. doi:10.1001/jama.2013.108769.

Meet Your New Assistant, Siri

Pearl, Robert. "The David and Goliath of Health Care: Apple's Siri vs. IBM's Watson." *Forbes.com*, October 31, 2013. Article provides additional information on the broader uses of medical technologies.

The Context of Age

Twenge, J. M., S. M. Campbell, B. J. Hoffman, and C. E. Lance. "Generational Differences in Work Values: Leisure and Extrinsic Values Increasing, Social and Intrinsic Values Decreasing." *Journal of Management*, March 1, 2010. doi:10.1177/0149206309352246.

Becton, John Bret, Harvell Jack Walker, and Allison Jones-Farmer. "Generational Differences in Workplace Behavior." *Journal of Applied Social Psychology*, January 14, 2014. doi:10.1111/jasp.12208.

The Almighty Dollar
O'Brien, Jim. "The Cost of Sepsis." *CDC's Safe Healthcare Blog*, September 8, 2015. https://blogs.cdc.gov/safehealthcare/the-cost-of-sepsis.
"Sepsis Alliance Responds to U.S. Government Findings That Most Expensive Condition to Treat in Hospitals Is Sepsis." Sepsis Alliance (news release), October 31, 2013. http://www.sepsisalliance.org/news/2013/sepsis_most_expensive_condition.

Why It's Hard to See the Problem
Weingarten, Gene. "Pearls Before Breakfast: Can One of the Nation's Great Musicians Cut Through the Fog of a D.C. Rush Hour?" *Washington Post Magazine*, April 8, 2007. https://www.washingtonpost.com/lifestyle/magazine/pearls-before-breakfast -can-one-of-the-nations-great-musicians-cut-through-the-fog-of-a-dc-rush-hour-lets -find-out/2014/09/23/8a6d46da-4331–11e4-b47c-f5889e061e5f_story.html.

Lessons from Uber
Isaac, Mike, and Leslie Picker. "Uber Valuation Put at $62.5 Billion After a New Investment Round." *New York Times*, December 3, 2015. http://www.nytimes.com /2015/12/04/business/dealbook/uber-nears-investment-at-a-62–5-billion-valuation .html.
Oremus, Will. "Silicon Valley Uber Alles: The Car-Service Start-up Is Worth Nearly as Much as Hertz and Avis Combined. How Is That Possible?" *Slate Magazine*, June 6, 2014. http://www.slate.com/articles/technology/technology/2014/06/uber_17 _billion_valuation_it_s_now_worth_nearly_as_much_as_hertz_and_avis.html.

CHAPTER THREE
"How One Young Family's Disaster Was Saved by Telemedicine." By the Council of Accountable Physician Practices (CAPP). Featuring Emma and Laura. *Better Together Health,* November 3, 2015. http://bettertogetherhealth.org/portfolio-posts/1-emma.
"See How Telemedicine Helped Felipe Get the Care He Needs with Ease." By the Council of Accountable Physician Practices (CAPP). Featuring Felipe and Juana. *Better Together Health,* November 3, 2015. http://bettertogetherhealth.org/portfolio -posts/2-felipe.

More Than Meets the Eye
Landry, Miles, Adriana C. Dornelles, Genevieve Hayek, and Richard E. Deichmann. "Patient Preferences for Doctor Attire: The White Coat's Place in the Medical Profession." *Ochsner Journal*, Fall 2013.

The Evolution of Fear
Berns, Gregory. *Iconoclast: A Neuroscientist Reveals How to Think Differently*. Boston: Harvard Business School Press, 2008.

In Doctors We Trust
Greenstone, Gerry. "The History of Bloodletting." *BCMJ*, January/February 2010. http://www.bcmj.org/premise/history-bloodletting.
Glazer, Sarah. "Therapeutic Touch and Postmodernism in Nursing." *Nursing Philosophy*, October 2001. doi:10.1046/j.1466-769x.2000.00061.x.

The Context of Health Care's Contradictions

Vyse, Stuart A. *Believing in Magic: The Psychology of Superstition*. New York: Oxford University Press, 1997.

Damisch, L., B. Stoberock, and T. Mussweiler. "Keep Your Fingers Crossed! How Superstition Improves Performance." *Psychological Science*, July 28, 2010. doi:10.1177/0956797610372631.

Kaptchuk, Ted J., and Franklin G. Miller. "Placebo Effects in Medicine." *New England Journal of Medicine*, July 2, 2015. doi:10.1056/nejmp1504023.

The President Is Having Heart Surgery

New York State Department of Health. "Cardiovascular Disease Data and Statistics." *Reports of Cardiovascular Disease Data and Statistics*. https://www.health.ny.gov/statistics /diseases/cardiovascular.

Sanghavi, Darshak. "Talk to the Invisible Hand." *Slate Magazine*, September 28, 2009. http://www.slate.com/articles/news_and_politics/prescriptions/2009/09/talk_to _the_invisible_hand.html.

Altman, Lawrence K. "Clinton Surgery Puts Attention on Death Rate." *New York Times*, September 6, 2004.

Baker, Peter. "Bill Clinton Undergoes a New Heart Procedure." *New York Times*, February 11, 2010. http://thecaucus.blogs.nytimes.com/2010/02/11/bill-clinton -hospitalized-for-chest-pains.

Wegener, Duane T., Richard E. Petty, Brian T. Detweiler-Bedell, and W. Blair G. Jarvis. "Implications of Attitude Change Theories for Numerical Anchoring: Anchor Plausibility and the Limits of Anchor Effectiveness." *Journal of Experimental Social Psychology*, January 2001. doi:10.1006/jesp.2000.1431.

Sanghavi, Darshak. "Disheartening Medicine: Even U.S. Presidents Don't Always Get the Best Cardiac Health Care." *Slate Magazine*, August 28, 2013. http://www.slate .com/articles/health_and_science/medical_examiner/2013/08/heart_procedures_in _presidents_problems_with_george_w_bush_barack_obama.html.

Building Patient Trust in a Digital World

Jamshed, Nayer, Fouziaf Ozair, Amit Sharma, and Praveen Aggarwal. "Ethical Issues in Electronic Health Records: A General Overview." *Perspectives in Clinical Research*, April/June 2015. doi:10.4103/2229-3485.153997.

Rodriguez, Leon. "Privacy, Security, and Electronic Health Records." *HealthIT Buzz* (blog), December 12, 2011. https://www.healthit.gov/buzz-blog/privacy-and -security-of-ehrs/privacy-security-electronic-health-records.

Makary, Martin A., and Michael Daniel. "Analysis: Medical Error—the Third Leading Cause of Death in the US." *BMJ*, May 3, 2016. doi:10.1136/bmj.i2139.

Caplan, Jeremy. "Cause of Death: Sloppy Doctors." *Time*, January 15, 2007. http:// content.time.com/time/health/article/0,8599,1578074,00.html.

Telling Patients the Truth

York, George. Subject matter appearing in this section ("Telling Patients the Truth") was based on a weekly internal newsletter York called "TheTermite," which is not in public circulation. However, some of its contents are based on the death on Anton Chekov, for which a citation is provided below.

Rayfield, Donald. *Anton Chekhov: A Life*. Evanston, IL: Northwestern University Press, 2000.

Harrington, Sarah Elizabeth, and Thomas J. Smith. "The Role of Chemotherapy at the End of Life." *JAMA*, June 11, 2008. doi:10.1001/jama.299.22.2667.

Weeks, Jane C., Paul J. Catalano, Angel Cronin, Matthew D. Finkelman, Jennifer W. Mack, Nancy L. Keating, and Deborah Schrag. "Patients' Expectations About Effects of Chemotherapy for Advanced Cancer." *New England Journal of Medicine*, October 25, 2012. doi:10.1056/nejmoa1204410.

Are You Getting Excellent Care?

Gawande, Atul. "Cowboys and Pit Crews." *New Yorker*, May 26, 2011. http://www.newyorker.com/news/news-desk/cowboys-and-pit-crews.

Gauthier, John. "Team-Based Care: Optimizing Primary Care for Patients and Providers." *Institute for Healthcare Improvement* (blog), May 16, 2014. http://www.ihi.org/communities/blogs/_layouts/ihi/community/blog/itemview.aspx?list=0f316db6–7f8a-430f-a63a-ed7602d1366a&id=29.

The Quality Conundrum

Morse, Susan. "Provider-Run Plans Lead Pack in NCQA Health Plan Ratings." *Healthcare Finance News*, October 18, 2016. http://www.healthcarefinancenews.com/news/ncqa-releases-2016-health-insurance-plan-ratings.

"CMS 2017 Star Ratings." Centers for Medicare and Medicaid Services (fact sheet), October 12, 2016. CMS.gov. https://www.cms.gov/Newsroom/MediaReleaseDatabase/Fact-sheets/2016-Fact-sheets-items/2016–10–12.html.

"Top Hospitals." Leapfrog, 2016. http://www.leapfroggroup.org/ratings-reports/top-hospitals.

"Health Plan Member Satisfaction Improves with Healthy Competition, Says J.D. Power Study." J.D. Power, March 17, 2016. http://www.jdpower.com/press-releases/2016-member-health-plan-study.

Who and What Matters to Your Doctor?

Ornstein, Charles, Lena Groeger, Mike Tigas, and Ryann Grochowski Jones. "Dollars for Docs: How Industry Dollars Reach Your Doctors." ProPublica, March 17, 2016. https://projects.propublica.org/docdollars.

"Editor's Choice: Food, Flattery, and Friendship." *BMJ*, May 29, 2003. http://www.bmj.com/content/326/7400/0.8.

Moynihan, Ray. "Who Pays for the Pizza? Redefining the Relationships Between Doctors and Drug Companies." *BMJ*, May 29, 2003. doi:10.1136/bmj.326.7400.1189.

"Open Payments." Centers for Medicare and Medicaid Services. 2016. http://www.cms.gov/openpayments/index.html.

Gupta, Reshma, Cynthia Tsay, and Robert L. Fogerty. "Promoting Cost Transparency to Reduce Financial Harm to Patients." *AMA Journal of Ethics*, November 2015. doi:10.1001/journalofethics.2015.17.11.mhst1-1511.

The Psychology of Choice

Morewedge, Carey K., Lisa L. Shu, Daniel T. Gilbert, and Timothy D. Wilson. "Bad Riddance or Good Rubbish? Ownership and Not Loss Aversion Causes the Endowment Effect." *Journal of Experimental Social Psychology*, July 2009. doi:10.1016/j.jesp.2009.05.014.

CHAPTER FOUR
The Legacy Player's Perspective
O'Donnell, Norah, host. "Transcript for Speaker Boehner." On CBS's *Face the Nation*, July 1, 2012. http://www.cbsnews.com/news/face-the-nation-transcripts-july-1-2012-speaker-boehner-senators-schumer-and-coburn-governors-walker-and-omalley/.
"Policy Basics: Where Do Our Federal Tax Dollars Go?" Center on Budget and Policy Priorities, March 4, 2016. http://www.cbpp.org/research/federal-budget/policy-basics-where-do-our-federal-tax-dollars-go.
Rubenstein, Grace. "New Health Rankings: Of Seventeen Nations, U.S. Is Dead Last." *Atlantic*, January 10, 2013. http://www.theatlantic.com/health/archive/2013/01/new-health-rankings-of-17-nations-us-is-dead-last/267045.
"US Health System Ranks Last Among Eleven Countries on Measures of Access, Equity, Quality, Efficiency, and Healthy Lives." The Commonwealth Fund, June 16, 2014. http://www.commonwealthfund.org/publications/press-releases/2014/jun/us-health-system-ranks-last.
"2016 Social Progress Index." Social Progress Imperative. 2016. http://www.socialprogressimperative.org/global-index.
Kantarjian, Hagop. "An Unhealthy System: Compared to Other Nations, Americans Overpay for Their Health Care and Get Little in Return." *U.S. News and World Report*, May 30, 2014. http://www.usnews.com/opinion/articles/2014/05/30/no-the-us-doesnt-have-the-best-healthcare-system-in-the-world.
"U.S. Spends Far More for Health Care Than Twelve Industrialized Nations, but Quality Varies." The Commonwealth Fund, May 3, 2012. http://www.commonwealthfund.org/publications/press-releases/2012/may/us-spends-far-more-for-healthcare-than-12-industrialized-nations-but-quality-varies.

Lead in the Water
Gupta, Sanjay, Ben Tinker, and Tim Hume. "'Our Mouths Were Ajar': Doctor's Fight to Expose Flint's Water Crisis." *CNN*, January 22, 2016. http://www.cnn.com/2016/01/21/health/flint-water-mona-hanna-attish/index.html.
Hernandez, Sergio. "The Poisoning of a City." *Mashable*, January 24, 2016. http://mashable.com/2016/01/24/flint-water-crisis.

Playing Favorites
Barlow, Rich. "BU Research: A Riddle Reveals Depth of Gender Bias." *BU Today*, January 16, 2014. http://www.bu.edu/today/2014/bu-research-riddle-reveals-the-depth-of-gender-bias.
Belle, Deborah, and Joyce Benenson. "Children's Social Networks and Well-Being." *Handbook of Child Well-Being*, January 2014. doi:10.1007/978-90-481-9063-8_55.
"Implicit Association Test." Project Implicit, Harvard University, 2011. https://implicit.harvard.edu/implicit/takeatest.html. To take the test referenced in this section, click the "Gender-Career IAT."

Zooming Out: Is Health Care a Human Right or a Privilege?
Akbareian, Emma. "The Blue and Black (or White and Gold) Dress: Actual Colour, Brand, and Price Details Revealed." *Independent*, February 27, 2015. http://www.independent.co.uk/life-style/fashion/news/the-dress-actual-colour-brand-and-price-details-revealed-10074686.html.

Grisham, Lori. "The Science Behind 'The Dress.'" *USA Today*, February 28, 2015. http://www.usatoday.com/story/news/nation-now/2015/02/27/dress-blue-black-white-gold-science/24113695.

Hamel, Mary Beth, David Blumenthal, Karen Davis, and Stuart Guterman. "Medicare at Fifty—Origins and Evolution." *New England Journal of Medicine*, October 29, 2015. doi:10.1056/nejmhpr1411701.

Blumenthal, David, and James Morone. "The Lessons of Success—Revisiting the Medicare Story." *New England Journal of Medicine*, November 27, 2008. doi:10.1056/nejmhpr0806879.

Mossialos, Elias, Martin Wenzl, Robin Osborn, and Dana Sarnak. "International Profiles of Health Care Systems, 2015." *Commonwealth Fund*, January 21, 2016. doi:10.15868/socialsector.25100.

Pains and Claims

"Medical Loss Ratio." The Center for Consumer Information and Insurance Oversight, 2016. http://www.cms.gov/CCIIO/Programs-and-Initiatives/Health-Insurance-Market-Reforms/Medical-Loss-Ratio.html.

"Explaining Health Care Reform: Medical Loss Ratio (MLR)." The Henry J. Kaiser Family Foundation, February 29, 2012. http://kff.org/health-reform/fact-sheet/explaining-healthcare-reform-medical-loss-ratio-mlr.

"Summary of the Affordable Care Act." The Henry J. Kaiser Family Foundation, April 25, 2013. http://kff.org/health-reform/fact-sheet/summary-of-the-affordable-care-act.

Hamel, Mary Beth, David Blumenthal, and Sara R. Collins. "Health Care Coverage Under the Affordable Care Act—a Progress Report." *New England Journal of Medicine*, July 17, 2014. doi:10.1056/nejmhpr1405667.

Bauman, Noam, Erica Coe, Jessica Ogden, and Ashish Parikh. "Hospital Networks: Updated National View of Configurations on the Exchanges." McKinsey on Healthcare, June 2014. http://healthcare.mckinsey.com/hospital-networks-updated-national-view-configurations-exchanges.

McQueen, M. P. "Less Choice, Lower Premiums: Many Exchange Plans Will Offer Narrow Networks." *Modern Healthcare*, August 17, 2013. http://www.modernhealthcare.com/article/20130817/MAGAZINE/308179921.

Terhune, Chad. "Anthem Sued over Limited Networks." *Los Angeles Times*, July 9, 2014. http://www.latimes.com/business/la-fi-anthem-suit-20140710-story.html.

Ebers, Paul Von. "Mega Health Insurance Mergers: Is Bigger Really Better?" *Health Affairs Blog*, January 22, 2106. http://healthaffairs.org/blog/2016/01/22/mega-health-insurance-mergers-is-bigger-really-better.

Potter, Wendell. "Health Insurers Watch Profits Soar as They Dump Small Business Customers." The Center for Public Integrity, January 26, 2015. https://www.publicintegrity.org/2015/01/26/16658/health-insurers-watch-profits-soar-they-dump-small-business-customers.

Whitman, Elizabeth. "Rising Costs of Medical Care, Health Insurance: Median Pay for CEOs in Health Care Companies Higher Than Any Other Industry, Analysis Finds." *International Business Times*, May 27, 2015. http://www.ibtimes.com/rising-costs-medical-care-health-insurance-median-pay-ceos-health care-companies-1938699.

Zooming In: The Inconsistencies of US Hospitals

Schneider, E. B., S. A. Hirani, H. L. Hambridge, E. R. Haut, A. R. Carlini, R. C. Castillo, D. T. Efron, and A. H. Haider. "Fighting the Weekend Trend: The Alarming,

Increased Mortality Among Elderly TBI Patients Admitted on Weekends." *Journal of Surgical Research*, February 2012. doi:10.1016/j.jss.2011.11.236.

Magill, Shelley S., Jonathan R. Edwards, Wendy Bamberg, Zintars G. Beldavs, Ghinwa Dumyati, Marion A. Kainer, Ruth Lynfield, Meghan Maloney, Laura Mcallister-Hollod, Joelle Nadle, Susan M. Ray, Deborah L. Thompson, Lucy E. Wilson, and Scott K. Fridkin. "Multistate Point-Prevalence Survey of Health Care-Associated Infections." *New England Journal of Medicine*, March 27, 2014. doi:10.1056/nejmoa1306801.

Peberdy, Mary Ann, Joseph P. Ornato, and Luke Larkin. "Survival from In-Hospital Cardiac Arrest During Nights and Weekends." *JAMA*, February 20, 2008. doi:10.1001/jama.299.7.785.

Zooming Out: Protecting Your Turf

Hamdy, Freddie C., Jenny L. Donovan, J. Athene Lane, Malcolm Mason, Chris Metcalfe, Peter Holding, Michael Davis, Tim J. Peters, Emma L. Turner, Richard M. Martin, Jon Oxley, Mary Robinson, John Staffurth, Eleanor Walsh, Prasad Bollina, James Catto, Andrew Doble, Alan Doherty, David Gillatt, Roger Kockelbergh, Howard Kynaston, Alan Paul, Philip Powell, Stephen Prescott, Derek J. Rosario, Edward Rowe, and David E. Neal. "Ten-Year Outcomes After Monitoring, Surgery, or Radiotherapy for Localized Prostate Cancer." *New England Journal of Medicine*, October 13, 2016. doi:10.1056/nejmoa1606220.

Järvinen, Teppo L. N., and Gordon H. Guyatt. "Arthroscopic Surgery for Knee Pain." *BMJ*, July 20, 2016. doi:10.1136/bmj.i3934.

Olson, Elizabeth G. "Medical Students Confront a Residency Black Hole." *Fortune*, April 1, 2013. http://fortune.com/2013/04/01/medical-students-confront-a-residency-black-hole.

More Is Not Better

"Supply-Sensitive Care." Dartmouth Atlas of Health Care. http://www.dartmouthatlas.org/keyissues/issue.aspx?con=2937.

Zooming Out: A Global Prescription

Gibson, C. Robert. "This Chart Reveals the Inhumanity of US Drug Prices Compared to Other Countries." *U.S. Uncut*, September 23, 2015. http://usuncut.com/news/us-drug-prices-in-the-us-are-literally-insane-when-compared-to-other-nations.

Johnson, Linda A. "Lack of Regulation, Little Competition, Research Costs Boost US Prescription Drug Prices." *U.S. News and World Report*, September 25, 2015. http://www.usnews.com/news/business/articles/2015/09/25/multiple-factors-cause-high-prescription-drug-prices-in-us.

Abelson, Reed. "Health Insurance Deductibles Outpacing Wage Increases, Study Finds." *New York Times*, September 22, 2015. http://www.nytimes.com/2015/09/23/business/health-insurance-deductibles-outpacing-wage-increases-study-finds.html.

Zooming In: US Drugs, Devices, and Destiny

Smetana, Kevin. "EpiPen Inventor Helped Millions and Died in Obscurity." *Tampa Bay Times*, September 24, 2009. http://www.tampabay.com/news/humaninterest/epipen-inventor-helped-millions-and-died-in-obscurity/1038756.

Popken, Ben. "Mylan CEO Salary Rose by 600 Percent as EpiPen Price Rose 400 Percent." *NBC News*, August 23, 2016. http://www.nbcnews.com/business/consumer/mylan-execs-gave-themselves-raises-they-hiked-epipen-prices-n636591.

Banerjee, Ankur, and Ransdell Pierson. "Mylan to Launch Generic EpiPen at Half the Price of Original." *Reuters*, August 29, 2016. http://www.reuters.com/article/us-mylan-nl-pricing-idUSKCN1140YF.

Fegraus, Laura, and Murray Ross. "Sovaldi, Harvoni, and Why It's Different This Time." *Health Affairs Blog*, November 21, 2014. http://healthaffairs.org/blog/2014/11/21/sovaldi-harvoni-and-why-its-different-this-time.

Anderson, Richard. "Pharmaceutical Industry Gets High on Fat Profits." *BBC News*, November 6, 2014. http://www.bbc.com/news/business-28212223.

Sanneh, Kelefa. "Everyone Hates Martin Shkreli. Everyone Is Missing the Point." *New Yorker*, February 5, 2016. http://www.newyorker.com/culture/cultural-comment/everyone-hates-martin-shkreli-everyone-is-missing-the-point.

Friedman, Megan. "Kim Kardashian's Morning-Sickness Pill Ad Was Actually a Massive Success." *Harper's Bazaar*, August 12, 2015. http://www.harpersbazaar.com/celebrity/latest/news/a11866/kim-kardashian-morning-sickness-diclegis-success.

The Illusion of Quality
Plassmann, H., J. O'Doherty, B. Shiv, and A. Rangel. "Marketing Actions Can Modulate Neural Representations of Experienced Pleasantness." *Proceedings of the National Academy of Sciences*, January 14, 2008. doi:10.1073/pnas.0706929105.

Our Prescription Addiction
Jones, Christopher M., Karin A. Mack, and Leonard J. Paulozzi. "Pharmaceutical Overdose Deaths, United States, 2010." *JAMA*, February 20, 2013. doi:10.1001/jama.2013.272.

Health Care as a Cultural Imperative
Magiorkinis, Emmanuil, Apostolos Beloukas, and Aristidis Diamantis. "Scurvy: Past, Present and Future." *European Journal of Internal Medicine*, April 22, 2011. doi:10.1016/j.ejim.2010.10.006.

CHAPTER FIVE

True, Kathryn. "The Politics of Health: Village-Run Health Programs in the Sierra Madre Region of Mexico." Context Institute, Fall 1994. http://www.context.org/iclib/ic39/werner.

Werner, David. "A Grassroots Struggle for Health and Rights in Rural Mexico." *Health Wrights*, 1994. http://www.healthwrights.org/content/articles/grassroots_struggle.pdf.

What We Can Stomach

Marshall, Barry, J. A. Armstrong, D. B. McGechie, and R. J. Glancy. "Attempt to Fulfill Koch's Postulates for Pyloric Campylobacter." *Medical Journal of Australia*, April 15, 1985.

"Interview: Barry Marshall." Academy of Achievement, May 23, 1998 (website revised September 23, 2010). http://www.achievement.org/autodoc/printmember/mar1int-1.

The Problem with Conventional Wisdom

Doitsh, Gilad, Nicole L. K. Galloway, Xin Geng, Zhiyuan Yang, Kathryn M. Monroe, Orlando Zepeda, Peter W. Hunt, Hiroyu Hatano, Stefanie Sowinski, Isa

Muñoz-Arias, and Warner C. Greene. "Cell Death by Pyroptosis Drives CD4 T-cell Depletion in HIV-1 Infection." *Nature*, January 23, 2014. doi:10.1038/nature12940.

Pearl, Robert. "HIV/AIDS Discovery Shows How Wrong Assumptions Can Be." *Forbes. com*, January 30, 2014. http://www.forbes.com/sites/robertpearl/2014/01/30/hivaids -discovery-shows-how-wrong assumptions-can-be. Article provides additional information on the medical discovery that overturned conventional wisdom.

Social Determinants of Health

"Social Determinants of Health: Know What Affects Health." Centers for Disease Control and Prevention. Page last reviewed: October 13, 2016. http://www.cdc.gov /socialdeterminants.

"What Are Social Determinants of Health?" World Health Organization, 2016. http:// www.who.int/social_determinants/sdh_definition/en.

Heiman, Harry J., and Samantha Artiga. "Beyond Health Care: The Role of Social Determinants in Promoting Health and Health Equity." The Henry J. Kaiser Family Foundation, November 4, 2015. http://kff.org/disparities-policy/issue-brief/beyond -healthcare-the-role-of-social-determinants-in-promoting-health-and-health-equity.

Smoking in America

Jensen, Christopher D., Douglas A. Corley, Virginia P. Quinn, Chyke A. Doubeni, Ann G. Zauber, Jeffrey K. Lee, Wei K. Zhao, Amy R. Marks, Joanne E. Schottinger, Nirupa R. Ghai, Alexander T. Lee, Richard Contreras, Carrie N. Klabunde, Charles P. Quesenberry, Theodore R. Levin, and Pauline A. Mysliwiec. "Fecal Immunochemical Test Program Performance over Four Rounds of Annual Screening." *Annals of Internal Medicine*, April 26, 2016. doi:10.7326/m15-0983.

"Cigarette Use Globally." The Tobacco Atlas/World Lung Federation. 2015. http:// www.tobaccoatlas.org/topic/cigarette-use-globally.

McCarthy, Justin. "In U.S., Smoking Rate Lowest in Utah, Highest in Kentucky." *Gallup.com*, March 13, 2014. http://www.gallup.com/poll/167771/smoking-rate-lowest -utah-highest-kentucky.aspx.

Obesity and Chronic Illness in America

Christensen, Clayton M., Jerome H. Grossman, and Jason Hwang. *The Innovator's Prescription: A Disruptive Solution for Health Care*. New York: McGraw-Hill, 2009.

Pearl, Robert. "Clayton Christensen: American Health Care Is Sick and Getting Sicker." *Forbes.com*, July 10, 2014. http://www.forbes.com/sites/robertpearl/2014 /07/10/clayton-christensen-american-healthcare-is-sick-and-getting-sicker. Article written following a comprehensive interview with Christensen in June 2014.

Gladwell, Malcolm. *David and Goliath: Underdogs, Misfits, and the Art of Battling Giants*. New York: Little, Brown, 2013.

Pearl, Robert. "Malcolm Gladwell on American Health Care: An Interview." *Forbes. com*, March 6, 2014. http://www.forbes.com/sites/robertpearl/2014/03/06/malcolm -gladwell-on-american-health care-an-interview. Article written following a comprehensive interview with Gladwell in February 2014.

Thaler, Richard H., and Cass R. Sunstein. *Nudge: Improving Decisions About Health, Wealth, and Happiness*. New Haven: Yale University Press, 2008.

Heath, Chip, and Dan Heath. *Switch: How to Change Things When Change Is Hard*. New York: Broadway Books, 2010.

Pearl, Robert. "'Decisive' Author Chip Heath on Doctors, Diets and the Dangers of Overconfidence." *Forbes.com*, May 8, 2014. http://www.forbes.com/sites/robertpearl/2014/05/08/decisive-author-chip-heath-on-doctors-diets-and-the-dangers-of-overconfidence. Article written following a comprehensive interview with Chip Heath in February 2014.

Werner, David. *Where There Is No Doctor: A Village Health Care Handbook*. Palo Alto, CA: Hesperian Foundation, 1977.

Stress, Depression, and Anxiety in America

Pearl, Robert. "Stress in America: Three Simple Treatments." *Forbes.com*, October 16, 2014. http://www.forbes.com/sites/robertpearl/2014/10/16/stress-in-america. Article written in collaboration with Dr. David Sobel, a primary-care physician and national expert in psychosocial factors in health, as the third and final installment in a series, "Stress in America."

Childhood Trauma: America's Silent Killer

"Adverse Childhood Experiences Questionnaire: Finding Your ACE Score." National Council of Juvenile and Family Court Judges, October 24, 2006. http://www.ncjfcj.org/sites/default/files/Finding%20Your%20ACE%20Score.pdf.

Felitti, Vincent J., Robert F. Anda, Dale Nordenberg, David F. Williamson, Alison M. Spitz, Valerie Edwards, Mary P. Koss, and James S. Marks. "Relationship of Childhood Abuse and Household Dysfunction to Many of the Leading Causes of Death in Adults." *American Journal of Preventive Medicine*, May 1998. doi:10.1016/s0749-3797(98)00017-8.

Intimate Partner Violence in America

"The National Domestic Violence Hotline." 1-800-799-SAFE (7233). http://www.thehotline.org.

"Together We Can End Domestic Violence and Sexual Assault." The NO MORE Project, 2016. http://nomore.org.

Pearl, Robert. "Domestic Violence: The Secret Killer That Costs $8.3 Billion Annually." *Forbes.com*, December 5, 2013. http://www.forbes.com/sites/robertpearl/2013/12/05/domestic-violence-the-secret-killer-that-costs-8-3-billion-annually. Citation provided to offer additional information and resources concerning the impact of domestic violence in America.

Social Inequities in America

"Quality Field Notes: Improving Equity in Health Care." Robert Wood Johnson Foundation, June 16, 2014. http://www.rwjf.org/en/library/research/2014/06/equity.html.

Pearl, Robert. "Why Health Care Is Different If You're Black, Latino or Poor." *Forbes.com*, March 5, 2016. http://www.forbes.com/sites/robertpearl/2015/03/05/healthcare-black-latino-poor. Article contains additional research, resources, and proposed solutions for disparities in American health care.

Solving Social Problems

Fletcher, Michael A. "What You Really Need to Know About Baltimore, from a Reporter Who's Lived There for over Thirty Years." *Washington Post*, April 28, 2015. https://www.washingtonpost.com/news/wonk/wp/2015/04/28/what-you-really-need-to-know-about-baltimore-from-a-reporter-who-lived-there-for-30-years.

"Baltimore's Leana Wen: A Doctor for the City." On NPR's *All Things Considered*, March 2, 2016. http://www.npr.org/sections/health-shots/2016/03/02/468893616 /baltimore-s-leana-wen-a-doctor-for-the-city.

"B'more for Healthy Babies Initiative Leads to Lowest Infant Mortality Rate on Record in Baltimore City." Johns Hopkins University, October 5, 2016. http://ccp.jhu .edu/2016/10/05/bmore-healthy-babies-initiative-leads-lowest-infant-mortality-rate -record-baltimore-city.

The Twenty-First-Century Gold Rush

"The CrunchBase Unicorn Leaderboard." *TechCrunch*, October 12, 2016. https:// techcrunch.com/unicorn-leaderboard.

The Young Bloods of Health Care

Carreyrou, John. "Hot Start-up Theranos Has Struggled with Its Blood-Test Technology." *Wall Street Journal*, October 15, 2015. http://www.wsj.com/articles/theranos -has-struggled-with-blood-tests-1444881901.

Herper, Matthew. "From $4.5 Billion to Nothing: Forbes Revises Estimated Net Worth of Theranos Founder Elizabeth Holmes." *Forbes Magazine*, June 21, 2016. http:// www.forbes.com/sites/matthewherper/2016/06/01/from-4–5-billion-to-nothing -forbes-revises-estimated-net-worth-of-theranos-founder-elizabeth-holmes.

Lapowski, Issie. "Theranos' Scandal Exposes the Problem with Tech's Hype Cycle." *Wired.com*, October 15, 2016. https://www.wired.com/2015/10/theranos-scandal -exposes-the-problem-with-techs-hype-cycle.

The Future of Genomics Isn't Now (Yet)

Boesveld, Sarah. "Can You Know Too Much About Your Genes? Jolie Has Turned a Spotlight on Testing, but It May Have Risks." *National Post* (Canada), May 17, 2013. http://news.nationalpost.com/news/canada/can-you-know-too-much-about -your-genes-jolie-has-turned-a-spotlight-on-genome-testing-but-it-comes-with -risks.

"Revolutionizing" Health Insurance

Farr, Christina. "Warning: Trying to Disrupt Health Insurance May Cause Headaches." *Fast Company*, January 26, 2016. https://www.fastcompany.com/3055700 /warning-trying-to-disrupt-health-insurance-may-cause-headaches.

Goldberg, Dan. "Oscar to Drastically Narrow Its Network in 2017." *Politico*, July 26, 2016. http://www.politico.com/states/new-york/city-hall/story/2016/07/oscar-to -drastically-narrow-its-network-104232.

The Wrist of the Story

Jakicic, John M., Kelliann K. Davis, Renee J. Rogers, Wendy C. King, Marsha D. Marcus, Diane Helsel, Amy D. Rickman, Abdus S. Wahed, and Steven H. Belle. "Effect of Wearable Technology Combined with a Lifestyle Intervention on Long-Term Weight Loss." *JAMA*, September 20, 2016. doi:10.1001/jama.2016.12858.

Why Big Ideas Lose Their Luster

Hingle, Susan. "Electronic Health Records: An Unfulfilled Promise and a Call to Action." *Annals of Internal Medicine*, September 6, 2016. doi:10.7326/m16-1757.

Jayanthi, Akanksha. "Physicians Rate Top EHRs for Use, Satisfaction, Vendor Support." Becker's Health IT and CIO Review, August 26, 2016. http://www

.beckershospitalreview.com/healthcare-information-technology/physicians-rate-top
-ehrs-for-use-satisfaction-vendor-support.html.

Gold in Health Care Rarely Glitters

Dubner, Stephen J., and Steven D. Levitt. "The Seat-Belt Solution." *New York Times Magazine*, July 10, 2005. http://www.nytimes.com/2005/07/10/magazine/the -seatbelt-solution.html.

"History of Seat Belts in the U.S." Bisnar Chase. http://www.bestattorney.com/auto -defects/defective-seatbelts/history-of-seat-belts.html.

"Policy Impact: Seat Belts." Centers for Disease Control and Prevention, January 21, 2014. http://www.cdc.gov/motorvehiclesafety/seatbeltbrief/index.html.

The Value of Vaccines

"Global Vaccine Action Plan 2011–2020." World Health Organization, 2016. http:// www.who.int/immunization/global_vaccine_action_plan/GVAP_doc_2011_2020 /en.

Wakefield, A. J., S. H. Murch, A. Anthony, J. Linnell, D. M. Casson, M. Malik, M. Berelowitz, A. P. Dhillon, M. A. Thomson, P. Harvey, A. Valentine, S. E. Davies, and J. A. Walker-Smith. "Retracted: Ileal-lymphoid-nodular Hyperplasia, Non-Specific Colitis, and Pervasive Developmental Disorder in Children." *The Lancet*, February 28, 1998. doi:10.1016/s0140-6736(97)11096-0.

"Measles Fact Sheet." World Health Organization. March 2016. http://www.who.int /mediacentre/factsheets/fs286/en.

The Boring Power of Prevention

Schieb, Linda, Sophia A. Greer, Matthew D. Ritchey, Mary G. George, and Michele L. Casper. "Vital Signs: Avoidable Deaths from Heart Disease, Stroke, and Hypertensive Disease—United States, 2001–2010." *Morbidity and Mortality Weekly Report* (*MMWR*), September 6, 2013. https://www.cdc.gov/mmwr/preview/mmwrhtml /mm6235a4.htm.

Schieb, Linda J. "Thousands of US Deaths from Stroke and Heart Disease Are Preventable." *JAMA*, November 6, 2013. doi:10.1001/jama.2013.280221.

CHAPTER SIX

Tversky, Amos, and Daniel Kahneman. "Judgment Under Uncertainty: Heuristics and Biases." *Science*, September 27, 1974. doi:10.1017/cbo9780511809477.002.

Kahneman, Daniel. *Thinking, Fast and Slow*. New York: Farrar, Straus and Giroux, 2013.

"Perceptions Are Not Reality: Things the World Gets Wrong." Ipsos MORI, October 29, 2014. https://www.ipsos-mori.com/researchpublications/researcharchive/3466 /Perceptions-are-not-reality-10-things-the-world-gets-wrong.aspx.

"Why the 'Ignorance Index' Matters." On CNN's *Global Public Square*, November 11, 2014. http://globalpublicsquare.blogs.cnn.com/2014/11/11/why-the-ignorance-index -matters.

To Have Not

"SNAP/Food Stamp Challenges." Food Research and Action Center. http://frac.org /initiatives/snapfood-stamp-challenges.

The Dawn of Health Care Reform
Mendell, David. *Obama: From Promise to Power*. New York: Amistad, 2007.
"Interview with David Mendell." PBS's *Frontline*, October 14, 2008. http://www.pbs
  .org/wgbh/pages/frontline//choice2008/interviews/mendell.html.
Obama, Barack. *Dreams from My Father: A Story of Race and Inheritance*. New York:
  Three Rivers Press, 2004.
Obama, Barack. *The Audacity of Hope: Thoughts on Reclaiming the American Dream*.
  New York: Crown Publishers, 2006.

Lessons from the Past
Morone, James A. "Presidents and Health Reform: From Franklin D. Roosevelt to
  Barack Obama." *Health Affairs*, June 2010. doi:10.1377/hlthaff.2010.0420.
Palmer, Karen S. "A Brief History: Universal Health Care Efforts in the US." Physicians
  for a National Health Program. 1999. http://www.pnhp.org/facts/a-brief-history
  -universal-healthcare efforts-in-the-us.
Starr, Paul. "The Hillarycare Mythology." *American Prospect*, September 13, 2007.
  http://prospect.org/article/hillarycare-mythology.
Schroeder, Steven A. "The Clinton Health Care Plan: Fundamental or Incremental
  Reform?" *Annals of Internal Medicine*, November 1, 1993. doi:10.7326/0003-4819
  -119-9-199311010-00014.
Wilson, Anthony. "Why 'HillaryCare' Failed and 'ObamaCare' Succeeded." *American
  Health Line*. http://www.americanhealthline.com/analysis-and-insight/features/why
  -hillarycare-failed-and-obamacare-succeeded.

Making the Case
Obama, Barack. "Remarks by the President to the Annual Conference of the American Medical Association." Transcript provided by the White House's Office of the
  Press Secretary. June 15, 2009. https://www.whitehouse.gov/the-press-office/remarks
  -president-annual-conference-american-medical-association.

A Policy Born of Political Reality
"Patient Protection and Affordable Care Act of 2010." Full text provided. May 1, 2010.
  http://housedocs.house.gov/energycommerce/ppacacon.pdf.
Obama, Barack. "Remarks by the President on the Affordable Care Act." Transcript provided by the White House's Office of the Press Secretary. April 1, 2014.
  https://www.whitehouse.gov/the-press-office/remarks-president-annual-conference
  -american-medical-association.

Big Bet 1: Covering the Forgotten
"Wage Statistics for 2015." Social Security Administration. https://www.ssa.gov/cgi-bin
  /netcomp.cgi?year=2015. Pertinent text: "By definition, 50 percent of wage earners
  had net compensation less than or equal to the median wage, which is estimated to
  be $29,930.13 for 2015."
Snyder, Michael. "Goodbye Middle Class: 51 Percent of All American Workers Make
  Less Than 30,000 Dollars a Year." *Washington's Blog*, October 21, 2015. http://www
  .washingtonsblog.com/2015/10/goodbye-middle-class-51-percent-of-all-american
  -workers-make-less-than-30000-dollars-a-year.html.

Chernew, Michael. "The Economics of Medicaid Expansion." *Health Affairs Blog*, March 21, 2016. http://healthaffairs.org/blog/2016/03/21/the-economics-of -medicaid-expansion.

"Where the States Stand on Medicaid Expansion." Advisory Board, January 13, 2016. https://www.advisory.com/daily-briefing/resources/primers/medicaidmap.

Diamond, Jeremy Scott, Zachary Tracer, and Chloe Whiteaker. "Why 27 Million Are Still Uninsured Under Obamacare." *Bloomberg*, October 19, 2016. http://www .bloomberg.com/graphics/2016-obamacare.

Big Bet 2: Covering the Excluded

Jost, Timothy. "The Supreme Court on the Individual Mandate's Constitutionality: An Overview." *Health Affairs Blog*, June 28, 2012. http://healthaffairs.org/blog/2012/06 /28/the-supreme-court-on-the-individual-mandates-constitutionality-an-overview.

Big Bet 3: Creating the Insurance Exchanges

"Health Insurance Marketplaces." The Center for Consumer Information and In- surance Oversight. http://www.cms.gov/CCIIO/Programs-and-Initiatives/Health -Insurance-Marketplaces/index.html.

"State Health Insurance Marketplace Types." Kaiser Family Foundation, 2016. http:// kff.org/health-reform/state-indicator/state-health-insurance-marketplace-types.

Big Bet 4: Caring for Seniors and Rewarding Excellence

Diamond, Dan. "10,000 People Are Now Enrolling in Medicare—Every Day." *Forbes. com*, July 13, 2015. http://www.forbes.com/sites/dandiamond/2015/07/13/aging-in -america-10000-people-enroll-in-medicare-every-day.

Shifting Perceptions Through Medicare Advantage

"Five-Star Quality Rating System." Centers for Medicare and Medicaid Services, 2016. http://www.cms.gov/Medicare/Provider-Enrollment-and-Certification/Certification andComplianc/FSQRS.html.

Big Bet 5: Integrating a Fragmented System

Haught, Randy, and John Ahrens. "Cost of the Future Newly Insured Under the Af- fordable Care Act (ACA)." Society of Actuaries, March 2013. http://cdn-files.soa.org /web/research-cost-aca-report.pdf.

Johnson, Carolyn Y. "Aetna Warned It Would Drop Out of Obamacare Exchanges If Its Merger Was Blocked." *Washington Post*, August 17, 2016. https://www .washingtonpost.com/news/wonk/wp/2016/08/17/aetna-warned-it-would-drop-out -of-obamacare-exchanges-if-its-merger-was-blocked.

The ACO Experiment

"Accountable Care Organizations (ACO)." Centers for Medicare and Medicaid Ser- vices, 2015. http://www.cms.gov/Medicare/Medicare-Fee-for-Service-Payment/ACO /index.html.

Zeitlin, Josh. "The Good—and Bad—News in the New ACO Results." Advisory Board, August 26, 2016. https://www.advisory.com/daily-briefing/2016/08/26/aco -results.

Pear, Robert. "Dropout by Dartmouth Raises Questions on Health Law Cost-Savings Effort." *New York Times*, September 11, 2016. http://www.nytimes.com/2016/09

/11/us/politics/dropout-by-dartmouth-raises-questions-on-health-law-cost-savings
-effort.html.

Big Bet 6: Finding a Meaningful Use for Technology

Rouse, Margaret. "What Is HITECH Act (Health Information Technology for Economic and Clinical Health Act)?" *TechTarget*, December 2014. http://searchhealthit
.techtarget.com/definition/HITECH-Act.

The Impact of Meaningful Use

Obama, Barack. "The Time Has Come for Universal Health Care." Speech delivered
at the Families USA Conference in Washington, DC, January 25, 2007. http://
obamaspeeches.com/097-The-Time-Has-Come-for-Universal-Healthcare-Obama
-Speech.htm.
"Step 5: Achieve Meaningful Use Stage 2." *HealthIT.gov*, August 23, 2012. https://www
.healthit.gov/providers-professionals/step-5-achieve-meaningful-use-stage-2.

Big Bet 7: Measuring Quality and Effectiveness

Frank, Lori, Ethan Basch, and Joe V. Selby. "The PCORI Perspective on Patient-Centered
Outcomes Research." *JAMA*, October 15, 2014. doi:10.1001/jama.2014.11100.
Gabriel, Sherine E., and Sharon-Lise T. Normand. "Getting the Methods Right—the
Foundation of Patient-Centered Outcomes Research." *New England Journal of Med-
icine*, August 30, 2012. doi:10.1056/nejmp1207437.

Will It Survive?

"Hydrocephalus Remains an Unsolved Medical Mystery." Hydrocephalus Association,
October 2009. http://www.hydroassoc.org/docs/Hydro_Why_FactSheet_v1.04.pdf.

Perception and Health Care Reform

Obama, Barack. "United States Health Care Reform." *JAMA*, August 2, 2016.
doi:10.1001/jama.2016.9797.

CHAPTER SEVEN
Pillar 1: Physicians Working Together on Your Behalf

Treacy, Michael, and Frederik D. Wiersema. *The Discipline of Market Leaders: Choose
Your Customers, Narrow Your Focus, Dominate Your Market*. Reading, MA: Addison-
Wesley, 1997.

The Advantages of Integration

Gawande, Atul. "The Hot Spotters: Can We Lower Medical Costs by Giving the Needi-
est Patients Better Care?" *New Yorker*, January 24, 2011. http://www.newyorker.com
/magazine/2011/01/24/the-hot-spotters.
"More Doctors Getting MBAs Can Lead to Innovation in Healthcare Industry." *Sound
Medicine* (public radio), January 20, 2015. http://sideeffectspublicmedia.org/post
/more-doctors-getting-mbas-can-lead-innovation-healthcare-industry.

The Death of Community Hospitals

Evans, Melanie. "Hospitals Face Closures as 'a New Day in Healthcare' Dawns."
Modern Healthcare, February 21, 2015. http://www.modernhealthcare.com/article
/20150221/MAGAZINE/302219988.

Thomas, Karen Kruse. "The Hill-Burton Act and Civil Rights: Expanding Hospital Care for Black Southerners, 1939–1960." *Journal of Southern History*, November 2006. doi:10.2307/27649234.

"What Hospital Executives Should Be Considering in Hospital Mergers and Acquisitions." Dixon Hughes Goodman, Winter 2013. http://www2.dhgllp.com/res_pubs /Hospital-Mergers-and-Acquisitions.pdf.

Fitzgerald, Kelly. "Mortality Rates at Rural Hospitals Unusually High." *Medical News Today*, April 3, 2013. http://www.medicalnewstoday.com/articles/258598.php.

The Resurrection of Primary Care

Forrest, Christopher B. "Primary Care in the United States: Primary Care Gatekeeping and Referrals: Effective Filter or Failed Experiment?" *BMJ*, March 29, 2003. doi:10.1136/bmj.326.7391.692.

Hing, Esther, and Chun-Ju Hsiao. "State Variability in Supply of Office-Based Primary Care Providers: United States, 2012." CDC's National Center for Health Statistics, May 2014. http://www.cdc.gov/nchs/products/databriefs/db151.htm.

Gawande, Atul. "The Cost Conundrum." *New Yorker*, June 1, 2009. http://www .newyorker.com/magazine/2009/06/01/the-cost-conundrum.

Integration Matters

Pearl, Robert. "Three Lessons in Rapid Change from an Unlikely Source: Health Care." *Forbes.com*, May 29, 2014. http://www.forbes.com/sites/robertpearl/2014 /05/29/3-lessons-in-rapid-change-from-an-unlikely-source-health care. Article was written in response to Chip Heath's request to outline the factors contributing to high performance and quality outcomes at Kaiser Permanente hospitals in Northern California.

Pillar 2: It's Better and Cheaper Not to Get Sick in the First Place

"HEDIS and Performance Measurement." National Committee for Quality Assurance (NCQA), 2016. http://www.ncqa.org/hedis-quality-measurement.

"Improving the Value of Specialty Care with a Focus on Joint Replacements: Action Steps for Purchasers." *California Joint Replacement Registry Issue Brief*, 2012. http:// www.pbgh.org/storage/documents/CJRR_IssueBrief_11.pdf.

Unleashing Digital Data

Suh-Burgmann, Elizabeth, and Walter Kinney. "Potential Harms Outweigh Benefits of Indefinite Monitoring of Stable Adnexal Masses." *American Journal of Obstetrics and Gynecology*, December 2015. doi:10.1016/j.ajog.2015.09.005.

Suh-Burgmann, Elizabeth, Yun-Yi Hung, and Walter Kinney. "Outcomes from Ultrasound Follow-up of Small Complex Adnexal Masses in Women over Fifty." *American Journal of Obstetrics and Gynecology*, December 2014. doi:10.1016/j.ajog .2014.07.044.

Unlocking Electronic Health Records

Mandl, Kenneth D., and Isaac S. Kohane. "Escaping the EHR Trap—the Future of Health IT." *New England Journal of Medicine*, June 14, 2012. doi:10.1056/nejmp 1203102.

Monegain, Bernie. "KLAS: Interoperability Progressing but Still Challenging Between Disparate EHRs." *Healthcare IT News*, October 12, 2016. http://www .healthcareitnews.com/news/klas-interoperability-progressing-still-challenging -between-disparate-ehrs.

Reinventing the House Call
Versel, Neil. "More Virtual Care than Office Visits at Kaiser Permanente by 2018."
  MedCity News, April 12, 2016. http://medcitynews.com/2016/04/virtual-care-kaiser
  -permanente.
"Majority of Americans Don't Use Digital Technology to Access Doctors." Nielsen and
  CAPP (Council of Accountable Physician Practices), 2015.

Disrupting Health Care
Christensen, Clayton M. "The Past and Future of General Motors." *Huffington Post*,
  May 25, 2011. http://www.huffingtonpost.com/clayton-m-christensen/the-past-and
  -future-of-ge_b_184780.html.
"The IHI Triple Aim." Institute for Healthcare Improvement. http://www.ihi.org
  /engage/initiatives/TripleAim/Pages/default.aspx.

Knowing When to Trust Your Gut
Gladwell, Malcolm. *Blink: The Power of Thinking Without Thinking*. New York: Little,
  Brown, 2005.

What Happens if Physicians and Hospitals Refuse to Change?
Tam, Eva, and Lukas Messmer. "Heart Surgeon Brings High-Tech Health Care to the
  World's Poor." *Wall Street Journal*, September 16, 2015. http://www.wsj.com/articles
  /heart-surgeon-brings-high-tech-healthcare-to-the-worlds-poor-1442391424.

CHAPTER EIGHT
Giamatti, A. Bartlett. "The Green Fields of the Mind." *Yale Alumni Magazine*, November
  1977. https://yalealumnimagazine.com/articles/3864-the-green-fields-of-the-mind.

On Care and Competition
Donohue, Julie. "A History of Drug Advertising: The Evolving Roles of Con-
  sumers and Consumer Protection." *Milbank Quarterly*, December 2006.
  doi:10.1111/j.1468-0009.2006.00464.x.
Scott, Dylan. "The Untold Story of TV's First Prescription Drug Ad." *STAT*, December
  11, 2015. https://www.statnews.com/2015/12/11/untold-story-tvs-first-prescription
  -drug-ad.
Shanafelt, Tait D., Omar Hasan, Lotte N. Dyrbye, Christine Sinsky, Daniel Satele, Jeff
  Sloan, and Colin P. West. "Changes in Burnout and Satisfaction with Work-Life
  Balance in Physicians and the General US Working Population Between 2011 and
  2014." *Mayo Clinic Proceedings*, December 2015. doi:10.1016/j.mayocp.2015.08.023.
Mata, Douglas A., Marco A. Ramos, Narinder Bansal, Rida Khan, Constance Guille,
  Emanuele Di Angelantonio, and Srijan Sen. "Prevalence of Depression and Depres-
  sive Symptoms Among Resident Physicians." *JAMA*, December 8, 2015. doi:10.1001
  /jama.2015.15845.

Fighting Words
Gibbs, Nancy. "Why Ebola Fighters Are *Time*'s Person of the Year 2014." *Time*, December 10, 2014. http://time.com/time-person-of-the-year-ebola-fighters-choice.

A Part of Life
McFadden, Robert D. "Giamatti, Scholar and Baseball Chief, Dies at Fifty-One." *New
  York Times*, September 2, 1989. http://www.nytimes.com/1989/09/02/obituaries
  /giamatti-scholar-and-baseball-chief-dies-at-51.html.

Opening Our Eyes

Zhong, Chen-Bo, Vanessa K. Bohns, and Francesca Gino. "A Good Lamp Is the Best Police: Darkness Increases Dishonesty and Self-Interested Behavior." *Psychological Science*, January 29, 2010. doi:10.1177/0956797609360754.

Kluger, Jeffrey. "Why Shady Deeds Are More Likely to Happen in the Dark." *Time*, March 3, 2010. http://content.time.com/time/health/article/0,8599,1969242,00 .html.

What's It Worth to You?

Shah, Avni M., Noah Eisenkraft, James R. Bettman, and Tanya L. Chartrand. "'Paper or Plastic?': How We Pay Influences Post-Transaction Connection." *Journal of Consumer Research*, November 6, 2015. doi:10.1093/jcr/ucv056.

Harris, Elizabeth. "Study: Paying Cash Is Painful, and Makes You Value Your Purchase More." *Forbes.com*, July 28, 2016. http://www.forbes.com/sites/elizabethharris/2016 /07/28/study-paying-cash-hurts-and-makes-you-value-your-purchase-more.

Abelson, Reed. "Health Insurance Deductibles Outpacing Wage Increases, Study Finds." *New York Times*, September 22, 2015. http://www.nytimes.com/2015/09/23 /business/health-insurance-deductibles-outpacing-wage-increases-study-finds.html.

A Complicated Mess

Kairinos, Nicolas, Kamlen Pillay, Michael Solomons, Donald A. Hudson, and Delawir Kahn. "The Influence Manufacturers Have on Negative-Pressure Wound Therapy Research." *Plastic and Reconstructive Surgery*, May 2014. doi:10.1097/prs .0000000000000130.

Cost: Make Health Care Affordable

Casey, Sean, retired software engineer. Interview by phone and e-mail, June to September 2016. Casey told of his experiences with Covered California and his mention in the president's speech on April 1, 2014.

Clinton, William J. "Statement on Signing the Health Insurance Portability and Accountability Act of 1996." Speech published by the American Presidency Project, August 21, 1996. http://www.presidency.ucsb.edu/ws/?pid=53211.

Palmer, Pat. "Why Is the 'Trauma Activation Fee' So Outrageous?" Medical Billing Advocates of America, March 24, 2014. https://billadvocates.com/trauma-activation -fee-outrageous.

Stein, Letitia, and Alexandra Zayas. "Florida Trauma Centers Charge Outrageous Fees the Moment You Come Through the Door." *Tampa Bay Times*, March 7, 2014. http://www.tampabay.com/news/health/florida-trauma-centers-charge-outrageous -fees-the-moment-you-come-through/2169148.

"2016 Employer Health Benefits Survey." From researchers at the Kaiser Family Foundation, NORC at the University of Chicago, and Health Research and Educational Trust, September 14, 2016. http://kff.org/health-costs/report/2016-employer-health -benefits-survey.

Islam, Ifrad. "Trouble Ahead for High Deductible Health Plans?" *Health Affairs*, October 7, 2015. http://healthaffairs.org/blog/2015/10/07/trouble-ahead-for-high -deductible-health-plans.

Rosenthal, Elisabeth. "Sorry, We Don't Take Obamacare." *New York Times*, May 14, 2016. http://www.nytimes.com/2016/05/15/sunday-review/sorry-we-dont-take -obamacare.html.

"Tragedy of the Commons." *World Heritage Encyclopedia*, 2013. http://self.gutenberg .org/articles/eng/Tragedy_of_the_commons.

Coordination: Reduce the Stresses of Medical Care
Watch How Care Coordination Helped Karen Through Her Cancer Journey. By the Council of Accountable Physician Practices (CAPP). Featuring Karen, her family, and care providers. Better Together Health, November 3, 2015. http://bettertogetherhealth .org/portfolio-posts/3-karen.

Two Paths
Gillon, Raanan. "White Coat Ceremonies for New Medical Students." *Western Journal of Medicine*, September 2000. doi:10.1136/ewjm.173.3.206.

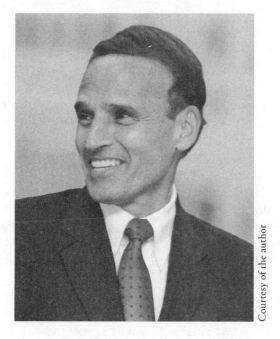

Robert Pearl, MD, is executive director and CEO of The Permanente Medical Group, responsible for the health care of 4.8 million Kaiser Permanente members, and he is the president and CEO of The Mid-Atlantic Permanente Medical Group. Selected by *Modern Healthcare* as one of the most powerful physician-leaders in the nation, Dr. Pearl keynotes around fifteen events per year for audiences of up to 10,000 people, hosted by organizations such as the *New England Journal of Medicine*. He is on the faculty of Stanford University and has taught at Duke University, the University of California–Berkeley, and Harvard University. His column on *Forbes.com* on the business and culture of health care includes articles such as a conversation with Malcolm Gladwell, which received up to 500,000 views. Dr. Pearl has been featured by media outlets including *Time*, ABC News, *USA Today*, and National Public Radio.